PENGUIN

THE DIE

Julia Ross, pioneering author an̲ᵈ _____, ____ _____
innovative counseling programs in the San Francisco Bay Area
since 1980. She is the executive director of Recovery Systems, a
clinic that treats people from all over the world for overeating
and mood problems, using an integrative program that emphasizes nutrient therapy and biochemical rebalancing. Julia trains
health practitioners throughout the United States and abroad.
Her work has been featured on many radio and television programs and in *Psychology Today*, *Health*, *Vogue*, and other magazines. The author of a second best seller, *The Mood Cure*, she lives
in Marin County, California. Learn more about Julia's work at
dietcure.com, moodcure.com, and recoverysystemsclinic.com.

The
Diet Cure

**The 8-Step Program to Rebalance
Your Body Chemistry and End Food Cravings,
Weight Gain, and Mood Swings—Naturally**

JULIA ROSS, M.A.

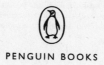

PENGUIN BOOKS

PENGUIN BOOKS
Published by the Penguin Group
Penguin Group (USA) Inc., 375 Hudson Street, New York, New York 10014, U.S.A.
Penguin Group (Canada), 90 Eglinton Avenue East, Suite 700, Toronto, Ontario, Canada M4P 2Y3
(a division of Pearson Penguin Canada Inc.)
Penguin Books Ltd, 80 Strand, London WC2R 0RL, England
Penguin Ireland, 25 St Stephen's Green, Dublin 2, Ireland (a division of Penguin Books Ltd)
Penguin Group (Australia), 250 Camberwell Road, Camberwell, Victoria 3124, Australia
(a division of Pearson Australia Group Pty Ltd)
Penguin Books India Pvt Ltd, 11 Community Centre, Panchsheel Park, New Delhi – 110 017, India
Penguin Group (NZ), 67 Apollo Drive, Rosedale, Auckland 0632, New Zealand
(a division of Pearson New Zealand Ltd)
Penguin Books (South Africa) (Pty) Ltd, 24 Sturdee Avenue, Rosebank, Johannesburg 2196, South Africa

Penguin Books Ltd, Registered Offices:
80 Strand, London WC2R 0RL, England

First published in the United States of America by Viking Penguin,
a member of Penguin Putnam Inc., 1999
Published in Penguin Books 2000
This revised edition published 2012

13 15 17 19 20 18 16 14

LIBRARY OF CONGRESS CATALOGING-IN-PUBLICATION DATA
Ross, Julia, M.A.
The diet cure : the 8-step program to rebalance your body chemistry and end food cravings,
weight gain, and mood swings—naturally / Julia Ross. — Rev. ed.
p. cm.
Includes index.
ISBN 978-0-14-312085-8 (pbk.)
1. Diet.   2. Diet therapy.   3. Food.   4. Nutritionally induced diseases.   5. Nutrition.   I. Title.
RA776.5.R685 2012
615.8'54—dc23
2011045720

Printed in the United States of America

Designed by Jaye Zimet

PUBLISHER'S NOTES
Neither the publisher nor the author is engaged in rendering professional advice or services to
the individual reader. The ideas, procedures, and suggestions contained in this book are not intended
as a substitute for consulting with your physician. All matters regarding your health require medical
supervision. Neither the author nor the publisher shall be liable or responsible for any loss or
damage allegedly arising from any information or suggestion in this book.

The recipes contained in this book are to be followed exactly as written. The Publisher is not responsible
for your specific health or allergy needs that may require medical supervision. The Publisher is not
responsible for any adverse reactions to the recipes contained in this book.

While the author has made every effort to provide accurate telephone numbers and Internet addresses
at the time of publication, neither the publisher nor the author assumes any responsibility for errors,
or for changes that occur after publication. Further, the publisher does not have any control over and
does not assume any responsibility for author or third-party websites or their content.

ALWAYS LEARNING   PEARSON

To
Frances Lillian Ross

and to the women and men
whose struggles have inspired us to find a better way

FOREWORD

Forty years ago, after I had completed my education at Harvard and the University of Pennsylvania and at the outset of my medical career, a foolish optimism gripped my profession. It was generally held that to improve the nation's health, all we had to do was make the existing health care more widely available.

It soon became painfully evident that more health care did not always lead to more health. In fact, the rapid advances of medical science seemed to be increasingly overpowered by the well-marketed culture of unhealthy consumption.

By the early 1980s, this alarming trend found many doctors seeking new ways to heal harmful habits. Twenty years ago, through my private practice and my work as a founding member of the American Holistic Medical Association, I was fortunate enough to become involved with the incredibly effective work of Julia Ross. Most of the patients with overeating and weight problems whom I sent to her clinic received major benefit. Eventually, I was so impressed that I signed on as their backup physician.

I am delighted that her unique approach, now in an updated edition, will be even more accessible. May it help guide you in your efforts toward greater health and well-being.

Richard Shames, M.D., author of
Felling Fat, Fuzzy or Frazzles?,
Thyroid Mind Power, and others
San Rafael, California
January 2012

AUTHOR'S CAUTIONARY NOTE

If you have a known or suspected medical condition, are taking medication of any kind, or have specific health concerns, you should consult a qualified health care provider before following any of the suggestions in this book. Supplement and pharmaceutical dosages are meant to be guidelines only, and dosage and results will vary according to the specific needs of each individual. The dietary guidelines, too, need to be tailored to each individual. Because this book cannot respond to individuals' needs and circumstances, as we do in our clinic, you should ask for a qualified health care professional to help you assess and apply *The Diet Cure*. Although we did our best to provide sound and useful information, we cannot and do not promise results to a reader. Neither the publisher nor the author is engaged in rendering professional advice or services to the individual reader. The ideas, procedures, and suggestions contained in this book are not intended as a substitute for consulting with your physician. All matters regarding your health require medical supervision. Neither the author nor the publisher shall be liable or responsible for any loss or damage allegedly arising from any information or suggestion in this book.

CONTENTS

PART III
YOUR MASTER PLAN FOR THE DIET CURE   243

The first edition of *The Diet Cure* was published in 1999. It has been a marvel from the start:

✦ The minute the book proposal hit the publishing houses, I began to get calls at my clinic from editors and publishers asking for personal help. When I came to New York, more publishers wanted to meet with me than with any other author my seasoned NYC agent had ever represented. Then there was a bidding frenzy. Why? Because the word was all over Manhattan that a truly new approach to the "weight problem" had arrived—the first since Atkins in 1972.

✦ After publication, grateful readers' reviews began to flood in. Out of dozens of similar postings, this is my favorite: "The chocolate cravings are gone! The ice cream cravings are gone! Refined carbs are not a part of my life anymore and I don't miss them. 6 weeks on *The Diet Cure* and I am down at least a size in clothing and I feel better than I ever have (EVER)." And twelve years later, they keep on coming.

✦ *The Diet Cure* keeps on selling—in both the United States and abroad. Take France, where, although obesity is relatively new, Parisian food writer Julien Tort had been struggling with it since childhood. One day, exploring American weight loss methods on the Internet, he discovered low-carb dieting. (This is big news in France, if you can imagine.) He went on Atkins and lost weight easily. He was thrilled. Until his willpower ran out and he reverted to pasta and bread. Back on the Internet he found *The Diet Cure*. Since then, he's lost seventy pounds, translated the book, and arranged its 2011 French publication.

✦ Many people buy multiple copies of *The Diet Cure* to give to friends and family. While I was at a spa celebrating a recent birthday, the masseuse started talking about a book she said had saved her life. She'd had cancer and had been treated, but could not stick to the cancer-recovery diet because her sugar cravings were so strong. (Sugar is the favorite food of cancer cells.) "Now," she said, "I'm four years sugar-free and six years cancer-free." When, intrigued, I asked her the name of the book's author, and then told her my name, the room became a screaming love fest, and she told me that she'd given away fifty copies of *The Diet Cure* as gifts.

More than ever before we need this gift: freedom from the unprecedented, diet-related plagues of the twenty-first century. *The Diet Cure* came out just before the first stunning reports of the obesity epidemic among adults, and then children, were released. Since then, this phenomenon has escalated to the point that even infant obesity has become a significant problem. The incidence of heart disease, kidney failure, and increased cancer risk has also skyrocketed, along with type 2 diabetes among both adults and children.

Why did things suddenly go so wrong? Because weight- and blood-sugar-destabilizing foods are much more plentiful in our diets now, and they are much harder to resist. Thanks to new research worldwide, and to former FDA chief David Kessler's 2010 exposé, we now know that the food industry's efforts to make its products more "palatable" have succeeded beyond even its wildest dreams. We're now officially a nation of food addicts, beyond the help of willpower or *any* diet. Our only hope is to locate a manual for dismantling that addiction. *The Diet Cure* is that manual.

So why a new edition? Since the book was first published, our clinic has worked with more than two thousand newly diagnosed overeaters. In the process, we have developed even better methods of correcting the biochemical imbalances that propel us into food addiction. My publisher and I agreed that it was time to send out a new lifeline—an even stronger edition of *The Diet Cure* that would include all of the clinical advances we've made and the research backing them up. To accomplish this, I have updated and streamlined almost half of the book—extreme measures for extreme times.

A few examples:

+ We've learned more about how to correct deficits in our brain's appetite chemistry, in our ability to handle stress, and in our sex hormone balance—three well-established triggers of the compulsion to overeat.
+ One of the most potent methods for eliminating afternoon, evening, and winter food cravings has only recently become available in the United States. We have it for you.
+ We know better how to test for and treat low thyroid function to improve metabolism and calorie burning.

✦ With diabetes now epidemic, we've found solid clinical research confirming our experience that saturated fat is safe, healthful, and the best blood sugar regulator of all.

✦ The Master Eating Plan has been completely reorganized and updated and includes a vital reevaluation of the facts on red meat, cholesterol, and vegetarianism.

✦ There are new nutrient supplement protocols, new lab tests, new books and CDs to recommend, new ways to find effective holistic practitioners, and more.

To all of you who have already read *The Diet Cure*: Trust me when I urge you to invest in this new edition. I've seen your dog-eared copies at my lectures and that many of you have even color-indexed them. But I promise that you will find treasures in the material I've added. (And I'm a better writer now, too!)

I wish you a successful escape from our twenty-first-century dietary disaster. Everything you'll need is packed and ready for you here in the new *Diet Cure*.

My best wishes to all of you!

8 Steps to the Diet Cure

This is not going to be like any diet book you have ever read. I won't mention calories except to forbid you to eat too *few*! I won't tell you to tune in to your "real" appetite because I know that if you could have you would have long ago. I won't tell you to discipline yourself because I know that your weight and eating habits are not the result of laziness, gluttony, or weak willpower.

You are trapped inside a body that is malfunctioning, and that body needs help. Years of dieting, psychotherapy, and the best pep talks about fitness can't help much when what you really need is a biochemical overhaul.

The clients who come to my clinic have already tried psychotherapy. If they haven't, or if they need more counseling, we provide it. We educate them about their health and encourage them to accept the body that their genes have programmed for them. But when that body is a wreck, psychological and educational approaches just aren't enough. Fortunately, we have now learned how to identify and repair the underlying physical imbalances that have been neglected for so long.

We used to think that dieting was the cure. Many of us still hope that the next diet will really "do it." But more of us have learned that dieting leaves us in worse shape than before we ever started. Our health, energy, mood, and weight have all deteriorated because of dieting. *And yet we can't quit.* We know no other escape from the weight gain that followed our last diet! We need to be cured of dieting. We need to find an entirely new way to deal with our weight problems.

And we have. You're about to learn it.

I discovered the Diet Cure while I was desperately looking for a cure for alcohol and drug addiction. At that time I was the director of a large treatment complex in the San Francisco Bay Area, Ohlhoff Outpatient Programs. We provided intensive counseling for addicted adults and adolescents and their families in three counties. In 1986, I began hearing that certain nutritional supplements could stop addicts' cravings for alcohol and even for cocaine. I asked my staff nutritionist to research and then to start offering these nutrients. They dramatically reduced our clients' drug and alcohol cravings within a week. Much to our surprise, they also cured the insatiable cravings for sweets and the thirty-pound weight gain that our clients typically suffered in early recovery.*

In 1988, I opened my own outpatient treatment program. Staffed with nutritionists and counselors, the Recovery Systems Clinic, in Mill Valley, California, is five minutes north of San Francisco. Initially, my clients at Recovery Systems were food addicts and others concerned about serious eating disorders and weight problems. Compulsive overeating and bulimia were their most common complaints. Some anorexics came to us, too, as well as people without any eating disorders, but with weight gain that was intractable. If these sound like tough problems, you're wrong. We rarely failed to help even our most severely impaired clients because we had the secret weapon. We tried the same nutrients with them that I had used with my drug- and alcohol-addicted clients. They were even more effective for eliminating food cravings and had the delightful side effect of eliminating mood swings, too.

As the word spread, we began to get many clients who did not have full-blown eating disorders but were looking for an escape from yo-yo dieting, low energy, moodiness, and a tendency to eat too much bread and ice cream. You can imagine how easy it was for us to help them, having already discovered nutrients that were powerful enough to "cure" the cravings and mood problems of bulimics and drug addicts. These miracle nutrients are called amino acids.

Amino acids are the key to the Diet Cure. They are stronger than willpower and more effective and safer than any appetite-suppressing drugs. Available in every health food store in America, these isolated protein fragments are the super-nutrients that your brain uses to make its most powerful pleasure chemicals: serotonin (our natural Prozac), catecholamines (our natural cocaine), endorphins (naturally stronger than heroin), and GABA (naturally more relaxing than Xanax). A brain

---

* For more on addiction, see *The Mood Cure* (Penguin Books, 2003).

that is fully stocked with these natural mood enhancers simply has no need for a sugar high.

What's more, you don't have to wait weeks or months to see changes: my clinic's clients consistently report that within twenty-four hours of taking amino acids, their food cravings disappear. Like them, you will no longer need to diet because you will have stopped overeating—*naturally*. These benefits soon become permanent. After three to twelve months you won't need the amino acids and other corrective supplements anymore. Instead, you will be permanently freed from cravings and easily able to follow the Diet Cure's satisfying eating suggestions for life.

THE EIGHT STEPS

At Recovery Systems, we have discovered specific steps to overcoming each of the eight physical, *bodily* handicaps that can lead directly to food cravings, overeating, and unnecessary weight gain.

Step One: Correcting BRAIN CHEMISTRY IMBALANCES to eradicate the negative feelings, like anxiety and depression, behind your "emotional" eating.

Step Two: Ending the LOW-CALORIE DIETING that inevitably leads to problems with mood, energy, overeating, and weight.

Step Three: Balancing UNSTABLE BLOOD SUGAR to eliminate the cravings for sweets and starches that propel us toward diabetes and adrenal exhaustion.

Step Four: Repairing LOW THYROID FUNCTION, a common cause of unnecessary weight gain and the fatigue that makes exercise impossible.

Step Five: Overcoming ADDICTIONS TO FOODS YOU'RE ALLERGIC TO and associated symptoms such as bloating, headache, constipation, and asthma.

Step Six: Calming HORMONAL HAVOC, which can induce food cravings and other distress, particularly during PMS and menopause.

Step Seven: Eradicating YEAST OVERGROWTH, which causes bloating and powerful cravings for sweets and starches.

Step Eight: Fixing FATTY ACID DEFICIENCY, the leading cause of cravings for rich, fatty foods.

Most of these imbalances, if they continue, can result in serious health problems. Whether you must take one, two, or all eight of these steps, you will be able to overcome your biochemical handicaps. You do *not* have to accept them. This book is a repair manual: It will help you to find and fix the physical malfunctions that have caused your particular eating, mood, or weight problem. Then you will drive away in your refurbished body and crave, binge, starve, and obsess no more.

HOW TO USE THIS BOOK

By using the techniques recommended in this book, you will be able to stop cravings and start to feel better in a matter of days, or even hours! The first step is to fill out the Quick Symptom Questionnaire, which follows this introduction. It will reveal which of the imbalances you probably have. Each of the eight biochemical imbalances has a chapter in Part I devoted to helping you recognize its symptoms. In Part II, you will find eight chapters that give you specific information on the steps needed to correct each of the imbalances discussed in Part I, including exactly which easy-to-find supplements and foods to use.

Once you have diagnosed your particular imbalances and know what steps you need to take to correct each one, turn to Part III. There you'll find many ways to make your Diet Cure easy, including a master supplement scheduler, menus and recipes, a food-mood log, and help in finding a holistic health professional, if you need one. The last chapter will take you through your first twelve weeks and set you on the road to a permanent cure.

It will take you a few weeks to study this book and design your supplement and food plan. But as soon as you start to follow your plan, you will see and feel the effects. Within twenty-four hours your mood and food problems should be notably improved, if not completely eliminated. Within three to twelve months you will be able to eliminate all but a few supplements for good.

You'll soon be used to eating for health and pleasure, neither starving nor bingeing, and enjoying permanent freedom from weight gain. As your body responds to special supplements and activating foods, you will become energized, craving-free, and a regular, happy exerciser. You will watch your body acquire its real, ideal shape and weight at a nice, steady pace.

Kate's Story

One of our clients, Kate, had all eight imbalances. Her story illustrates how these imbalances can intertwine and how she was able to successfully address them all.

A creamy-skinned blonde who wrote children's books, Kate had suffered from chronic childhood earaches caused by an allergy to dairy products. As a result, she was given many courses of antibiotics, which created an intestinal yeast overgrowth, causing her to bloat, overeat sweets, and gain weight. Her mother put her on a diet when she was 8 years old.

Kate's energy had never been robust, but it dropped even lower, and she began to gain more weight after she started her period. This was partly the result of a low thyroid problem she had inherited from her mother and maternal grandmother. There was diabetes in the family as well, and Kate's inherited tendency toward unbalanced blood sugar was intensified by her early overeating of sweets. Consuming sweets also contributed to her severe PMS: before her periods, Kate's food cravings were at their worst. By age 15 she had become a perpetual yo-yo dieter, gaining more weight and eating more after every diet. As the child of an alcoholic father, she had inherited mood problems, which she soothed by eating. Her Swedish father had also passed on his genetic need for special fats—so Kate craved rich, fatty foods as well as sweets and starches.

What happened to Kate, who had every imbalance that we address in *The Diet Cure*? Just one week after starting on the targeted supplements and foods, she lost interest in her Reese's peanut butter cups and her pasta Alfredo. Her PMS and yeast overgrowth were gone in three months. By that time her thyroid had been tested and treated, raising her energy and allowing her to exercise moderately four times a week. Because she was actually enjoying healthy food, and plenty of it, she did not feel deprived without her sweets, and it was easy for her to continue with her improved diet permanently. She lost forty-five pounds in the first year, stayed there for six months, and then lost the last thirty pounds in nine months. She said that she even enjoyed her six-month plateau, because she had never been able to keep weight off in the thirty years she had been dieting.

If, like Kate, you have multiple imbalances to overcome, you will be taking many supplements for several months. However, because they work so quickly and are needed only temporarily, you will be able to tolerate them. After all, you have probably done much harder things—like eat nothing but hard-boiled eggs for months! And this time your efforts will go toward building, not stripping, your health. Remember this: a healthy, balanced body cannot have chronic mood and weight problems.

The Quick Symptom Questionnaire

My goal in this book is to stop your food cravings, address your eating and weight problems, and eliminate your mood swings and negative obsessions about your body. But first we have to determine what is causing these problems.

Our clinic asks clients to fill out an extensive symptom questionnaire so that we can isolate the causes of their problems. The questionnaire here is similar to the one we administer at Recovery Systems. Its eight sections will help you to identify your particular physical imbalances. Circle the number next to any symptom that applies to you, and follow the directions at the end of each section to calculate your score. If you are uncertain whether you might have a particular imbalance, please turn to the more complete symptom lists found in the corresponding chapters.

1. Is it your brain's depleted appetite-and-mood-chemistry?

4 Eating is a reward or for pleasure, comfort, or numbness
4 Sensitivity to emotional (or physical) pain; cry easily
4 Worry, anxiety, phobia, or panic
4 Difficulty getting to sleep or staying asleep
3 Difficulty with focus, attention deficits
2 Low energy or drive
4 Obsessive thinking or behavior
4 Difficulty relaxing after tension, stress
3 Depression, negativity

4   Low self-esteem, lack of confidence
4   More mood and eating problems in winter or at the end of the day
3   Irritability, anger
4   Use alcohol or drugs (including antidepressants) to improve mood or sleep

Total Score _____ If your score is over 10, please turn to chapters one and nine.

2.   Are you suffering because of low-calorie dieting?

4   Increased cravings for and focus on food; overeating
4   Regain weight after dieting, more than was lost
3   Increased moodiness, irritability, anxiety, or depression
3   Less energy and endurance
3   Usually eat less than 2,100 calories a day
3   Skip meals, especially breakfast
3   Eat mostly low-fat carbohydrates
2   Constantly think about weight
2   Use aspartame (NutraSweet) or other diet sweetener daily
2   Take Prozac or similar serotonin-boosting drugs
2   Have become vegetarian
3   Decreased self-esteem
4   Have become bulimic or anorexic

Total Score _____ If your score is over 12, please turn to chapters two and ten.

3.   Are you struggling with blood sugar instability or high stress?

4   Crave a lift from sweets or alcohol, but later experience a drop in energy and mood after ingesting them
4   Family history of diabetes, hypoglycemia, or alcoholism
3   Nervous, jittery, irritable, headachy, weak, or teary on and off throughout the day; calmer after meals
3   Mental confusion, decreased memory, hard to focus or get organized
4   Frequent thirst or urination
3   Night sweats (not menopausal)
5   Light-headed, especially on standing up
4   Crave salty foods or licorice

4 Often feel stressed, overwhelmed, and exhausted
4 Dark circles under eyes or eyes sensitive to bright light
4 More awake at night
Total Score _____ If your score is over 10, please turn to chapters three and eleven.

4. Do you have unrecognized low thyroid function?

4 Low energy
4 Easily chilled (especially hands and feet)
4 Other family members have thyroid problems
4 Can gain weight without overeating; hard to lose excess weight
3 Have to force yourself to do even moderate exercise
4 Find it hard to get going in the morning
3 High cholesterol
3 Low blood pressure
4 Weight gain began after going on antidepressant or antipsychotic medication
3 Hair loss (in females) or sparse eyebrows
3 Use food, caffeine, tobacco, and/or other stimulants to get going
Total Score _____ If your score is over 15, please turn to chapters four and twelve.

5. Are you addicted to foods you are actually allergic to?

3 Crave milk, ice cream, yogurt, cheese, or doughy foods such as pasta, bread, and cookies, and eat them frequently
3 Experience bloating after meals
4 Gas, belching
3 Digestive discomfort of any kind
3 Chronic constipation and/or diarrhea
4 Respiratory problems, such as asthma, postnasal drip, congestion
3 Low energy or drowsiness, especially after meals
4 Allergic to milk products or other common foods
3 Undereat or often prefer beverages to solid food
3 Avoid food or throw up food because bloating after eating makes you feel fat or tired
4 Can't gain weight
3 ADHD

    3 Severe headaches, migraines
    4 Food allergies in family
Total Score _____ If your score is over 12, please turn to chapters five and thirteen.

6. Are your hormones unbalanced?

    4 Premenstrual, perimenopausal, or menopausal mood swings or food cravings
    4 Irregular periods or migraines
    3 Experienced a miscarriage, an abortion, or infertility
    4 Use(d) birth control pills or hormone replacement
    3 Uncomfortable periods or cramps, lengthy or heavy bleeding, or sore breasts
    4 Peri- or postmenopausal discomfort (e.g., hot flashes, weight gain, sweats, insomnia, or mental dullness)
    3 Skin eruptions with period, or PCOS (polycystic ovary syndrome)
Total Score _____ If your score is over 6, please turn to chapters six and fourteen.

Note: Some men experience "male menopause" as a result of hormonal imbalance. Men, please see the box on page 84 if you are experiencing weight gain and emotional stress.

7. Do you have yeast overgrowth triggered by antibiotics, cortisone, or birth control pills?

    4 Often bloated, abdominal distention
    3 Foggy-headed
    2 Depressed
    4 Yeast infections
    4 Used antibiotics extensively (at any time in life)
    4 Used cortisone frequently or birth control pills for more than one year
    4 Have chronic fungus on nails or skin, or athlete's foot
    3 Recurring sinus or ear infections as an adult or child
    3 Chronically fatigued
    4 Rashes
    3 Stool unusual in color, shape, or consistency
Total Score _____ If your score is over 12, please turn to chapters seven and fifteen.

8. Do you have fatty acid deficiency?

4 Crave chips, cheese, and other rich foods more than, or in addition to, sweets and starches

4 Have ancestry that includes Irish, Scottish, Welsh, Scandinavian, or coastal Native American

3 Alcoholism and depression in the family history

4 Feel heavy, uncomfortable, and "clogged up" after eating fatty foods

3 Had your gallbladder removed

4 History of hepatitis or other liver or gallbladder problems

4 Light-colored stool

4 Hard or foul-smelling stool

4 Pain on right side under your rib cage

Total Score _____ If your score is over 12, please turn to chapters eight and sixteen.

After you have finished tallying your symptoms in the questionnaire and reading the corresponding chapters, you will create your own Master Plan for the Diet Cure. This plan will include supplements, foods, and special support. When your Diet Cure Master Plan is completed, you will be ready to launch into week one, Detox Week.

If you have any questions about your scores, check the more detailed symptoms lists within the first eight chapters. Even if you have only a few key symptoms in a section, they may well indicate an imbalance that you should explore.

If you have so many high scores that you feel overwhelmed, just concentrate on your top-scoring imbalance. Go right to the corresponding action chapters in Part II. Seeing quick progress in that area will encourage you to move on to the next-highest-scoring imbalance. It will get much easier as you go along.

The
Diet Cure

Part I

Identifying the
Eight Imbalances

ONE

Depleted Brain Chemistry

The Real Story Behind "Emotional" Eating

Almost everyone who has ever come into my office has felt like a failure. "I just don't seem to have the willpower to stay on a diet anymore," or "I can never stick to the maintenance part of the plan." Mostly, this is because they crave sweets or starchy carbs and can't do without them for long. They start with "just a little" and end up eating a lot more than they feel they should. Often their spouses or other family members criticize them, saying, "Why don't you just try harder?" or "If you'd just limit yourself to one . . . ," which only serves to make them feel even worse about themselves. "I guess they're right," they say, "I just don't have enough self-discipline." Yet oddly, these same people are usually doing well in every other aspect of their lives. They are effective at work, they keep the bills paid and the checkbook balanced, they organize their children's lives beautifully. They mastermind professional projects while keeping their households and personal lives functioning. They are actually models of willpower.

We point this out. We remind them that they *have* lost weight— dozens, sometimes hundreds of times. Truly, there is nothing harder than dieting. Most of those critical spouses and family members could never stand the course of even *one* diet.

So if it's not lack of willpower, what *is* wrong with you? Are you an emotional basket case who can't get by without comfort food? If you had more strength, could you power through your problems without overeating? Should you feel ashamed of yourself for needing emotional sustenance from food? No! I hope to help you understand why you are using food as self-medication. *It's not because you are weak willed; it's because you're low in certain brain chemicals.* You don't have enough of the brain chemicals that should naturally be making you feel emotionally strong and complete.

These brain chemicals are thousands of times stronger than street drugs such as heroin. And your body *has* to have them. If not, it sends out a command that is stronger than anyone's willpower: "Find a druglike food to briefly substitute for our brain's missing comfort chemicals. We cannot function without them!" Your depression, tension, irritability, anxiety, and cravings are all symptoms of a brain that is deficient in the mood-enhancing and pleasure-promoting chemicals called neurotransmitters.

WHAT HAPPENED TO YOUR NATURAL MOOD AND APPETITE REGULATORS?

Something has interfered with your neurotransmitters' production. What is it? It's obviously not too unusual, or there wouldn't be so many people using food to feel better, or taking antidepressants for depression relief. Actually, there are several common problems that can result in your feel-good brain chemicals becoming depleted, and none of them are your fault![1]

✦ *You may have inherited deficiencies.* We are learning more all the time about the genes that determine our moods and other personality traits. Some genes program our brains to produce certain amounts of mood-enhancing chemicals. But some of us inherited genes that undersupply some of these vital mood chemicals. That is why some of us are not emotionally well balanced and why the same emotional traits seem to run in families. If your mother always seemed to be on edge, and had a secret stash of chocolate for herself, it should come as no surprise that you, too, need foods such as candy or cookies to calm yourself. Parents who have low supplies of naturally stimulating and sedating brain chemicals often produce depressed or anxious children who use food, alcohol, or drugs as substitutes for the brain chemicals they desperately need.

✦ *Prolonged stress "uses up" your natural sedatives, stimulants, and pain relievers.* This is particularly true if you have inherited marginal amounts to begin with. The emergency stores of precious brain chemicals can get used up if you continually need to use them to calm yourself. Eventually your brain can't keep up with the demand. That's why you start to "help" your brain by eating foods that have druglike effects on it.

✦ *Regular use of druglike foods such as refined sugars and flours and regular use of alcohol or drugs (including some medicines) can inhibit the production of any of your brain's natural pleasure chemicals.* All of these substances can plug into your brain and actually fill up the empty places, called receptors, where your natural brain drugs—the neurotransmitters—should be plugging in. Your brain senses that the receptors are already full, so it further reduces the amounts of neurotransmitters that it produces. As the amounts of these natural brain chemicals drop (remember, they can be thousands of times stronger than the hardest street drugs), more and more alcohol, drugs, or druglike foods are needed to fill newly emptied brain slots. This vicious cycle ends when these substances you ingest are unable to fill the bill any longer. Now your brain's natural mood resources, never fully functional, are more depleted than they ever were, and you still crave your mood-enhancing drugs—whether it's sugar or alcohol and cocaine.

✦ *You may be eating too little protein.* In fact, you almost certainly are if you've been dieting or avoiding fatty foods, many of which are high in protein, too. Your brain relies on protein—the only food source of amino acids—to make all of its mood-enhancing chemicals. If you are not getting enough protein, you won't be able to manufacture those crucial chemicals. A little later in this chapter and in chapter eighteen, you'll learn about complete and incomplete proteins, and what is "enough" protein for you. Eating the equivalent of three eggs, a chicken breast, or a fish filet at every meal should get you enough protein to keep your brain in good repair.

EATING FOR ALL THE WRONG REASONS

At Recovery Systems, we treat people who use food to remedy a variety of negative emotional states. Here are the stories of some typical clients.

♦ Monica ate for comfort. She needed a treat to get through the day. A pastry in the morning, chocolate in the afternoon, and a rich dessert after dinner made her life worth living, especially on bad days.

♦ Sharon ate at night to get to sleep. She couldn't fall asleep by ten or eleven o'clock, even on nights when she was not upset. Being upset made it worse. But a few bowls of cold cereal with milk and sugar would unravel her tension pretty reliably and help her fall asleep.

♦ Paul ate because he was depressed. He ate more in the wintertime and during his lonely nights. Bread, pasta, and late-night bowls of ice cream were his antidepressants.

♦ Brenda ate because she needed an energy boost. She needed sweets first thing in the morning to get her going and throughout the rest of the day to keep her going, especially during her afternoon energy dip at work.

♦ Dinah ate to numb her painful memories. She had been sexually assaulted often as a child, and food had become her ally, something she could always count on to soothe her and literally kill the pain.

♦ Brandon ate when he was angry. He stuffed himself with candy bars to keep from losing his temper, or after he'd finally exploded inappropriately, again.

♦ Andrea "got high" by starving. When she ate, it not only made her feel fat and bloated, but she lost her elevated mood.

Our counselors found that with clients like these, no amount of therapy seemed to stop this "emotional" eating. I wondered if there could possibly be a physiological cause for this intractable behavior. Eventually, I would find my answer, but it would come from an unexpected source.

THE TOP CAUSE OF EMOTIONAL EATING

In the early 1980s, I became the director of a large San Francisco addiction treatment program. Our clients were very serious about getting sober, and we gave them the most intensive treatment available anywhere. Yet they could not stop using. Eighty to ninety percent relapse rates or worse were standard then, and still are, in the alcohol- and drug-addiction treatment field. Take the much-admired U.S. drug court program. A national study of seventy-six drug courts found a 10 percent success rate.[2] Contrast that with a Sacramento, California, drug court program designed along Diet Cure lines, which has an 83 to 87 percent success rate according to two different studies and saved its county $20 million in its first ten years.[3]

As I studied the heartbreaking relapses, I began to see a pattern. Our clients had stopped drinking, but they had quickly developed a heavy addiction to sweets. Sugar and alcohol are highly refined, simple substances that are instantly absorbed, not needing digestion (complex carbs, like whole grains, need time to be digested). Both sugar and alcohol instantly (and temporarily) raise levels of several potent mood chemicals in the brain. This high would be followed by a low, of course. So, just as when they were using alcohol, our sugar-bingeing clients were often moody, unstable, and full of cravings. Since alcohol usually works even faster than sugar does, at some point, caught in a particularly low mood, they would break down and have a drink. One drink would become a full-blown relapse.

I began hiring nutritionists to help solve this disturbing relapse problem. They suggested to our clients that they quit eating sweetened foods, foods made from refined (white) flour, and caffeine, and that they eat more whole grains and vegetables. Unfortunately, these nutritional efforts didn't pay off. For reasons that we understood only later, our clients just couldn't stop eating the sweets and starches that eventually led them back to alcohol. For six years we struggled with finding a solution. Then, in 1986, we found one.

The solution came from Dr. Joan Mathews Larson, the director of a nutritionally oriented alcoholism-treatment center in Minneapolis. This brilliant pioneer, the author of *Seven Weeks to Sobriety*, introduced me to a technique that was quickly eliminating her alcoholic clients' cravings and raising her center's long-term success rate from 20 percent to 80 percent! The technique, based on the exciting research of neuroscientist Kenneth Blum, Ph.D., involved the use of specific amino acids that could rapidly feed the addicted brain exactly the type of protein that it needed to naturally fill up its empty neurotransmitter sites. This amino acid therapy revolutionized the work at our clinic, too, dramatically raising our success rates with alcohol- and drug-addicted clients. But our most spectacular successes were with our food-addicted clients: more than 90 percent of the compulsive overeaters we have treated with amino acid therapy have been freed from their food cravings within twenty-four hours.

USING AMINO ACIDS TO
END FOOD ADDICTION

When psychological help does not clear up emotional eating, we need to look at the five brain chemicals that regulate our appetites and moods. They are:

1. Glucose; adequate levels keep our blood supplies stable (that means fewer cravings and less moodiness)
2. Endorphins, our natural comfort chemicals
3. Serotonin, our natural antidepressant and sleep promoter
4. GABA (gamma-aminobutyric acid), our natural tranquilizer
5. Catecholamines, our natural energizers and mental focusers

If we have enough of all five, our emotions are stable. When they are depleted or out of balance, what we call "pseudo-emotions" can result. These false moods can be every bit as distressing as those triggered by abuse, loss, or trauma. They can drive us to relentless overeating.

For some of us, certain foods, particularly ones that are sweet and starchy, can have a druglike effect, altering our brains' mood chemistry and fooling us into a false calm or a temporary energy surge. We can eventually become dependent on these druglike foods for continued mood lifts. The more we use them, the more depleted our natural mood-enhancing chemistry becomes. Substituting amino acid supplements for these drug foods can have immediate and dramatic effects.

Toni, a 26-year-old Native American, was referred to our clinic because she was exhausted, profoundly depressed, anxious, and suffering lifelong trauma from the physical and emotional violence of her family.

Toni drank alcohol and ate sweets to cope. She went regularly to her scheduled counseling sessions but was unable to rouse herself to communicate with her counselor. She had volunteered to come to Recovery Systems, hoping that a new approach would help. Toni had already been through three long-term treatment programs for alcohol addiction. Clearly, she was motivated to solve her problem.

When we saw Toni's condition, the nutritionist and I conferred and decided to give her amino acids on the spot. I asked her to tell me one thing: What was the worst thing she was experiencing at that moment? She said, "I'm soooo tired." Her slumped body and still, dull eyes confirmed this.

Our goal? To treat her lack of energy and depression by raising her levels of catecholamines, the body's natural energizers. We gave her our smallest dose—500 milligrams of L-tyrosine. While we waited and hoped for an effect, I spoke about how and why amino acids can be helpful.

After about ten minutes, Toni said, "I'm not tired anymore."

"Great!" I said. And then I asked my next question: "What is the worst thing you are experiencing, now that your energy is better?"

She answered by bending over and grasping herself around the stomach. "I'm really uptight."

We then gave Toni the smallest dose of GABA—100 milligrams— a natural Valium-like chemical. We suspected that this supplement would help relieve her tension and allow her to relax—and it did. She stretched her legs out in front of her and then stood up, got a glass of water, and went to the bathroom. While she was gone, her counselor came in and happened to tell me that Toni was in a lot of emotional pain because of the chronic alcoholic violence in her family. When her family members drank alcohol, they all became different people, vicious and cruel. And they had never been able to stay away from alcohol.

When Toni returned, I asked her, "Can we give you something to help you endure the emotional pain that you are in?" She said yes, so I gave her a supplement containing 300 milligrams DL-phenylalanine (DLPA) and 150 milligrams L-glutamine. (DLPA is the amino acid used to alleviate emotional pain by raising endorphin levels. Glutamine balances mood by leveling out blood sugar.)

In ten minutes I asked Toni how she was feeling, and she smiled and said, "Just right."

I was incredulous. How could these small amounts really be helping her? Our European-American clients usually need two to four times as much of each type of amino acid to get such dramatic effects.

I asked if she would like any more of any of the aminos I had already given her for energy, relaxation, mood and pain relief. Her answer: "Just right," and a shake of her head.

By this time Toni's eyes were sparkling. Weeks later her counselor reported that by continuing with the amino acids she had first used in our office, Toni was actually talking for the first time in their counseling sessions, was being praised at work, was being noticed for the first time by men, and was staying sober and sugar-free without effort.

MOOD FOODS: HOW AMINO ACIDS FEED YOUR BRAIN

The four key neurotransmitters are made of amino acids. There are at least twenty-two amino acids contained in high-protein foods such as fish, eggs, chicken, and beef, including the nine amino acids that are considered essential for humans. Other foods, such as grains and beans, have fewer aminos, so they need to be carefully combined to provide complete protein (for example, rice and beans, or corn and nuts). Even then these foods contain much less protein, and the carb content is much higher.

If you are eating three meals a day, each meal including plenty of protein (most people with eating and weight problems are doing neither), your positive moods and freedom from cravings can be maintained. But most people need to kick-start the brain's repair job, using certain key amino acids. This will allow you to actually enjoy eating protein and vegetables instead of cookies and ice cream. After a few months, you will be getting all the aminos you need from your food alone and won't need to take amino acids as supplements any longer.

Amino Acids Help Post-Optifasters[4]

In a study published in October 1997, University of North Texas researcher Kenneth Blum and colleagues monitored two groups of dieters for two years after they had completed a medically monitored fast. The fasters had used the product Optifast, a powdered nutritional drink containing various vitamins and minerals, which dieters use to replace one, two, or even three meals a day. In Dr. Blum's study, 247 Optifast graduates were divided into two equal groups. One group took the amino acids listed in this chapter. The other group took no amino acids. As we know from Oprah Winfrey's highly publicized experience with Optifast and from the 1992 Senate investigation of Optifast and Nutrisystem, a quick regain of weight after a liquid fast is to be expected in more than 90 percent of cases. However, this did *not* happen to Dr. Blum's amino-acid-taking group.

At the end of two years, the amino-acid takers showed:

+ a twofold decrease in percent overweight for both males and females;
+ a 70 percent decrease in cravings for females and a 63 percent decrease for males;
+ a 66 percent decrease in binge eating for females and a 41 percent decrease for males;

> ✦ the experimental group regained only 14.7 percent of the
> weight they had lost during fasting, while the control
> group regained 41.7 percent of their lost weight.

Restoring depleted brain chemistry sounds like a big job—but it isn't. Three of the four key neurotransmitters are made from just a single amino acid each! Because biochemists isolate these key amino acids and extract them from special yeasts, you can easily add the specific ones that may be deficient. These "free form" amino acids are instantly bioavailable (in other words, they are predigested), unlike protein powders from soy or milk, which are harder to absorb. Hundreds of research studies at Harvard, MIT, and elsewhere have confirmed the effectiveness of using just a few of these targeted amino acid precursors to increase the key neurotransmitters, thereby eliminating depression, anxiety, and cravings for food, and even alcohol, and drugs. You can find out more about aminos and behavior in my book *The Mood Cure*.

STOPPING CARBOHYDRATE CRAVINGS CAUSED BY BLOOD SUGAR DROPS

It may sound impossible, but you might be able to stop your food cravings almost instantly with just one amino acid supplement. Any absence of fuel for your brain's functions is perceived correctly by your body as a code-red emergency. Powerful biochemical messages then order you to immediately eat refined carbohydrates to quickly refuel your brain. There are only two fuels that the brain can readily use:

1. Glucose, which is blood sugar made instantly from sweets or starches (fats and protein can also be broken down to make glucose slowly and steadily)
2. Glutamine, an amino acid protein made from foods (and available as a supplement carried in all health food stores)

Glutamine reaches the starving brain within minutes and can often immediately put a stop to even the most powerful sweet and starch cravings. The brain is fueled by glutamine when glucose levels drop too low. Don't be intimidated by the strong effects of supplementation. Glutamine is a natural food substance; in fact, it's the most abundant amino acid in our bodies. It serves many critical purposes: stabilizing our mental functioning, keeping us calm yet alert, and promoting good digestion.[5]

DO YOU USE SUGAR, CHOCOLATE, OR CAFFEINE FOR ENERGY AND FOCUS?

When your brain is adequately fueled with its backup supplies of glutamine, you are ready to rebuild your four key neurotransmitters, starting with the catecholamines, your natural caffeine. Without these natural brain stimulants, you can be slowed down and have a hard time concentrating. You're less animated and enthusiastic. Your physical as well as your mental energy can drop without adequate catecholamines. The amino acid that provides this jet fuel is the nutritional powerhouse L-tyrosine, which produces the four catecholamines—L-dopa, dopamine, adrenaline, and norepinephrine—and it goes to work in minutes.

DO YOU EAT WHEN STRESSED?

The next key mood-enhancing chemical is GABA (gamma-aminobutyric acid), our natural Valium. GABA acts like a sponge, soaking up excess adrenaline and other by-products of stress and leaving us relaxed. It can drain the tension and stiffness right out of knotted muscles. GABA can even smooth out seizure activity in the brain. Think what it can do for garden-variety stress and uptightness and the urge to eat when stressed (which more than 60 percent of us do).

How Effective Are L-tyrosine and GABA?

A young couple came into my office for help with a big problem. She had discovered that her husband was using speed (methamphetamine) on a daily basis. Her father had just died of alcoholism, and she had come home from the funeral to discover her husband with his drugs laid out on the kitchen table. She was distraught and furious (she had always been tense and edgy, anyway) and stuffing herself with candy. She told him he had three days to assemble a recovery plan or move out. He threw his drugs away and made an appointment to see me. He had started to use speed on the road as a performer when his energy had started to sag years before. Over the years, he found himself always tired unless he was on speed. He'd been secretly using it daily for years. When he got to me, he had used no speed in two days, and he was exhausted, trying hard to stay awake and craving sugar.

As they sat together, the husband was slumped dejectedly back into his chair, and his wife was ramrod straight on the edge of hers. I left to consult briefly with our nutritionist and came back with 1,000 milligrams of L-tyrosine for the husband and 100 milligrams of GABA for his wife. Within twenty minutes, the wife was sitting back, relaxed and smiling, while her husband was straight-backed and alert. Correcting their brain chemistries helped enormously in getting their marriage back on track: He left the next day for an inpatient treatment program; she went home with her GABA. Now, fifteen years later, he has not used drugs since. He is back on stage and his energy is fine without drugs, largely because of the L-tyrosine that he used for six months to rebuild his own brain energy system. His wife relaxes with her GABA whenever she needs to. Neither overeats.

DO YOU EAT FOR COMFORT?

For many people, overeating helps compensate for a depletion of our powerful natural pain relievers, the endorphins. Life's pain can be unendurable without adequate amounts of these buffer chemicals. Some of us (for example, those of us from alcoholic families) may be born with too little natural pain tolerance. We are overly sensitive to emotional (and sometimes physical) pain. We cry easily. Like our alcoholic parents, we need something to help us endure our daily lives, which seem so painful. Others of us use up too much endorphin through chronic pain, trauma, or stress. We just run out, especially if we were born short on endorphins to begin with. When our comfort chemicals run low, we turn to comfort foods.

If you need food as a reward and a treat, or to numb your feelings, your natural pleasure enhancers, the pain-killing endorphins, are probably in short supply. Foods that elevate your endorphin activity can easily become addictive. If you "love" certain foods, those foods are firing a temporary surge of endorphins—the "love" chemicals that are thousands of times stronger than heroin. Endorphins can do more than kill pain; they provide the sensation of pleasure, too. Sex releases a surge of endorphins. Euphoria, joy, the "runner's high"—these are all feelings produced by endorphins. Some people have so much natural endorphin that they smile all the time and get great pleasure from everyday life. Of course, we all endure suffering and loss. But with enough endorphins, we can bounce back.

For anorexics and bulimics, the trauma of starving and vomiting can trigger an addictive endorphin high, because trauma of any kind can set off an automatic burst of soothing endorphins. You may know of people who felt no pain for hours after a terrible physical injury. Runners don't get their big endorphin high until they have run past "the wall of pain." At that point, they have run too far![6]

LOW SEROTONIN: WHEN YOU USE CARBS FOR ANXIETY, DEPRESSION, OR INSOMNIA

This can be the easiest deficiency of all to develop. Very few foods are high in the amino acid tryptophan, which is the only nutrient that the body can use to make serotonin. According to a 1997 study in the UK's top medical journal, *The Lancet*, tryptophan is one of the first nutrients to be depleted by weight loss dieting. If, in addition to dieting, you inherited low serotonin levels or experience a lot of stress, your levels can fall low enough to set off regular carb cravings in the afternoon and evenings to soothe worry, depression, fear, anger, insomnia, and more.

Restoring your serotonin levels can be a life-or-death matter: Suicides and violent crimes are closely associated with deficiencies of serotonin. The sometimes-fatal obsessions and self-hate of bulimics and anorexics are clearly linked to inadequate or disturbed serotonin function as well.[7]

Obsessive fears and phobias are common among people with low serotonin levels. Do you have any obsessions that might be caused by low serotonin? The men and women I have worked with who report obsessive behavior tend to be "neatniks" and suffer from negative obsessing about their physical appearance. As we all know, anorexics are driven to obsessively control their food intake.

It may be a difficult adjustment for you to begin to view symptoms such as perfectionism, fear, and low self-esteem as biochemical problems and not just psychological ones. But the success of antidepressants like Prozac has already alerted us to the biochemical nature of many symptoms that don't respond to psychological help alone.

Drugs like Prozac are called selective serotonin reuptake inhibitors (SSRIs), because they keep whatever serotonin we have active. But they do not actually provide *additional* serotonin. For this reason, most people using SSRIs often continue to have some low-serotonin symptoms. Before there were SSRIs, the pharmaceutical compound L-tryptophan was commonly used to increase serotonin levels. For more than twenty years, psychiatrists and health food stores enthusiastically recommended it for relieving depression and food cravings and normalizing sleep without side effects. Many people found that their symptoms were eliminated permanently after only a few months of L-tryptophan use.

In 1989, a single bad batch of L-tryptophan, which killed several people and made many more very sick, prompted the Food and Drug Administration (FDA) to ask for a voluntary ban on U.S. sales. One Japanese company, Showa Denko, had produced this contaminated batch. Showa Denko has never made tryptophan again. Despite evidence that no other manufacturer has ever made a problem batch, until 2005 the FDA recommended that L-tryptophan not be sold as a supplement. (Interestingly, it has made no effort to stop the sale of infant formula, most of which contains added L-tryptophan.)[8]

With L-tryptophan unavailable, drugs such as Prozac, Zoloft, and Celexa have become our primary tools for combating the crippling symptoms of low serotonin. Unfortunately, these drugs provide only temporary and incomplete benefits, and often have uncomfortable or dangerous side effects, including weight gain and diabetes. Fortunately, in 1998 a different version of tryptophan called 5-HTP (5-hydroxytryptophan) became available over the counter. The positive effects of 5-HTP on appetite and weight loss have since been documented.[9]

In 2005, L-tryptophan, which converts into 5-HTP as well as other important biochemicals like niacin, was made available again, with FDA approval, online and in stores. Both forms work beautifully to stop afternoon, evening, and winter carb cravings. They both help tremendously with insomnia. Since insomnia is closely correlated with weight gain (and many other problems), this is an important added benefit. Note: tryptophan is often best when insomnia is a particularly serious problem.

Whatever mood-enhancing brain chemicals may be in short supply can be replenished quickly, easily, and safely. Chapter nine will provide instructions on how to create an amino supplement plan individualized for your unique brain chemistry needs.

For much more on this fascinating subject, see my second book, *The Mood Cure.*

TWO

Malnutrition Due to Low-Calorie Dieting

The Number Two Cause of Overeating, Weight Gain, Bulimia, and Anorexia

Have you ever dieted? Do you skip meals for any reason? Do you try to eat fewer than 2,100 calories a day? Of course you do; you're a twenty-first-century American trapped in a weight gain spiral. Dieting seems the obvious solution. . . . Too bad it's only made things worse.

In fact, America really is on a killer diet. Although low-calorie dieting has demonstrated no long-term success rate (and despite low-calorie dieting, the majority of Americans are now overweight for the first time in history), the lure of dieting continues to be irresistible. We are dieting more frequently, more radically, and at younger ages every year. In 1964, a Harris poll found that 15 percent of adults were dieting. By 1992, 70 percent of women and 50 percent of men were dieters, as were 80 percent of seventh-grade girls.[1] The result: an unprecedented epidemic of overweight, obesity, and diabetes.

Food restriction has since become an established fact of dietary life for most Americans. In the twenty-first century, though, a new kind of dieting has evolved: Although many dieters still take stabs at formal programs such as Weight Watchers or South Beach, most tend to create their own weight loss regimens. In the process, the distinction between dieting and healthy eating is becoming ever more confused. For instance, we have normalized skipping meals (especially breakfast); we substitute coffee, diet soda, iced tea, and energy drinks for real food; we favor low-fat and low-cal products; and we snack instead of eating complete meals.

The Failure of Low-Calorie Dieting

✦ The results of a 12-month study of four popular diets: All had 50–60 percent drop-out rates, and those who continued achieved an average weight loss of only 5.5 pounds in twelve months.[2]

✦ A government review of 55 studies found no sustained weight loss at all after 12 months.[3]

✦ Two-thirds of dieters soon regain more weight than they ever lose.[4]

✦ The more weight initially lost, the greater the rebound weight gain.[5]

As you'll see in this chapter, any style of low-calorie dieting guarantees *weight increase* over time and contributes significantly to the general decline in physical and mental health that we are facing now in the United States, and that you, personally, are probably experiencing.

THE CALORIE CONTROVERSY

Unfortunately, low-calorie dieting just adds up to starvation. Your body can't tell the difference between Jenny Craig's packaged meals and concentration-camp fare. It's a startling comparison to make, but the consequences of depriving yourself of food are always the same, whether the deprivation is voluntary or not.

If you have been a serious dieter, your average daily caloric intake has frequently dropped below the amount provided at the Nazi concentration camp at Treblinka: 900 per day. When I give this figure to female high school and college students, they gasp. They think of 900 calories as generous and regard 2,500 calories per day as "gross." You may agree with them. Yet the U.S. Department of Agriculture (USDA) standards indicate that 2,500 calories is the *minimum* amount of calories an adolescent or adult woman needs to get the minimum amounts of life-sustaining nutrients such as iron. Men need at least 2,800 calories a day. But it's not just the calories we need; eating 2,500 to 2,800 calories of junk food won't protect us from malnutrition, either. We need plenty of vegetables, fruits, proteins, and fats, as well as healthy carbohydrates, for our bodies to function properly.

Frankly, uniform caloric recommendations don't seem to exist. Even the *Nutrition Desk Reference* (*NDR*), a hefty, 672-page tome, offers no comment on calories at all. It uses a phrase that's found everywhere: "If the daily caloric intake is 2,000 . . ." You'll notice that the serving sizes on almost all packaged foods are based on the mysterious 2,000-calorie number.

Fortunately, the World Health Organization (WHO) has solved our problem through its experience with worldwide emergency food shortages. It has established that *starvation begins at fewer than 2,100 calories per day*. The organization uses this calculation as a basis for determining its guidelines for emergency food aid: 2,300 calories for women and 2,500 for men.

There are two things that nutrition experts all agree on:

1. *Junk-food calories are hazardous.* Sugar, white flour, and junk fats, while high in calories, are health hazards that offer nutritional depletion instead of nourishment. Unfortunately, they account for most of our calories, yet they do nothing to supply the essential food and nutrients our bodies need. Obviously, junk foods are the worst promoters of unneeded weight gain.

2. *U.S. women don't eat enough food.* On any given day, half eat fewer than 1,500 calories. That makes our average intake less than 1,800 calories per day.[6] All sources agree: this is not enough food to keep our calorie furnace going. The more food you eat, the faster you burn calories (unless you have a thyroid impairment or you overeat). Are you skipping meals, cutting calories whenever you can, and eating too much fast food? It's that easy to move into malnutrition. Like so many of us, you are probably too rushed to prepare fresh, whole foods—which, as you will learn in chapters eighteen, nineteen, and twenty, is crucial and not as difficult as you may think. Fast and packaged foods you choose for convenience contain few nutrients. Most of the essential vitamins and minerals you need have been destroyed in processing (such as the refining of sugar or flour) and are not adequately supplied by the few synthetic nutrients that may have been added back in.

We all need nutrient-rich calories. They do not typically add unneeded weight, even if we eat lots of them. Please, try to stop counting calories and fat grams. If you follow your individualized Diet Cure program and eat foods that make you feel strong and energetic, you'll be doing fine; you will lose unneeded pounds and settle into your body's own ideal weight. Chapter eighteen will give you the details of how to get the best calories; how many calories just doesn't seem to matter much. Our clinic has almost never had a problem with clients eating too many calories (only too few), as long as the calories were high quality. The truth is that low-calorie dieting not only doesn't work; it's actually surprisingly dangerous. This chapter will explain how it may have harmed you. Chapter ten will tell you what you can do about it.

A FEW OF THE HEALTH CONSEQUENCES OF LOW-CALORIE DIETING

✦ Gallstones caused by liquid fasting and diets under 800 calories a day; 25 percent of very-low-calorie dieters must have their gallbladders removed
✦ Increased risk of developing diabetes
✦ Bone loss at hip and spine[7]
✦ Thyroid suppression (slowed metabolism, fatigue)
✦ Decreased sexual interest
✦ Loss of muscle and exercise capacity[8]
✦ Increased depression and anxiety
✦ Mental dullness (lower scores on intelligence tests)
✦ Stroke, caused by diet pills
✦ Binge eating and bulimia
✦ Anorexia (20 percent death rate)
✦ Decreased life expectancy

Dieters and Drugs

Dieters know that hunger pangs can be powerful, and rather than listen to their bodies' cries for more food they often pacify themselves with drugs that will silence those pleas. Some of these drugs seem relatively benign at first; however, dieters can become more and more dependent on them. For years, dieters have recognized the power of cigarettes in squelching hunger. The vast majority of fashion models smoke, and cigarettes are often packaged for women with subtle messages about being "long" and "slim." Many people have come to rely on caffeine, either in coffee, colas, or over-the-counter diet pills. Amphetamines can be an alluring appetite suppressant as well.

Then, too, sometimes people indulge in drugs to alter their moods and perceptions, to loosen up and feel better about themselves, or for an energy pickup (a need you'll experience quite often if you aren't eating right). Often they think that since their use is "casual," they don't have to worry about the physical toll these drugs are taking on them, much less the possibility of addiction. I truly hope that if you are using any of these drugs, you are not yet addicted to them. Ask yourself the following:

✦ Am I drinking more caffeine—either as coffee or in diet sodas—or more alcohol to satisfy my need for more food?

✦ Have I ever used harder drugs to stifle hunger pangs?

✦ Am I using drugs, such as Phentermine, Dexatrim, or stronger stimulants to stay thin?

If you answer yes to any of these, you're skating on thin ice. I can't tell you when the ice will crack beneath you, but I can tell you that you'll need to get help escaping from the danger zone of addiction once you've entered it. It will be important to find therapeutic support in the form of counseling and twelve-step programs. You should also read chapters one and nine on brain chemistry, since brain chemistry imbalances are responsible for cravings for street (and pharmaceutical) drugs. And read my second book, *The Mood Cure* (Penguin Books, 2003), which gives detailed information on effectively using nutrition to escape addiction.

THE LEGACY OF THE 1970S:
THE DIETING AND JUNK-FOOD GENERATIONS
GROW UP MALNOURISHED

The malnourishment of the typical American female started with the baby boomers, who grew up after World War II. With plenty of food available, and with access to vitamin-fortified grains and milk and iodine-enriched salt, they grew up with no fear of malnutrition and its related diseases. They didn't worry about pellagra (caused by vitamin B_3/niacin deficiency) or beriberi (caused by B_1/thiamine deficiency), which were real threats to previous generations, killing and crippling millions worldwide. Perhaps as a result, the boomers easily fell for the Twiggy look, popularized by the famous emaciated model who appeared in the magazines of the early 1960s. The thin, boyish look for women was suddenly in, while natural womanly curves and body fat were out. Starving—low-calorie dieting—was now sophisticated and glamorous. By the seventies, dieting had become an entrenched (and immensely profitable) enterprise. Since then, on any given day, more than half the adult and adolescent females in the United States can be found restricting their caloric intake. Men have latched onto the dieting craze, too, especially young men and gay men.

Dieting is particularly dangerous because it radically diminishes what we now know are marginal nutrient resources. USDA household food consumption surveys in 1965 showed that three basic nutrients were seriously deficient in American food: vitamins A, C, and B_6. By 1990, adequate amounts of thirteen basic nutrients had been lost to the typical American diet: vitamins A, C, B_6, thiamine, riboflavin, and folic acid; and the minerals calcium, iron, magnesium, zinc, copper, manganese, and chromium![9]

Diseases of malnutrition that haven't been seen in generations are starting to crop up again. Scurvy, a severe vitamin C deficiency marked by a rash and bleeding into the skin and mucous membranes, is normally seen only in countries in which starvation is common. But in 1993, a 14-year-old girl in Detroit was diagnosed with full-blown scurvy. It wasn't that she wasn't eating; it was that she had junk-food malnutrition. Though high in calories, her entire diet consisted of burgers, shakes, fries, candy, and soda pop.

British expert Mervat Nasser documents the effects of U.S.-style fast food in Egypt, the UK and elsewhere in her book *Culture and Weight Consciousness*. Poor-quality, highly addictive food appears to be causing weight increases and diabetes worldwide. This is followed by dieting, which leads to perpetual weight struggles and eating disorders.[10]

CHILDREN AND TEENS BEGIN DIETING
IN LARGE NUMBERS

I am particularly concerned about people who dieted as children. A 1981 report on levels of twelve basic nutrients found that dieting girls 15 to 18 years old were seriously deficient in eleven of them! Why? Largely because since the 1960s, young girls have become regular dieters. Like so many of them, did you begin to diet because you were terrified by the weight gain that is normal in puberty? Prepubescent girls' bodies are only 10 to 15 percent fatter than boys', but they are genetically programmed to eventually develop twice as much fatty tissue in their breasts, hips, thighs, and stomachs. As your body grew natural and healthy curves in your teens, did you start dieting as a way of life? Did dieting become totally confused with normal eating for you, as it has for most American girls, and for perhaps most American adults as well?

The fact is that when children and teens diet, their fat cells double in size and increase in number. Their already naturally escalated fat production can double, sending them off on a lifetime of unnecessary dieting.

As the first baby boomers' children, born in the 1960s, reached puberty in the 1970s, a bizarre and tragic consequence of dieting became apparent. A new wave of eating disorders, directly linked to low-calorie dieting, was building toward what has become an epidemic in the 1990s. A significant 1991 study identifying the risk factors for developing an eating disorder found that a history of dieting and being born after 1960 topped the list.[11]

Skipping meals, food restricting, low-calorie dieting, fasting, excessive exercise, and diet pill use have become the norm among American females of all ages. It is not a big step from these "casual" dieting practices to bulimia and anorexia. More and more girls, women, and, increasingly, men are crossing this line every day.

ANOREXIA AND BULIMIA:
THE DIRECT CONSEQUENCES
OF NUTRIENT RESTRICTION

Has deliberately skipping meals evolved into occasional all-day fasting and eventually become compulsive fasting—or anorexia? You may have found how easily you can get rid of the food consumed during a "pig-out" by vomiting or taking diet pills or laxatives. The use of these purging methods can become more frequent as bulimia and addiction to diet pills and laxatives take over.

The high school and college girls who come to my lectures report that 60 to 80 percent of all the girls at their schools binge, purge, and starve on a regular basis. It is discussed openly; there is no real stigma left. In fact, many girls *want* to be anorexic. They are disappointed if they can't throw up and become bulimic. In a 1995 University of Michigan study, 86 percent of the 557 incoming freshmen women were dieters. Three percent were bulimic. Within six months, an additional 19 percent of the dieters had become bulimic. In total, 22 percent of freshmen girls were bulimic within six months of entering college. Although this study ended at six months, we can assume a continued increase in bulimia and the emergence of anorexia among these dieting students over time. In fact, dieters are *eight times* more likely than non-dieters to develop eating disorders, according to the head of psychiatry at Tufts University and eating disorder expert L. K. George Hsu, MD.[12]

Puberty and adolescence are especially dangerous times for undereating, because the body is still growing. During this critical period, rapidly developing bodies already require at least 2,500 high-quality calories per day, yet many girls at this age, if not most, try to limit themselves to fewer than 1,000 calories a day, and often those are junk-food calories. This starvation dieting can quickly develop into compulsive eating, bulimia, and anorexia. In fact, two 14-year-old anorexic girls came to the Recovery Systems Clinic recently. Their eating disorders had started after their very first diets.

As with anorexia, bulimia is rooted in the dieting mentality. Miranda's story is a sadly typical one. A 24-year-old beauty with a well-proportioned and muscular body, Miranda found herself close to the upper weight limit for her height. (Muscle is heavier than fat.) She had never dieted in her life, but when she went to flight attendant training school, she noticed that most of the other trainees were regular dieters. At the school, which served fast food, she did not get her usual nutritious food or her usual exercise. She found herself gaining a little weight. Concerned that she might go over the weight limit, she began skipping meals. Soon her starving had turned to bingeing and vomiting. By the time she left the training, only two months later, she had developed unbearable sweet cravings and was bingeing and purging at least once a day. Even back home on her exercise program and healthy diet, she could not shake the cravings. Her bulimia progressed. Miranda came to our clinic at age 27, obsessed and miserable, bingeing and purging three to five times per day. I'm happy to say that through using the supplements outlined in chapter ten and following the Diet Cure plan, many bulimic women like Miranda have been able to return to their original weight and health.

Why is it so easy to become a bulimic? One reason is that both binge-ing and vomiting can trigger waves of potent brain chemicals, the endorphins. The release of these natural heroin-like brain chemicals helps establish the powerful compulsions that bulimics are helpless to fight. When we develop false ideas about what we "should" weigh and begin dieting, we open ourselves up to the possibility of developing an eating disorder, just as Miranda did.

A growing number of women—and men—are forced by the dieting mentality into the danger zone of anorexia. They have literally lost their appetites as well as weight. No longer protected by healthy rebound food cravings, they never get to the point where they "just *have* to have a steak." When low-calorie dieting becomes a way of life, so does the descent through the levels of starvation.

A few months into her first-ever diet, 14-year-old Courtney developed most of the symptoms of full-blown anorexia. She was chronically sick with colds and flu, lost her period, and was too weak to exercise. She quit going out with her friends and just stayed at home. She developed radical mood swings that included irritability, hysteria, and insomnia. Soon it became easy for her to starve; an apple could last her all day.

Courtney's symptoms are classic signs of malnutrition. In the concentration camps, the starving prisoners made tiny amounts of food last all day, too. How do the starving survive? How do anorexics endure working out for hours each day in the gym, like the Nazis' slave laborers?

Most of the anorexics whom I have worked with *actually get high on starvation*. Anorexia triggers the same kind of powerful high that opiates like heroin trigger in drug users. How do we know? When anorexics are given drugs that prevent opiates from affecting them, they go into sudden withdrawal, just as heroin users do. Their highs are cut off. It turns out that anorexic starvation, like bulimic vomiting and bingeing, is a traumatic experience that can stimulate a deep survival mechanism: The release of endorphins, the powerful, natural druglike chemicals that allow us to experience pleasure. They also kill pain and ease stress. If your body has become addicted to these natural opiates and you resume normal healthy eating, you will miss the endorphin highs. Like laboratory monkeys who pull the lever that gives them heroin in preference to food or drink until they die, an anorexic will ferociously defend her refusal to eat for powerful biochemical reasons. Bulimics binge and refuse to keep food down with a similar ferocity, and for the same reasons. This obsessive behavior is actually caused by nutritional deficiencies—which, thankfully, we now know how to address.

HOW VITAMIN AND MINERAL DEFICIENCIES
CAN LEAD TO ANOREXIA

Let's take just two vitamin and mineral deficiencies commonly caused by low-calorie dieting and trace their course as they trigger the symptoms of eating disorders.

Vitamin B$_1$ (thiamine). Easily depleted by undereating, this is one of the nutrients that your body cannot make itself, so you must get B$_1$ from foods, primarily the whole foods that chronic dieters and people with eating disorders rarely eat enough of: beans, whole grains, seeds, meats, and vegetables.

Common Early Symptoms of Thiamine Deficiency

+ Loss of appetite
+ Reduced weight
+ Abdominal discomfort
+ Constipation
+ Chest pain
+ Anxiety
+ Sleep disturbance
+ Fatigue
+ Lack of well-being
+ Depression
+ Irritation

At some point in your dieting, your B$_1$ levels may have dropped into the danger zone. You were still the same person, but one day you had just enough B$_1$, the next day you didn't, and the symptoms of anorexia began to erupt, like sores do on the skin of people with vitamin C deficiency. Anorexia actually just means "loss of appetite." When a condition such as vitamin B$_1$ deficiency kills your appetite, you eat less, particularly if you are dieting to begin with. Suddenly, dieting becomes easy. You aren't fighting a normal appetite anymore. You lost it when you lost too much vitamin B$_1$ from dieting. We literally are what we *don't* eat. You can't control what is lost in a diet. It isn't just your body fat that is lost; it's your muscle and bone, and brain tissue, too. Anorexics have empty spaces that show up on brain scans where they have literally lost brain weight.

Zinc. This mineral is hard to find in foods, even when we are not dieting. Red meat, egg yolk, and sunflower seeds are high in zinc. But these are fatty foods, and red meat has a bad name, so they are not likely to be included in dieters' meals. According to eating disorders specialist and nutrition researcher Alex Schauss, Ph.D., study results from Stanford University, the University of Kentucky, and the University of California, Davis, agreed that most anorexics and many overeaters and bulimics were zinc deficient.[13] The influential mineral zinc is the second most abundant trace element in the body. *A classic symptom of zinc deficiency is loss of normal appetite.* Without enough zinc, the body can register only extreme sweetness, saltiness, or spiciness as having any taste. Simple, healthy food becomes unappetizing. In anorexics, little or no appetite remains at all. Other common zinc-deficiency symptoms are apathy, lethargy, retarded growth, and interrupted sexual development. One five-year study, reported by Dr. Schauss, showed an astounding 85 percent recovery rate for anorexia in patients given zinc supplementation. It concluded: "The zinc supplementation resulted in weight gain, better body function and improved outlook."[14] At Recovery Systems we, too, have had success using zinc (along with other nutrients) to help stop the cravings of overeaters and bulimics as well as the appetite loss of anorexics. Clients report that junk foods actually begin to be repellent, sweets are "too sweet," and vegetables and other formerly "boring" foods taste much better once they have taken enough zinc.

It's especially important for teens to get enough zinc. During puberty, reproductive development is at its height. Zinc is crucial for reproductive function as well as appetite, immune function, and mental clarity. If dieting reduces the supply of zinc and other minerals at this nutrient-demanding growth stage, not only can appetite disappear but eventually a girl's menstruation may taper off, along with her mental function, as an eating disorder sets in. In boys and men, zinc is a key ingredient in sperm and protects against prostate problems as well as weak immunity.

Fortunately, these deficiencies are easily addressed with supplements and foods. In chapter ten you will find specific nutritional suggestions to help you if you are anorexic or bulimic.

IS THERE AN IDEAL WEIGHT?

Finding the ideal weight is a dilemma for most women—and increasing numbers of men—in this country and abroad. It's heartbreaking that so many people are caught in this terrible bind: On the one hand, the food industry urges us to eat unhealthy, addictive foods that make it impossible for us to stay at our optimal, genetically programmed weights. On the other hand, the diet and fashion industries and the media torture us with images of bodies that most people really should not have, that can be created only by starving or "carving."

There are as many ideal weights as there are people. You may have heard of the three body types known as ectomorph (thin), mesomorph (medium, muscular build), and endomorph (stocky). In India, these same three types have been recognized for six thousand years and are called *pitta*, *vata*, and *kaffa*. Many studies warn us that it is actually more dangerous to have a low weight for your body type than a heavier weight. In his book *Big Fat Lies*, exercise physiology professor Glenn A. Gaesser makes it clear that fitness (that is, good health status) has little or nothing to do with low weight. Weight loss, for any reason, raises the rate of premature death by 240 percent, according to fifteen studies cited by Gaesser.

As you try to answer the weight question for yourself, keep in mind that the obesity epidemic has resulted in an unprecedented mass distortion of our ancient genetic weight programming. Prior to the 1970s, when our weight began to fluctuate and gradually excalate, the average healthy woman worldwide was 5'4" tall, weighed 145 pounds, and had almost 29 percent body fat. (The average man had 11 percent body fat at age 20 and 25 percent at age 60.)

Weight and body mass index charts never were an accurate gauge of healthy body weight; the numbers on these charts have been yo-yoing for years as various groups fought over what is "normal" weight. For example, if you were a 5'5" woman, according to the Metropolitan Life Insurance Company chart of 1959, depending on your frame (measured at your elbow) you could be between 111 and 143 pounds and be considered healthy. In 1983, those numbers were bumped up—now you could weigh between 117 and 155. Then again, in the 1990s, the USDA said that the healthy weight range for a 5'5" woman is 114 to 150, depending not on your frame but on your age. Meanwhile, the task force of the National Institutes of Health said that, based on body mass, a 5'5" woman is overweight if she's above 144 pounds, though until last year its figures said you could have weighed as much as 156.

So what *should* you weigh? It is your body's job to maintain its genetically programmed features, including its weight. (Try changing your eye color.) Yet we have been conducting a terrible experiment in weight alteration for more than fifty years. When I was growing up in the sixties, before this started, most women were at their genetically programmed, ideal weights; in other words, their *true* weights. Movie stars and even models were much heavier than they are now. Marilyn Monroe varied from a size 10 to size 14 and was always considered gorgeous, as were equally voluptuous stars such as Jayne Mansfield and Rita Hayworth. All of us felt pretty good about our bodies then, unless we were *under*weight! Being considered skinny, thin, or scrawny was a death blow to self-esteem and social status.

Then came the high-carb, low-fat 1970s, and our weights started to go up. We started to diet en masse, yet our weights continued to go up. Then even more addictive foods containing high fructose corn syrup and damaged vegetable oils such as soy and corn oil were introduced. Most sweets contain two forms of sugar: sucrose and fructose. It turns out the fructose is even more damaging than sucrose. That's why high fructose corn syrup, introduced in the 1970s, is now so closely correlated with diabetes and obesity. In all of human history, these kinds of weight-distorting foods had never before been consumed. They have now totally overwhelmed our genetic appetite and weight programming. Their addictive power is currently undisputed (except by the sugar industry). How can we just say no to a substance that's more potent than cocaine? (Yes, the research cited in chapter eighteen confirms it.) We've tried going to the opposite extreme, but low-cal dieting throws our genetic weight programming off in yet another way, by slowing our natural metabolic rates, as you'll see. We cannot get back to the bodies we were intended to inherit—our *true* bodies at their *true* weights—without being able to give up addictive carbs for good and substitute adequate amounts of *true* food. It's a good thing you have *The Diet Cure* in your hands. Hold on tight and it will guide you out of this deadly dilemma.

HOW DIETING CAUSES WEIGHT *GAIN*

Up to 83 percent of those who start formal weight loss programs drop out because: (1) they can't stop eating; (2) they can't lose weight; or (3) they continue to gain weight while sticking to their diet plan! Some dieters are neither overweight nor overeaters to begin with. But after enough dieting attempts, dieters progressively gain more weight and are apt to become overeaters. Those who are already compulsive eaters know that they tend to lose all control after a monitored fast or more gradually lose control after less extreme diets; most dieters gain back any weight they lose within two years after a diet. But many have regained more than they ever lost to begin with. It is typical for dieters to become progressively heavier and weigh more than they ever would have been had they never dieted. Has rebound weight gain set off a panic that propelled you into more dieting, more rebound weight gain, or, eventually, an eating disorder?

DIETING SLOWS METABOLISM: THE FLAME GOES OUT

One reason dieters gain weight is that they do not get enough protein and calories to build and maintain muscle tissue. Instead of using carbohydrates to make glucose, the body's fuel, your dieting body starts burning its own muscle, just as someone in an isolated cabin might run out of firewood and have to burn furniture for warmth. Sure, the fuel "works," but you really don't want to get to this point. Since muscles burn calories and keep your metabolism high, this loss of muscle causes the calories you eat to be stored as fat rather than burned as energy. This is why it's important to keep your muscles well fed and toned through moderate exercise.

Loss of muscle mass isn't the only reason for rebound weight gain after a diet. After the trauma of dieting, your body adds extra pounds to protect against what it correctly perceives as the danger of future famines (in other words, more diets!). It does this by lowering the metabolic flame; levels of T_3, the thyroid hormone that raises your metabolic thermostat, begin to drop within hours of calorie deprivation and continue to fall until the body receives more calories. Why? Because the body knows it is starving. This is a law of nature. Rats that are allowed to feed only two hours per day, rather than eat freely all day as they normally do, end up 30 percent heavier.

Let me offer a specific example of how dieting causes weight gain. Francine, a 40-year-old cashier, came to Recovery Systems five years after starting a medically monitored fast that included a mere 400 calories plus one hour of exercise per day. Within a year on that diet, she dropped from her top weight of 300 pounds to 150 pounds. At the end of the year, she was taken off the fast. By the time we met her she had gone from 150 to 500 pounds. It had taken her thirty years to gain 300 pounds gradually, but only four years to gain 350 additional pounds because of dieting. In fact, she went on the fast two more times during this period, with no weight loss at all!

Francine, like many people who diet, began with a slow-burning metabolism. As a child she had been heavy and had lower energy than her sisters. She had a low-functioning thyroid gland. Through medical testing, medication, and nutritional support, we turned up her metabolic flame so that her calories began to burn at a normal rate, and she slowly began to lose weight once and for all.

REBOUND OVEREATING:
THE DIETER BECOMES A FOOD ADDICT

We know that one half to two thirds of people who begin dieting are not overeaters. This includes those with significant weight problems. But what about the rest? One third to one half of those on formal diet programs do eat compulsively, and may have developed food cravings as strong as any alcoholic's or drug addict's cravings.

Some people have been food cravers since childhood. They are the most easily catapulted into binge eating caused by dieting. Others probably never craved, hid, or stole food in their lives until they began to diet. But after a diet, they may have discovered that the body had a second way of preserving its ideal weight: it didn't just burn calories more slowly; it also fought back against starvation by escalating food cravings until they were strong enough to overwhelm the will to diet. In one study, this rebound overeating was evident just a few weeks after starting a low-calorie diet.[15] These powerful cravings may not stop when weight is regained. This is why I call dieting Russian roulette. We don't know which diet will trigger food cravings that will not stop. Chapter one explained that the brain chemistry of overeating is very similar to that of alcohol and drug addiction. As you crave and consume more refined carbohydrates (sweets and starches), these "drug foods" can create a false high in the brain. You may have become helplessly dependent on junk foods that you began to overeat only because of a diet.

One of my clients, Sharon, a 49-year-old physical therapist, had uncontrollable food cravings that had suddenly erupted four years previously, after the first of six medically monitored fasts she had endured. A runner, she'd quit smoking and had gone from 170 pounds up to 225. On the first fast, she lost 100 pounds but gained it back in six months. Within that first year she lost her gallbladder and got cancer. The next year Sharon began another fast, and over the years found that with each fast she developed more cravings and weight gain until she reached 250 pounds. Sharon had never been a compulsive eater in her life, until she began to fast, and she had never before experienced quick weight gain. The good news is that her cravings and weight gain stopped in the first week on our program.

If you are an overeater, you may consume thousands of calories of sugar, starch, and fat, and yet be almost as malnourished as an anorexic. Healthy, whole foods rarely inspire binges. Fish, chicken, beef, beans, vegetables, whole grains, fruit—all these sources of real nourishment are missing from most compulsive overeaters' diets. The empty calories in junk food are like black holes, using up valuable nutrients. For example, the mineral chromium, deficient in almost all our diets, is further depleted by eating sweets. Chromium is critical for preventing blood sugar swings. Without it, your sweet cravings can grow ever stronger. Other valuable vitamins and minerals are wasted and lost in the stress of trying to digest junk food. As you start to overeat junk food after a diet and to undereat *real* food, especially vegetables and protein, you become even more malnourished. With junk-food eaters, starvation is real—it just may not show.

HIDDEN RISKS OF LOW-CALORIE DIETING

Low-calorie dieting doesn't just lead to weight gain. It can also cause major nutritional deficiencies: overconsumption of carbohydrates, diabetes, and addiction to artificial sweeteners and drugs such as tobacco and appetite suppressants. Let's see if you might be suffering from any of these common problems caused by not eating enough good food.

FAT DEFICIENCY

It's hard to think of fat as a nutrient, because for years we have all been hearing so much about fat as a health hazard. While we fear and vilify fat, we have forgotten how essential it is to our health. Here are some real fat facts for you:

+ A Harvard study of forty thousand nurses found that the 20 percent with the lowest fat intake had the highest rate of cancer.
+ Eskimos had normal cholesterol levels for thousands of years on a diet containing 75 percent sea-animal fat.
+ Mediterraneans, too, are notably free of heart disease, although they consume diets containing 40 percent fat.
+ Scandinavians, the Celtic Irish, and north coast Native Americans, among others, have high genetic requirements for the fats that they traditionally got from their original fish-based diets. Depression and alcoholism are two conditions that they suffer now that their diets are much lower in fish and the natural fats that fish contain.
+ We all need the essential fat-soluble vitamins D, A, and E that low-fat diets jeopardize. Some of the most important functions of these vitamins are to maintain our immune systems and our eyesight and to protect against stroke, liver disease, diabetes, and osteoporosis.

✦ Every cell in the body is protected by a lining of fat.
✦ The brain is 60 percent fat.

The fact is, fats (or fatty acids, as they are biochemically known) play an essential role in the entire body's function. Our recent low-fat mania has yielded many adverse results.

The Low-Fat Experiment That Failed. You may remember that in the 1970s the Pritikin Institute (now called The Pritikin Longevity Center and Spa), the nation's first low-fat diet center, electrified the country. Nathan Pritikin's program was designed for people with severe and chronic health problems, primarily heart disease. His therapeutic diet became mainstream before any long-term evaluation of the Pritikin approach had been done. The extraordinary media attention that the Pritikin Diet quickly received eventually led to what has become a national fat phobia.

Former Pritikin Institute nutritionist and respected health writer Ann Louise Gittleman tells us in her book *Beyond Pritikin* that there was indeed an initial weight loss and health gain for those who came to the Pritikin Institute. But later many of these same people, on the same low-fat regimen, gained back at least as much weight as they had lost. Although their heart problems cleared up, they began to regain unneeded weight and developed new health problems, such as arthritis, chronic yeast infections, and increased PMS, as a result of their low-fat, high-carb diets. Our current nationwide low-fat experiment has produced the same effect: fat consumption has dropped (the average American now consumes 34 percent of his or her calories as fat),[16] yet weight has gone *up* over the past ten years. Instead of eating fats, we're overeating carbohydrates. For millions who do not have heart disease, and who never overate fat to begin with, low-fat, high-carb dieting has become a menace.

Fat Deficiency Causes Fat Cravings. Although many of our clients have avoided fat, overeating sweets and starches instead, some are addicted to fatty foods, such as cheese, peanut butter, fries, and potato or corn chips. When we add certain healthy oils to their diets, they lose excessive interest in rich roods and their weights drop. Low-fat dieting depletes our bodies of essential invaluable fatty nutrients. In reaction, our bodies signal us via cravings to eat more fats. But the kinds of fats in the junk food that we binge on in response to those cravings do not satisfy our fundamental nutritional needs, and we actually put on weight as we become fat deficient. When we eat the specific fats we need, which we can get from animals, fish, nuts, and plants, our fat cravings cease. (If this sounds like you, turn to chapter eight to see if you have fatty acid deficiency.)

Fatty foods such as avocado, salmon, and olives are profoundly nourishing, and a few handfuls of nuts a week actually cut the risk of heart disease. Organic butter and coconut oil are highly nutritious, stable, and safer to cook with than any other fats.

PROTEIN DEFICIENCY

Low fat typically means low protein. What are the healthy protein-rich foods that you may be trying to avoid because of their fat content?

- eggs
- chicken with skin
- red meat
- nuts
- seeds
- cheese

Take a close look. Many of the best sources of protein have become suspect. When you throw this baby out with the bathwater, you are headed for protein malnutrition. Remember, protein is the only food that can be used to create new muscle. Like most dieters, you may be avoiding protein-rich foods because they also contain fat. "I don't want to use up my calories for the day on a steak, because it's too fatty!" you tell yourself. "I'd rather use them on ice cream." Protein is a food that few people crave (a hallmark of a healthy food!), so it's easy to dispense with.

Protein Malnutrition Causes Brain-Power Outage. As the activity of the brain decreases with dieting, the brain's mental and emotional stability can falter—even fail. The brain itself shrinks. (You can recognize brain chemistry deficiency by its very specific symptoms, such as depression, anxiety, irritability, obsessiveness, and low self-esteem.) My clients who are dieters or have eating disorders always suffer from mood problems, caused primarily by protein malnutrition. The four brain chemicals that dictate your moods are all derived from the amino acids in protein foods. Even nondieters who tend not to eat enough protein can suffer from low-protein brain drain.

TRYPTOPHAN DEPLETION: THE PATH TO DEPRESSION, LOW SELF-ESTEEM, OBSESSION, AND EATING DISORDERS

Serotonin, perhaps the most well known of the brain's four key mood regulators, is made from the amino acid L-tryptophan. Because few foods contain high amounts of tryptophan, it is one of the first nutrients that you can lose when you start dieting. Studies show that serotonin levels can drop too low within seven hours of tryptophan depletion. Let's follow this single essential protein (there are nine all together) as it becomes more and more depleted by dieting, to see how decreased levels of even one brain nutrient might turn you toward depression, compulsive eating, bulimia, or anorexia.

When our serotonin levels drop, so do our feelings of self-esteem, regardless of our actual circumstances or accomplishments. These feelings can easily be the result of not eating the protein foods that keep serotonin levels high. As their serotonin-dependent self-esteem drops, girls tend to diet even more vigorously. "If I get thin enough, I'll feel good about myself again!" Tragically, they don't know that they will never be thin enough to satisfy their starving minds. Extreme dieting is actually the worst way to try to raise self-esteem, because the brain can only deteriorate further and become more self-critical as it starves. More and more dieters worldwide are experiencing this miserable side effect of weight reduction on the brain.

When tryptophan deficiency causes serotonin levels to drop, you may become obsessed with thoughts you can't turn off or behaviors you can't stop. Once this rigid behavior pattern emerges in the course of dieting, the susceptibility to eating disorders is complete. Just as some low-serotonin obsessive-compulsives wash their hands fifty times a day, some young dieters may begin to practice a constant, involuntary vigilance regarding food and the perfect body. They become obsessed with calorie counting, with how ugly they are, and with how to eat less and less. As they eat less, their serotonin levels fall further, increasing dieters' obsession with undereating. As their zinc and vitamin B_1 (thiamine) levels drop low as well, their appetite fades. This can be the perfect biochemical setup for anorexia.

Control, which so many therapists and researchers have observed as the central issue of anorexia, often comes down to this: tryptophan (and serotonin) deficiency results in an outbreak of the obsessive behavior that we call "controlling." There may be psychological elements in the picture, too, but a low-serotonin brain is ill equipped to resolve them. Several large international studies of the causes of anorexia have concluded that the cause is a genetic serotonin-related mood disorder, *not* a psychological one.[17]

TRYPTOPHAN, SEROTONIN, COMPULSIVE OVEREATING, AND BULIMIA

For reasons we don't entirely understand, some dieters whose serotonin levels drop lose self-esteem and become obsessed with weight loss, but do *not* lose their appetites. On the contrary, their appetites expand. In the late afternoon and evening, especially in winter and during PMS (low-serotonin times for all of us), these dieters can become ravenous and binge on sweets and starches.

One of our clients ate regular breakfasts and lunches but dreaded her evenings, when she would binge on ice cream and cookies, whether she had eaten a normal dinner or not. Terrified of weight gain, she would throw up as soon as she ate.

In several studies, bulimics were deprived of the single protein tryptophan. In reaction, their serotonin levels dropped and they binged more violently, ingesting and purging an average of 900 calories more each day.[18] In another study, adding extra tryptophan to the diet reduced bulimic binges and mood problems by raising serotonin levels. Most recently, a University of Oxford researcher, Katherine Smith, reported that even years into recovery, bulimics can experience a return of their cravings and mood problems after only a few hours of tryptophan depletion. She concluded, "Our findings support suggestions that chronic depletion of plasma tryptophan may be one of the mechanisms whereby persistent dieting can lead to the development of eating disorders in vulnerable individuals."[19]

Note that most compulsive eaters do not vomit. They keep it all down. But dieting can lower their serotonin levels, too, causing the same wild cravings and self-hate that bulimics suffer.

As we trace the fate of only one depleted nutrient, tryptophan, and the brain chemical made from it, serotonin, you can again see how easily a dieter can develop an eating disorder. If you consider how many other critical brain and body chemicals are depleted through dieting, you have a more profound appreciation of the dangers you are risking on low-calorie diets.

We have just looked at the important nutrients that we *lose* on low-fat diets. Now let's talk about what foods are left. The foods that contain no fat fall into one category: they are all carbohydrates.

THE LOW-FAT, HIGH-CARB RECIPE FOR FOOD ADDICTION AND DIABETES

Carbohydrate foods made from white flour, like pasta, bagels, and bread, are likely to be your first choice on a low-fat diet. You will probably also consume lots of sweets. Grains in their natural, whole form contain some protein, vitamins, minerals, and fats. Unrefined sweets, like fruit and sugarcane, also contain valuable nutrients. But you probably eat the refined, stripped forms of these sweet and starchy carbohydrates. Most low-fat dieters reach for cookies, muffins, pastries, pasta, cereal, and similar foods made from a combination of white flour and white sugar. Addiction researcher Forest Tennant, M.D., draws the biochemical parallel between the effects of eating these high-carbohydrate foods and the elevating effects of alcohol and cocaine. Pointing out that these foods can trigger powerful brain-chemical releases, he calls alcohol the ultimate carbohydrate drug. Refined from high-carbohydrate foods like grains and grapes, alcohol contains three more calories per gram than its original high-carbohydrate sources.[20] When we ask sweets and starch addicts how these foods affect their moods, like alcoholics they often say that the substances make them feel happy, energized, comforted, or relaxed. Over time it takes more carbohydrates to deliver the druglike effect, leading to stronger sweet cravings, more and bigger binges, faster weight gain, and higher blood sugar. If you are bulimic, you probably began vomiting at this stage to empty out, so you could quickly start bingeing again. You may also have started to alternate between periods of abusing alcohol and abusing food.

What about the risk of diabetes? Many of us fear developing diabetes but don't realize that most diabetes (or chronically high blood sugar) is caused just by eating too many refined carbohydrates. Rates of diabetes are skyrocketing parallel to average weight gain. Although as a nation we reduced our consumption of fat, our consumption of carbohydrates continues to rise. Each of us now eats an average of more than one hundred pounds of various sugars, including high fructose corn syrup, every year, in contrast to the twenty-five pounds we ate in 1900.

Because refined carbohydrates made from sugar and white flour rapidly increase insulin levels, they can permanently exhaust the pancreas (the insulin-producing organ), causing diabetes. Another factor that contributes to diabetes is mineral malnutrition. Eating sugar in large quantities can cause loss of minerals, most notably chromium, which is particularly important for blood sugar regulation.

Because pregnant mothers are eating so many carbs, we now have obese and diabetic toddlers! Diabetes is the ultimate eating disorder that can result from low-cal dieting. Diabetic food addicts are unable to stop eating sweets and starches, even though they know that these substances are literally killing them. In chapter ten I'll be talking about how diets lower in carbohydrates and adequate in fat and calories, particularly Atkins, avoid all of these problems and yet promote healthy weight loss. The research is clear!

THE ARTIFICIAL SWEETENER TRAP

Billie drank a pot of black tea from a lovely handmade teapot in a special corner overlooking her garden. She sweetened each cup with several packets of NutraSweet (aspartame). She was a compulsive eater, so she felt that using a diet sweetener was a good, healthy choice for her. When I asked her to give up her black tea because of its caffeine content, she wept. So I relented and said, "Okay, keep the tea for a week. Just stop using NutraSweet." She happily agreed. Two days later I got a phone call from her. "I hate black tea!" she said. She thought it was the tea she craved, but she had actually been an aspartame addict for years, without even knowing it. She experienced the longest drug withdrawal cravings I have ever seen when she stopped using her NutraSweet. For months, she could not satisfy her thirst with any liquid because her body so sorely missed the aspartame.

Most dieters, and even many of you who are not serious dieters, use diet drinks and diet foods to avoid high-calorie sweeteners. Before coming to me, my clients have typically been drinking quarts of diet soda, even cases of it, every day, bingeing on junk food and washing it down with Diet Cokes. Artificial sweeteners contribute to compulsive eating for some users. You may have noticed that your cravings for sweets and fatty foods, and your weight, have increased along with your aspartame use. Several studies have confirmed this ironic fact in both animals and humans.[21] Richard Simmons, the diet and fitness guru, announced that he had given up diet soda after years of addiction and suddenly lost ten pounds!

The amino acid phenylalanine, which is a component of aspartame, can be quite stimulating, especially when combined with caffeine. It and aspartame's other ingredients compete with tryptophan. They block its conversion into the calming, antidepressant brain chemical seratonin. This is one important way that aspartame impedes recovery for those of you who are anorexics and bulimics, even when you try to begin eating normally again. Artificial sweeteners can also make you feel bloated and fat, further discouraging real food consumption. You may avoid food or purge it.

So far, more than ten thousand aspartame users have reported over one hundred adverse symptoms, compiled by the FDA. They include everything from menstrual changes, weight gain, and headaches to severe depression, insomnia, and anxiety attacks.

Aspartame is not the only chemical sugar on the market you should avoid. Saccharin is not only linked with cancer, but, like aspartame, it can cause an increase in the consumption of sweets.[22] Sucralose can have side effects, too, and people are even starting to report side effects from using stevia, despite the fact that it is derived from a plant.

Fortunately you'll lose your sweet cravings on the aminos and won't need these sweeteners anyway.

VEGETARIANS' SPECIAL CHALLENGES AND RISKS

Vegetarian diets can lead to malnourished states and, eventually, eating disorders, even when the vegetarian had no intention of reducing weight by eliminating meat. Flesh foods—like red meat, poultry, and fish—are high-protein foods that contain all of the essential amino acids. Avoiding these foods can weaken many crucial body functions, including muscle and brain strength. Both are dependent on adequate protein. It is possible to get enough protein from vegetarian sources, but it takes careful study and planning. Many vegetarians eat little else but carbohydrates and become quite addicted to sweets.

What may be most difficult to get from a vegetarian diet is iron. Twenty percent of women generally are iron deficient. Iron deficiency is a particularly common problem among female athletes. Iron status is also closely linked with mental and emotional functioning. When dieting depletes iron levels, the result is the mental and emotional fog so characteristic of eating disorders. Very similar symptoms result from zinc deficiency, which is also easy for vegetarians to develop. Red meat is one of the few reliable and easily digestible sources of both zinc and iron (it's harder to metabolize the zinc and iron found in foods like raisins, kale, and spinach).

Fifty percent of anorexics are vegetarian. One of my favorite colleagues, sports medicine specialist Al Loosli, M.D., treats many female high school and college athletes who are vegetarian. According to Dr. Loosli, these vegetarians often suffer from loss of periods, bone mass deterioration and fractures, general weakness, and reduced endurance. Many of them have full-blown eating disorders.[23]

Many of my vegetarian clients have supplemented with iron and zinc successfully, and increased protein from plant sources. Others have reluctantly added fish to their diets several times per week and felt much stronger. Still others have had to accept that their bodies were not built to thrive on a vegetarian diet and have added back red meat and poultry. Several recent books have linked blood type with optimal diet and found that blood type O, in particular, requires animal protein. In chapters ten and eightteen you will find specific suggestions for how to be a vegetarian without becoming depleted in B vitamins, iron, zinc, and protein. I appreciate the idealism of ethical vegetarians, but I also admire the courage it can take to question this popular trend.

Whatever problems you've developed as a result of restricted eating, please read chapter ten, "Nutritional Rehab for the Chronic Dieter," to start supplying your critical nutritional needs. Then, Part III of *The Diet Cure* will help you to develop, perhaps for the first time, a holistic plan for using food, supplements, exercise, and other support that will allow you to recuperate from the effects of low-calorie dieting and reach your own ideal, *healthy* weight.

Unstable Blood Sugar

Carb Addiction, Hypoglycemia, Diabetes, and Adrenal Exhaustion

---

A Special Note Regarding Insulin-Dependent Diabetes

If you are diabetic and taking insulin, you will need to monitor your insulin levels often and work very closely with your M.D. to keep your levels optimal. Insulin levels will come down as your diet improves, once you start taking the supplements. But this low-sugar and -starch diet will drop your glucose levels too fast if your meds aren't reduced at the same time.

You probably know by now whether your own insulin-producing capacity has become irreversibly damaged. If so, you will not be able to stop your medicine, but you will "manage" it much more easily. I highly recommend *Dr. Bernstein's Diabetes Solution*, by Richard K. Bernstein, M.D., as a guide to managing severe diabetes with a diet like the one we recommend (with less carb and more protein and healthy fat than the usual diabetic diet) and excellent, practical suggestions for exercise and medication management.

Sweets and starches are both carbohydrates. You may have discovered that they are equally addictive. If you could stop eating them permanently, on your own, you probably wouldn't be reading this book. You have tried "just saying no." You have probably stopped eating them for short periods during a diet, but I want you to be able to walk away from them, for life, *easily*. And I don't mean you should shift over to health-food cereals, granola bars, and honey-sweetened cookies. Although these products do contain some nutritious ingredients, their first or second ingredient is usually sugar, fruit juice concentrate, or some other sweetener.

Some people successfully quit sugar in a roundabout way by gradually substituting healthier and healthier foods. But weaning yourself from sugar can take years, if it works at all. Many people are so sensitive to concentrated carbohydrates that they really can't do this. They can't stop eating dried fruit any more than others can stop eating Oreos. Brown sugar and honey, like their refined white cousin, can be highly addictive substances.

Most of you can be freed from your sugar cravings in just twenty-four hours. How? First, take your aminos; second, quit undereating; and third, balance your blood sugar.

THE BLOOD SUGAR BLUES

Your body and brain are built of protein, water, fat, minerals, and vitamins. Like auto parts that must be made from very specific materials such as metal and rubber, body parts—muscles, hormones, nerves, bones—must be made from water and solid nutrients like protein, minerals, and fat. Without them, your body doesn't have the building blocks to replenish itself and replace worn-out cells. Carbohydrates have a very different function. They are the fuel that your body uses. Yes, they're important, but just as you cannot build an engine or a tire out of gasoline, you cannot make muscles or bones out of carbs. Imagine a car that did not get its oil replaced or its tires repaired. How far could it go on gasoline alone?

Your body does need high-quality carbohydrate "gas," but the amount depends on how much "driving" your body is doing. Athletes and fast metabolizers need more carbohydrates. Less active people need fewer. And not just any carbohydrate will do the job. You need *high-quality* ones, like vegetables, beans, and fruit; not low-quality carbohydrates that are highly sweetened with sugar, or starchy ones such as white bread or bagels and pasta, *which are converted into sugar in seconds in your mouth*.

If you are a carbo junkie, you are frequently running low on glucose, the blood sugar fuel made from carbs that keeps your brain and body going. But if glucose is made from carbohydrates and you are regularly eating lots of sweet and starchy carbs, how can you be running so low on blood sugar? Paradoxically, it's *because* you are eating so many high-carbohydrate foods! Your body can't tolerate the amount of carbohydrates in highly processed foods such as soda, candy, or cookies, especially if you eat your carbohydrates without lots of balancing protein, fiber, and fat. If you had lox and cream cheese on your bagel, you'd be all right. If you ate a steak every time you had a candy bar, you'd probably be okay, too! But you don't, of course. And some people are so sensitive to sweets that no matter what they eat with them (even if they eat a full meal), they'll get a headache and feel irritable after the initial pleasure injection wears off.

So what happens to all the sweets and starches you eat? Many turn into blood sugar (glucose)—in seconds!—while still in your mouth, shocking and alarming your whole system. "Get rid of it, fast!" shrieks your body. Out rushes insulin, made by your pancreas for just such occasions. Insulin knocks every bit of that glucose high out of your bloodstream and quickly stores it as fat, where it gathers in your body, crowding your muscles and clogging your arteries. As you gain excess fatty weight around your middle from consuming too many carbohydrates, insulin gets less effective. The more carbs you eat, the more fat you store in your abdomen, and the more insulin you need. Meanwhile, your pancreas is running out of the protein it needs to meet the escalating demand for insulin, because you aren't eating much protein. You're filling up on those addictive carbs instead. Often, the end result of all this is diabetes—when, in a sense, your gas tank just fills up with sugar.

THE ADRENALS RUSH TO HELP

But before you get to that point, while you still have plenty of insulin, your problem is that, too often, you don't have *enough* glucose. Either you go too long without anything but a cup of coffee, or the high-carb items you consume force an insulin surge that sweeps your glucose away, or both. At this point your adrenal glands, your emergency stress team, are mobilized to handle the situation. Blood sugar that drops too low can drop you into a coma because your brain is particularly vulnerable to any absence of blood sugar. So, like firefighters with a safety net, the adrenal hormones are sent out to "catch" your blood sugar before it falls too low. They boost it with emergency stores of a special sugar called glycogen.

If this stressful scenario repeats itself too often, your adrenals will get overwhelmed. That's because they are simultaneously taking care of all of the other stresses that are affecting you. So, sooner or later, your adrenals will be unable to make the save as effectively. You'll start feeling worse faster after your sweet or starchy highs. As you feel the increasing need to raise your blood sugar back up, you'll run to the nearest candy machine more often. This low blood sugar, or hypoglycemic, distress is one of the most common problems that we see at our clinic.

Common Symptoms of Low Blood Sugar (Hypoglycemia), in Order of Frequency

- ✦ Craving sweets or starches
- ✦ Nervousness
- ✦ Headaches
- ✦ Weakness
- ✦ Faintness, dizziness
- ✦ Frequent feelings of overstress and/or feeling overwhelmed
- ✦ Irritability, anger, rage
- ✦ Depression
- ✦ Drowsiness
- ✦ Tremors, cold sweats
- ✦ Forgetfulness
- ✦ Lack of concentration, ADHD
- ✦ Unprovoked anxiety and worry
- ✦ Confusion
- ✦ Sensation of trembling in the abdomen
- ✦ Heart palpitations, rapid pulse
- ✦ Muscle pains
- ✦ Numbness
- ✦ Indecisiveness
- ✦ Crying spells
- ✦ Lack of sex drive (women)
- ✦ Lack of coordination
- ✦ Leg cramps
- ✦ Insomnia
- ✦ Blurred vision
- ✦ Muscle twitching and jerking
- ✦ Itching and crawling skin sensations
- ✦ Sighing and yawning
- ✦ Unconsciousness[1]

IS YOUR BLOOD SUGAR RISING OR FALLING?

If you are in the first, hypoglycemic stage of the blood sugar roller-coaster ride, then much of the time your pancreas is still hardy, punching out the insulin to stop sugar shock. But you may be beginning to show signs of impending diabetes: your pancreas can't keep up the pace and release enough insulin indefinitely. Your pancreas was built for the occasional shock, not for daily or hourly carbo overload.

Eventually your pancreas will falter in its job of keeping up your insulin supply. As a result, your blood sugar can eventually rise too high, for too long, too often. You become diabetic. People with the more common type 2 diabetes have all been hypoglycemic and addicted to refined carbohydrates to the point that their pancreas's capacity to cope with high blood sugar has been exhausted.

All diabetics or prediabetics would love to manage their blood sugar problem with diet and exercise, and they try, but they cannot. They are unable to eat healthy food because they are too heavily addicted to carbohydrates. Realistically, their cravings for carbs have to be dealt with before they can begin to exercise and eat in a healthier way.

PREDIABETES? DIABETES?

The high-fructose sweets developed in the United States have created an epidemic of adult and child diabetes that is now circling the world. Here are the signs:

Common Symptoms of Diabetes
- ✦ Overweight
- ✦ Lowered resistance to infection
- ✦ Boils and leg sores
- ✦ Lesions and cuts take a long time to heal
- ✦ High blood pressure
- ✦ Craving for sweets, but eating sweets does not satisfy
- ✦ High sugar in urine and blood
- ✦ Extreme systemic acidity
- ✦ Severe itching
- ✦ Rapid weight loss without dieting
- ✦ Constant hunger
- ✦ Elevated cholesterol
- ✦ Heart and kidney disease

+ Increased thirst and urination
+ Failing eyesight
+ Fatigue

LOW BLOOD SUGAR AND CARB ADDICTION

Most low and high blood sugar problems are caused by overeating sweets and starches. How did you get addicted? It could have started with any or all of the imbalances that I discuss in this book: brain-chemical imbalances, dieting, food allergy, hormonal imbalances, yeast overgrowth, or, as we'll see later in this chapter, too much stress.

But your first problem may be that you were born or now reside in the United States. Diseases of sugar addiction such as hypoglycemia and diabetes are almost unknown in countries that are too "primitive" to import our fancy high-fructose sodas and other sweets. In the United States, per capita we each consume an average of more than one third of a pound of this super-sugar per day! That is a big habit, and it's getting bigger. And this doesn't include the junk-food starches, like chips, pasta, and white bread, that the body can't distinguish from sugar.

The Pimas, a Native people who live on both sides of the border between the United States and Mexico, are among the most vulnerable people in the world to "carbo-drugs" (as I like to call them). In the United States, where they have unlimited access to junk carbohydrates, they have one of the highest rates of obesity and diabetes in the world. But the Mexican Pimas across the border, who still eat mostly whole corn, beans, vegetables, fruit, eggs, chicken, and meat, have neither diabetes nor obesity!

Every ethnic group that comes to the United States (except the English, who may eat as poorly as we do) experiences a drastic reduction in health in the first and certainly by the second generation from exposure to our "diet."[2] That's because essentially we have stopped eating food here; we mostly eat chemicals and carbo-drugs. Products made from them are cheap, overly available, and addictive—of course we eat them! And then we can't stop. Some of us, like the Pimas, are addicted more easily. (Fortunately, the very quality that makes Native Americans so vulnerable to drugs such as sugar, white flour, and alcohol also makes them respond instantly to the nutritional supplements that I describe in chapter eleven.)

A California Native tribal member came to me at age 47 with diabetes so bad that he had become impotent and lost his wife. He had such low energy that he could hardly get up in the morning or stay awake after dinner to visit with his children. Worse, he was losing his eyesight. He knew he had to do something about his health—quickly. I offered him four capsules of a multiple vitamin–mineral formulation designed to stop blood sugar swings. The next day he reported that after taking the first two capsules the night before he had stayed alert until ten P.M. (he usually dozed from seven o'clock on), that he woke up alert (unheard of), and that after taking the second two capsules he had felt fine all the next day. Within two months, he was no longer impotent. Now, I have rarely seen people of other ethnic backgrounds respond this quickly and dramatically to supplements designed to balance blood sugar levels. But people of all ethnicities do respond to this same approach—it just takes days rather than hours.

If you have chronic low blood sugar or are diabetic, staying on a low-carb diet and getting some moderate exercise works miracles. Blood sugars even out quickly, and health, energy, and weight normalize. Simply staying away from sugary foods can usually stop symptoms such as headaches, dizziness, and irritability immediately.

So why don't people with unbalanced blood sugar "just do it"? Most people suspect that it's because diabetics and hypoglycemics are too self-indulgent and have no willpower, or that they just don't care. But they're wrong. Their only problem is that they are up against a biochemical power much stronger than they are. They are caught in the jaws of a relentless biological mechanism that demands that they continue to eat carbs.

Fortunately, it's easy to disarm this biochemical monster. All we typically need are one mineral, an amino acid, and a few vitamins. These natural substances can turn off the carb cravings in just a few minutes. (In chapter eleven, you'll get the exact details of this monster-taming protocol.)

Although most of our clients have been hypoglycemic, we have also worked with many type 2 diabetics, as well as a few type 1 diabetics. We have been able to help them all successfully avoid sweet and starchy carbs. But they do need extra help if (1) they are diabetic and the damage to their pancreas has been too great; or (2) their adrenal glands have become too exhausted by sugar and stress.

Any Doubts About How Addictive Sugary Foods Can Be?

Many clients have told me that they got hooked the very first time they got a high from ice cream, sodas, or cookies. Personally, I think of refined sugar as a drug. When white sugar was first introduced to Europe in the sixteenth century, it was kept under lock and key, because of its potency. It was worth its weight in silver and they even called it "crack"! Just because sugar is legal, cheap, and easily available doesn't mean that it isn't dangerous. Remember, cocaine was once the key ingredient in Coca-Cola, and available to adults and children all across America. The job of the food industry is to addict us!

ARE YOU OVERSTRESSED?
DO YOUR ADRENALS NEED HELP?

Because almost everyone who comes to Recovery Systems has a low blood sugar problem, we are very familiar with the symptoms of hypoglycemia. But it took years for us to realize that many of the symptoms of hypoglycemia are identical to the symptoms of adrenal exhaustion.

As explained earlier, the adrenals are your stress-defense team. One of their primary duties is to handle any blood sugar slumps. In case of a sudden emergency, like when blood glucose drops after insulin has made a sugar sweep in reaction to a Snickers bar, the adrenals release adrenaline, which is why eating sweets can make you nervous, jittery, and irritable. That jolt of adrenaline is intended to get you out of a potentially dangerous fix by forcing the release of a backup fuel supply called glycogen. It's hard work for the adrenals each time they have to perform this emergency procedure. And if you eat sweets and starches a lot, especially without balancing them with protein, you are eventually going to exhaust them. This is true if you diet a lot, too, because your blood glucose is always low when you diet. Dieting is a big strain on the adrenals. There is no greater strain than impending death, which is what the adrenals perceive starvation dieting to be. (Adrenal production of the chief stress hormone cortisol becomes wildly overactive during any low-calorie dieting,[3] and even more so during anorexia.) But *any* extreme or prolonged stress can overtax them.

THE STAGES OF STRESS EXHAUSTION

No matter how much stress we endure, we have just two little glands to fight it for us: the adrenal glands. In periods of profound stress—a divorce, drug addiction, low-calorie dieting, an eating disorder, a major illness or injury—we can go into adrenal overdrive. Our adrenals can get stuck in the "on" position, pushing our whole system into chronic fight-or-flight mode. The chemicals the adrenals release to accomplish this are adrenaline and cortisol: adrenaline is needed for short blasts (when you're approached by a mugger or an angry boss); cortisol bolsters us in the longer-lasting stresses (like the flu or a divorce). As this state of adrenal alarm progresses, other systems try to compensate: The thyroid may turn down its hormonal activity in an attempt to reverse the adrenal overdrive. This can make us tired and heavy as our metabolic rate slows. DHEA and other adrenal hormones can alter their functions, too, as the adrenals become depleted. Often we don't get the relaxation and rest that would allow us to repair and rebound. So we get sick more often, or we have trouble sleeping. Eventually, this cortisol overdrive wears out our produciton capacity. Then we start running too low on cortisol and feel tired, sick, and stressed more often. In the third stage we are quite low most of the day, in cortisol, DHEA, thyroid, and other hormones, like testosterone, estrogen, and progesterone. In this stage we are always tired and cannot cope at all well with even minor stress. PMS and the increasingly common symptoms of perimenopause (irregular menstrual cycles, more cramping, and moodiness, which can all occur for up to fifteen years before menstruation ceases) and menopause can also become severe.

Where are you in the stages of adrenal stress exhaustion? See if you have any of the typical symptoms on the following page.

A story on stress, reported in the *New York Times*, included the interesting results of a survey showing that 68 percent of those questioned felt stressed most or all of the time.[4]

A survey of more than 1,000 adults found that 79 percent of women and 69 percent of men reported stress eating of sweets, particularly chocolate.[5]

Common Symptoms of Adrenal Exhaustion

+ Sensitivity to exhaust fumes, smoke, smog, petrochemicals
+ Inability to tolerate much exercise, or feel worse after exercising
+ Feeling of being mentally, emotionally, and physically overstressed
+ Rapid mood or energy changes
+ Dark circles under the eyes
+ Dizziness upon standing
+ Lack of mental alertness
+ Tendency to catch colds easily when weather changes
+ Headaches, particularly migraines
+ Breathing difficulties
+ Edema (water retention)
+ Salt cravings
+ Trouble falling asleep or staying asleep
+ Feeling of not being rested upon awakening
+ Feeling of tiredness all the time
+ Low blood sugar symptoms
+ Low tolerance of loud noises and/or strong odors
+ Tendency to startle easily, panic
+ Recurrent chronic infections
+ Light-headedness
+ Tendency to get upset or frustrated easily
+ Tendency to get a second wind (high energy) late at night
+ Low or high blood pressure
+ Inability to feel excited by challenges
+ Sensitivity to bright light
+ Sweating or wetness of hands and feet
+ Chronic heartburn
+ Cravings for alcohol
+ Lack of appetite
+ Infrequent urination
+ Lack of thirst
+ Clenching and/or grinding of teeth, especially at night
+ Chronic tension in the lower neck and upper back
+ An excessively low cholesterol level (below 150 mg/dl)
+ And more

As you're considering these symptoms, think about the other stressors, beyond too many carbs, that may have led you to adrenal exhaustion. What have your emotional, financial, and work stress levels been? Do your parents or other family members cope well with anxiety and troubles? A weak adrenal response to stress can be passed on genetically. This is often the case in addictive families in which tranquilizing drugs, like alcohol and tobacco, are used when stress becomes too overwhelming.

ALCOHOL, COFFEE, TOBACCO, SALT, AND YOUR ADRENALS

Alcohol is a super-sugar that can be enormously stressful to the adrenals. Coffee (especially with sugar) can spike your blood sugar, too, then crash it. Cigarettes, which are liberally laced with sugar (up to 90 percent!), can have the same effect.[6] Yet most smokers describe tobacco as "calming." Somehow, tobacco seems to counter the effects of the adrenaline that carbs, caffeine, and stress all stimulate. The more "calming" tobacco you need, the more concerned you should be about the condition of your adrenal glands.

Do you crave salty foods such as chips, pretzels, or olives? Do you crave sweet foods like cookies, gummy candy, or ice cream? When you crave salty and sweet foods at the same time, you can be sure that your adrenals are overworked, because they are in charge of keeping the levels of both sodium and glucose in your system balanced.

The adrenals can become really overwhelmed and worn out if you alternate dieting and overeating sweets and starches. That leaves them less able to help you with illness, trauma, allergies, injury, and daily stress. High doses of pharmaceutical cortisone (such as prednisone) can also shut down your adrenals.

In chapter eleven, I'll give you the details on exactly what to take to restore your adrenal function. If your basic supplements and improved diet do not relieve your symptoms of adrenal exhaustion, you must test your adrenal function with an accurate, inexpensive, and painless saliva test. It is all too easy to become stressed beyond what simple remedies can handle. Depending on the stage of adrenal exhaustion that your symptoms and test results show you to be in, you can take adrenal-restorative supplements, natural hormones, or medications to quickly rebuild your stress-coping capacity. If your symptoms don't improve, you should consult a physician for additional help.

Then you can look at your lifestyle and de-stress it. You'll need to be careful not to overexercise—that demands too much of your adrenals. Learn to give in to relaxation at least twice a day. Breathe quietly. Get plenty of rest. Learn yoga or other stretching-to-relax exercises, or just make the time to participate in your favorite relaxing activities (see chapter twenty-one for more advice on how to relax) and get whatever counseling you might need to help you de-stress. Be nice to yourself—everything depends on it.

LEANNE'S STORY

Leanne was a client who suffered unknowingly from adrenal burnout. After fifty years of overeating sweets and many years of smoking tobacco (she quit alcohol when she turned 40), Leanne, an office manager, was one hundred pounds overweight and an oversensitive powder keg. She blew up at everything. She tried to relax, but she never seemed to be able to. Her adrenal-stress profile (obtained through a saliva test) showed her dangerously low in the essential stress-coping chemicals cortisol and DHEA. The lab technicians retested her specimen three times because they could not believe her score.

Why was Leanne so stressed? Her addiction to sweets started when she was a little girl, and she had a genetic thyroid problem, so she gained weight easily. By age 7, she was enduring regular diets and was being dragged to the scale and beaten by her parents because she did not (*could* not!) lose weight. Leanne had even tried living at a weight loss center for months at a time. Until she finally "gave up" in her 40s, she had tried every diet and fast imaginable. Starvation dieting had stressed her out, she said, as had her heavy sugar and tobacco (and former alcohol) use. Constant family criticism and inner self-hate stressed her terribly as well, but a temperamental boss and long hours had finally taken her over the top.

A few days after she began using nutritional supplements, Leanne stopped overeating sweets. She had no trouble eating well and was finally chocolate-free. She lost forty-five pounds in her first year. In counseling, Leanne was able to detach from the early abuse and stop hating herself. She became less irritable. But after a year and a half, she felt that she was still too easily stressed, and her weight had not dropped for six months, though this was the first time in her life that she had not regained weight after a weight loss. We decided to test her adrenal function. Before we got the results, we had given her extra nutrients to support her adrenals. But after we got the results, we agreed with her doctor that she needed more aggressive care. In addition to suggesting

DHEA, the doctor put her on three small daily doses (2.5 to 5 milligrams) of cortisol (Cortef) per day. In short order, she was feeling stronger and less reactive. She could really relax at last, and she began to lose weight again. After four months, she was able to go off of the medication entirely. Her own adrenals had rested up and were working again on their own.

Leanne is a good example of someone whose adrenals are too worn out to be restored by an improved diet and supplements alone. I suspect that many of you are in this category because of the terribly high stress levels that we are all living with these days. I consider the adrenal saliva tests (which you can even order yourself) and treatments among the most exciting new developments in health care since the 1980s.

Now it's time to go into action with the specific supplements, foods, and tests that you'll use to treat the blood sugar and adrenal blues. If you are panicking about changing your entire eating style, don't forget that you can always go back to sweets. As the rabbis say, "Your health is the most important thing. You can always kill yourself later." Just turn to chapter eleven and try my advice for killing your sweet tooth instead.

FOUR

Unrecognized Low Thyroid Function

Tired, Cold, and Overweight

"Overweight people are lazy gluttons." If there's any myth I would like to debunk, it's that one. No one volunteers for unneeded weight gain. I have never met people who try harder at anything than the people who come to our clinic for help in losing excess weight. I *do* see many people who are too tired to exercise or even cut up vegetables. They always say, "I'm just lazy. I'm not trying hard enough." But over the years I've seen that their "laziness" miraculously disappears as a result of a successful restoration of their thyroid function. As for gluttony, like everyone else, I used to think that weight gain was always the direct result of overeating. But then I learned how to help people stop overeating by eliminating low-calorie dieting, increasing the quality of their food, and using amino acids and other nutrients. Some of my clients immediately lost the weight they needed to lose, but others either lost very slowly or not at all. They did immediately quit gaining additional weight, but they were frustrated to be eating so well, so effortlessly, with little or no weight *loss*. Inevitably, their thyroid was the problem.

If you have a thyroid disorder that has forced you to gain weight, you have probably been subjected to ridicule, humiliation, and contempt for years, even for life. And yet you have tried everything to stop the weight gain. You have been willing to pay almost any price to lose weight. You are disciplined. You may be keeping your calories at starvation levels on a daily basis, while forcing yourself to exercise despite your low energy, trying to prevent more weight gain, even if you have lost hope of ever losing weight. Still, your doctors tell you that you aren't trying hard enough. You are tired and easily chilled. Your body seems unable to burn calories briskly, to keep your weight at appropriate levels for your body type. Sounds like a thyroid problem—yet in your annual physicals you are told, "Your thyroid has always tested normal and it is again this year."

Some of my heaviest clients are not food cravers or overeaters at all. They eat normally. In fact, many of them chronically *undereat*, because moderate eating, even combined with exercise, has resulted in continued weight gain! Some of them actually gain weight on starvation diets or medically monitored fasts. When I looked into the research on this, I found that fully half of people entering formal weight loss programs do not overeat. The dropout rate for these programs runs as high as 85 percent,[1] partly because so many dieters just cannot lose weight by cutting calories.

As you learned in chapter two, dieting (or starvation) may have triggered your weight increase, shutting down your thyroid and causing calories to be stored rather than burned. For most of you, dieting just makes an already sluggish thyroid even more sluggish. But identifying and correcting a low-functioning thyroid can make all the difference.

How do you know your fatigue and weight gain are due to a thyroid problem? There are other key signals that this gland is the culprit. Constantly having cold hands and feet (do you wear socks to bed?) is one. Having gained weight after a big hormonal shift such as getting your first period, having a miscarriage or baby, or entering menopause is another. Having family members with thyroid problems also is a big red flag, as is overreliance on caffeine or other stimulants.

To help you further understand why your thyroid isn't functioning properly, let's look at how it is supposed to work.

THE FUNCTION OF THE THYROID

Where is your thyroid? It sits like a butterfly on your vocal cords, just below your Adam's apple.

What does your thyroid do? This remarkable master gland affects every cell in your body, regulating cell metabolism like a thermostat. Your body needs a constant level of heat to perform its functions vigorously. There's a huge difference in how your cells function, depending on whether they are cold or warm. When your thyroid function is low (what is called a "sluggish" thyroid), it doesn't produce enough active hormones, or your own immune system is fighting your thyroid and preventing the hormones from getting to the cells, so your whole system becomes more inert. And that is the way you tend to feel if your thyroid is not able to do its job well. Literally every part of your body, from your skin to your heart, head to toe, is diminished when the thyroid is not functioning well. Because the thyroid regulates the burning of calories, your weight tends to go up as your thyroid function goes down.

SYMPTOMS AND CAUSES OF LOW THYROID FUNCTION

First, and most important: if you suspect you may have a thyroid problem, look at your symptoms and your history carefully, *yourself.* I have found that nothing is more important than your sense about how your own body is working—or *not* working. At the Recovery Systems Clinic, we always look first at symptoms of thyroid problems instead of relying only on tests, as most medical doctors do. Our doctors do a physical examination of the thyroid, test reflexes, review a temperature log, and order blood tests. Yet if symptoms strongly suggest there may be a thyroid problem, the doctors may ignore negative test results entirely and try a monitored trial of medication. Keep in mind as you look at this list of symptoms that you don't have to have all of them, but if you have several that are severe, you should definitely read this chapter.

Most Common Symptoms and Risk Factors of Low Thyroid Function

- ✦ Uncomfortably heavy since childhood
- ✦ Family history of thyroid problems
- ✦ As a child, played quietly rather than vigorously
- ✦ Weight gain began when you got your period, had a miscarriage, gave birth, or began menopause
- ✦ Low energy, fatigue, lethargy, need lots of sleep (more than eight hours), trouble getting going in the morning
- ✦ Tendency to feel cold, particularly in hands and feet
- ✦ Tendency toward excessive weight gain or inability to lose weight
- ✦ Hoarseness, gravelly voice
- ✦ Depression (including postpartum)
- ✦ Low blood pressure/heart rate
- ✦ Menstrual problems, including excessive bleeding, severe

cramping, irregular periods, severe PMS, scanty flow; early or late onset of first period; premature cessation of menstruation (amenorrhea)

+ Reduced sexual drive
+ Poor concentration and memory
+ Swollen eyelids and face, general water retention
+ Thinning or loss of outside of eyebrows
+ Tend to have a low temperature (under 97.8)
+ Headaches (including migraines)
+ High cholesterol
+ Lump in throat, trouble swallowing (e.g., pills)
+ Slow body movement or speech

Other Common Symptoms of Low Thyroid Function

+ Miscarriage
+ Goiter; enlarged, swollen, or lumpy thyroid (look at the base of your throat, below your Adam's apple)
+ Coarse, dry hair
+ Hair loss
+ Infertility, impotence
+ Weak, brittle nails
+ Anemia, low red-cell count
+ Dry, coarse, or thick skin
+ Overuse of caffeine or other stimulant drugs

In addition, low thyroid function can cause these symptoms, which may be more common in older women:

+ Pale skin
+ Hypoglycemia
+ Constipation
+ Hair loss
+ Labored, difficult breathing
+ Swollen feet
+ Nervousness, anxiety, panic
+ Enlarged heart
+ Premature graying
+ Gallbladder pain
+ Pain in joints
+ Angina
+ Heart palpitation, irregular heartbeat
+ Muscle weakness

✦ Atherosclerosis (hardening of arteries)
✦ Strong-smelling urine
✦ Tongue feels thick
✦ Vision and eye problems
✦ Excess ear wax

Note: Autoimmune conditions often associated with thyroiditis include diabetes, rheumatoid arthritis, multiple sclerosis, lupus, Addison's disease, allergy, and pernicious anemia.

SLUGGISH THYROID, SLUGGISH MOOD

If your thyroid has been sluggish, you have probably not been able to get the complete benefits from the foods you have consumed or even the nutritional supplements that you have taken. This low-thyroid malnutrition may have been going on for years, leading to depression. Depression is not necessarily caused by low thyroid, but whenever I see it, particularly when the client wants to sleep all day, has trouble getting up in the morning, has a low libido, and is generally tired and apathetic, I investigate the thyroid.

At the clinic, we became particularly aware of low-thyroid depression because it would not respond as well to our amino acids, which are usually so helpful so quickly. If I suspect that low thyroid is the cause of their depression, I often suggest that patients start taking the amino acid L-tyrosine immediately. I have learned that if they don't feel more energetic in ten to fifteen minutes, or they only have a brief or subtle response, they are likely to need medical treatment for a thyroid problem. Once the thyroid is running well, the depression lifts.*

HOW COULD YOUR THYROID DEVELOP A PROBLEM?

For most people, there is more than one trigger for low thyroid function.

Genetics. This may be the most common cause of thyroid problems. You may have relatives who have been diagnosed and treated for low thyroid. More often, and more tragically, they may never have been properly di-

---

* If you have depression characteristic of low serotonin and your thyroid function is low, you may not respond to tryptophan or 5-HTP until your thyroid is repaired.

agnosed or treated. Review this chapter's symptom questionnaire with your relatives in mind, and interview your family members. You may be surprised by what you learn.

Brid, one of our clients, took her 70-year-old mother, Mae, to her M.D. after she herself had been successfully treated by him for severe problems caused by thyroiditis (a surprisingly common allergic reaction to her own thyroid). Brid had, as a result of her thyroid problem, allergy, energy, sleep, and mood problems. She knew Mae had been disabled by similar symptoms since age 35 (after she had given birth to two children). Indeed, Mae reported that she was deeply exhausted and anxious, and had suffered extreme weight gain. She also had a nodule on her thyroid that could be seen from across the room.

When I asked her whether she'd ever tested her thyroid function, she said she had been given the standard thyroid blood test (TSH) many times and that the results were always in the normal range. No other test had been given to her, nor had a doctor ever examined her thyroid. But when Brid's M.D. tested Mae more thoroughly, her scores on another kind of thyroid test were astronomically high, indicating that she definitely had a thyroid problem. Now that Mae has been successfully treated she is happy, energized, and at her normal weight. What's more, it turned out that Mae's mother had had almost identical symptoms, down to a thyroid nodule that visibly protruded from the same spot in her throat!

Low-Calorie Dieting and Nutrient-Deficient Diets. These also reduce thyroid function, as well as other body functions. Slowing down the thyroid early on in the process of starvation actually helps the body hold on to its nutritional resources until the ordeal (the famine, or diet) is over. Within hours of restricting calories, the thyroid will slow down and remain slow until the restriction is lifted. Many dieters suffer a metabolic decline that never ends until the condition is treated with thyroid hormone replacement. For them, the resulting permanent slowdown of calorie burning results in the familiar post-diet rebound weight gain.

Hormonal Events. When your menstrual period first began, did you begin to diet, fast, and skip meals in an effort to stop sudden excessive breast development or general weight gain? Until I ask clients what was going on when their dieting started, many have never taken their first hormonal body changes seriously. "I just started dieting at around fourteen," they say, as if this had no significance. But the beginning of adolescent body changes is often the crucial moment when thyroid problems begin. Dieting at this point can further depress your thyroid, which has probably already begun to falter, causing excessive weight gain and early breast development. If this happened and you continued with yo-yo dieting, your thyroid would have become unable to rebound.

Hormonal events throw many vulnerable people into low-thyroid states. Even if you passed through puberty normally, a miscarriage, abortion, or pregnancy may have depressed your thyroid function. "I never lost all of the weight after my last baby" is a common complaint of our clients whose thyroids gave out after giving birth. Postpartum depression is the next possible signal of a troubled thyroid. The final hormonal trigger, often confused with what we, probably mistakenly, assume is natural aging, is the menopausal thyroid sag.

Vegetarian Diets. Eating a vegetarian diet can cause you to become pale and listless because the body lacks iron, which is needed for vigorous thyroid function, along with other nutrients such as selenium and zinc. These nutrients are found plentifully in red meat but are more difficult to get from foods on a vegetarian eating plan, especially if you are a vegan (no animal products of any kind).

Soy. Soybean products such as tofu can have a powerfully negative effect on your thyroid, actually inhibiting its ability to produce its primary hormone, T_4. Many studies are showing other harmful effects as well. If you are a vegetarian, losing this primary protein source will leave you in a particularly difficult spot: you'll have to weigh the risk of using tofu against your need to adhere to nonanimal protein sources. (See chapter fourteen for information on the effects of soy on hormones, and see chapter eighteen for more on the problems with soy.)

Anorexia. People with anorexia typically have starvation-triggered low thyroid function. If they have no major genetic thyroid problem, anorexics usually bounce back just by being given more food and supplements—particularly certain minerals and the amino acid L-tyrosine—that the thyroid needs to make its hormones.

The Adrenal Link

Because adrenal malfunction can reduce thyroid function, it is crucial to test your adrenals as well as your thyroid. Many of my clients have exhausted adrenal glands as well as malfunctioning thyroids. If you have been under continual stress, your adrenals may be the cause of your thyroid problem. Fatigue and low body temperature are symptoms common to both low adrenal and low thyroid function.

If the adrenals become overactive during chronic stress, the thyroid may slow down to try to calm the system. If the adrenals are diverted (by chronic stress) from their job of regulating the immune system, thyroiditis can result. In thyroiditis, the thyroid becomes inflamed. This inflammation can scar and eventually destroy your thyroid gland. Your own best anti-inflammatory is the natural cortisone your adrenals would make if they weren't otherwise occupied. The adrenals are energizing partners of the thyroid. If the thyroid fails, the adrenals can get overworked and run down. The result is a stressed—tired, but wired—sensation that won't go away. If you have adverse reactions to thyroid medication, such as jitteriness and palpitations, be sure to check your adrenals. (See pages 48 and 163.)

It you have been diagnosed with thyroid disease and treated with thyroid hormone and the treatment does not seem to be working (you continue to have symptoms), your adrenals may be exhausted. Unless both the thyroid and adrenals are functioning well, your energy, weight, and general health cannot be optimal.

Physical Injury or Severe Illness. A 1995 study of adverse effects of physical injury on the thyroid reviewed the convincing evidence showing that head injuries often adversely affect the thyroid. One of our trusted medical advisers, Richard Shames, M.D., author of *Thyroid Power* and *Thyroid Mind Power*, says that whiplash, which drastically affects the throat (where the thyroid sits), often seems to affect thyroid function. The shock of a major illness can also depress your thyroid's effectiveness.

Intolerance to Wheat, Rye, Barley, and Oats. This family of grains contains a thyroid-irritating substance called gluten. Gluten intolerance is a common cause of thyroiditis, a serious autoimmune condition that often clears up when victims stop eating breads, pastas, pastries, etc. *More on Hashimoto's later in this chapter.*

Prescription Drugs. The most popular thyroid-inhibiting drugs are SSRI antidepressants like Zoloft and Lexapro. Estrogen (including the estrogen in birth control pills) and lithium are the most well-known thyroid-inhibiting drugs. Sulfa drugs and antidiabetic drugs also slow thyroid function.[2] But there are many more thyroid inhibitors. Review any drugs you are taking with a pharmacist and your physician. Study the information on the enclosure that comes with the package, or ask the pharmacist to give you a copy. If you are on an SSRI, read *The Mood Cure* Chapter 11 "Natural Alternatives to Antidepressant Drugs."

Chemicals in Our Water, Fish, and Teeth That Suppress Thyroid. Fluoride and various forms of chlorine (including perchlorate in pools and chewing tobacco) and fluoride can suppress thyroid function. Perhaps this is why so many people seem to have low-thyroid symptoms nowadays; most water supplies are treated with both these chemicals. There are also harmful hydrocarbons in unfiltered water that have been shown to suppress the thyroid. (See page 284–85 for information on unadulterated water.) No wonder so many of our low-thyroid clients have been swimmers. The nitrates in so many prepared meats are also thyroid suppressors, as is the mercury in our seafood, which has reached dangerously high levels. Large fish, like tuna and swordfish, contain the highest levels of mercury. The mercury contained in 'silver' amalgam dental fillings can expose us to even more toxicity, according to many reports, including one by the FDA in 2011.[3] The combined impact can suppress thyroid function. A recent client was able to go off his thyroid medication after testing positive for excessive mercury and then having it removed. Check GotMercury.org for fish info and discuss mercury testing with a holistic practitioner.

The Iodine and Salt Controversies. Our thyroid hormones are composed of tyrosine and iodine. Tyrosine is easy to find in all animal- and in many vegetable-protein sources. Iodine is harder to find; iodine deficiency became epidemic in the United States and abroad when our soils became depleted of it by the early 1900s. Thyroid deficiency symptoms, most notably disfiguring goiters (swellings at the neck), and mental retardation became commonplace as a result. Iodized salt, bread, and milk came to the rescue, and goiter and retardation rates rapidly diminished. Unfortunately, a marked increase in autoimmune thyroiditis also ensued and has continued to be a modern plague worldwide wherever salt has been iodized.

Is it the amount added? The daily minimum requirement for survival is 150 micrograms per day. One quarter teaspoon of iodized salt delivers 130 micrograms. Most people consume much more salt than this each day and get more from their food, if they eat seafood, the occasional seaweed, and organic food grown on enriched soil.

Too much iodine triggers thyroiditis. It can also cause both hyperthyroidism and hypothyroidism. Doctors sometimes use high doses to suppress thyroid function in those with hyperthyroidism. Some people have violent hyperthyroid reactions to the iodine in medications or water purification tablets. The Japanese, who eat lots of high-iodine foods such as fish and seaweed, have high rates of thyroid cancer.

Sea salt, which has become very popular in recent years, contains many other minerals, but almost no iodine, while iodized salt has been stripped of most minerals. Customers love the variety of the colors and tastes in natural salts. Many restaurants and processed-food producers are even cooking with sea salt or other non-iodized salts.

Are we getting enough iodine if we use only sea salt? One quarter of males and up to half of females (especially pregnant or lactating women) are now deficient—even more so since the 1970s when bread and milk ceased to contain added iodine. Some companies (e.g., Hain) are producing iodized sea salt. This may be a good answer.

Keeping consumption of iodized and non-iodized salt in balance is a challenge. If you eat high-iodine foods such as seaweed and kelp regularly, you might stick to just sea salt at home since you will probably also be getting plenty of iodized salt when you eat out.

In holistic medicine now, there is a huge interest in iodine therapy. One of our clinic's staff members had a thyroid problem she had inherited from her mother. It got much worse in her forties and she tried every possible medication. All gave her insomnia, even in tiny doses. Then she tried iodine therapy and had quick weight loss and relief from all her other low-thyroid symptoms as well. However, many of our clients have tried it with no benefit, while others have been harmed by it.

The key is to watch your thyroid symptoms carefully and attempt to get enough but not too much iodine. Monitor your symptoms even more closely if you try taking supplemental iodine. Watch especially for insomnia, palpitations, or rashes.

TESTING YOUR THYROID FUNCTION

Once you are certain about your symptoms and clear on whether you or anyone in your family has experienced symptoms of low thyroid, it's time to gather more information to determine once and for all if, indeed, you do have low thyroid function. Armed with this information, you can work with your health care professional to determine whether you need thyroid medication (which I will discuss in detail in chapter twelve).

TEST RESULTS THAT LIE

The most common test for thyroid function is the TSH (thyroid-stimulating hormone) test. The TSH measures the thyroid stimulating hormone sent by the pituitary gland in the brain, which relays orders to the thyroid gland about how much thyroid hormone the body needs at a given time.[4] The ideal range, according to many U.S. doctors and British thyroid expert A. P. Weetman, M.D.,[5] is between one and two. TSH levels greater than two indicate that the body needs more thyroid hormone than it is getting and that the pituitary gland is sending a message to the thyroid to encourage it to produce more. However, TSH is not the most accurate indicator of a thyroid problem. Christine, a 50-year-old financial adviser, was a prime example of a person with a thyroid problem that went undiagnosed because of the unreliability of the TSH test. Christine, chubby as a child, had become quite heavy as an adolescent after she began to get unusually profuse and painful periods at 11 years old. She slimmed down briefly as a teenager and met her husband-to-be. Before her wedding a few years later, because her weight had started to go up again, she used diet pills for the first and only time. As soon as she quit the pills, her weight really surged, and she was on the dieting roller coaster for life.

A sensitive and lovely woman, Christine had been beaten raw by the contempt she had encountered everywhere. Most particularly she had been hurt by her husband (one of the wiry, eats-anything body types), who had never stopped complaining about her weight and berating her for "not trying harder." He tended to blame her weight for all of the problems in their marriage—this despite the years of self-torture he had witnessed as she struggled through one diet after another.

Christine said she had never been a sweets lover, though she enjoyed wine several evenings a week. Since menopause, she had developed a taste for fatty foods for the first time. But she had never been a binger.

After menopause began, she stopped being able to lose any weight at all, even with her most austere and punishing diet standby, liquid fasting. She finally just gave up and let the weight come on, until she heard about our program. As she and I reviewed her symptoms and history, a textbook case of hypothyroidism took shape. I kept exclaiming, "Not that symptom, too?!" In addition to all the classic ones, she had some symptoms that I had only seen listed in books—never in a person—such as excessive ear wax and an enlarged heart. Christine told me that she had always felt that she might have a thyroid problem. She said that she had mentioned this to every doctor that she had ever seen and they had all shrugged and said, "Sorry, we've checked it, and your thyroid is doing fine." TSH tests confirmed that she was in the "normal" range. She never thought to ask any further questions. If she had, she would really have been "fine" years before.

More extensive lab testing, as well as ankle reflex and temperature tests, confirmed that her thyroid was indeed malfunctioning. As a result, her doctor started her on a treatment protocol, in her case, a prescription for glandular thyroid hormone replacement Armour, which solved the problem. We have heard this same story at our clinic countless times: the TSH test failed to reflect the true state of thyroid affairs. If the TSH test does not show abnormality, most doctors refuse to proceed further. They insist that their patient is lying about how much she or he eats, and then give lectures about how only increased self-discipline will achieve weight loss. Yet time after time I have seen a more complete workup (with up to eight tests included) show results that correspond with the actual experience of the person tested. In Christine's case, a more thorough thyroid assessment led to needed treatment. The results: normalized weight and energy at last, without dieting.

THREE MORE HELPFUL TESTS

These three additional tests can help detect a thyroid problem: the basal temperature test, which you can do at home; the thyroid gland exam; and the ankle reflex test, which your doctor can do.

Measuring Your Basal (Underarm) Temperature. This home-testing method has been used for many years by physicians. A study confirming its accuracy, conducted by Dr. Broda Barnes on one thousand patients, was first published in the *Journal of the American Medical Association* in 1942.[6]

1. You can order a Geratherm Hypothyroid Basal Thermometer at MFASCO Health & Safety (mfasco.com or 800-221-9222). Digital thermometers are not as accurate as the old mercury ones, but they are safer.
2. Place the thermometer in your armpit ten minutes after awakening but before you get out of bed. Turn the light on. Keep your eyes open.
3. Leave it there for ten minutes.
4. Do this for three mornings, or more, to get an average temperature. If you are menstruating, basal temperature testing is most accurate during your period. Ovulation causes the temperature to rise, which is why women can use the basal temperature for pregnancy planning as well as measuring thyroid function. Even if you are having hot flashes, your basal temperature will not be distorted. If the axial (underarm) temperature is consistently subnormal (below 97.8 degrees), your thyroid function is probably low.

Testing Your Thyroid Gland and Ankle (Achilles Tendon) Reflex. Your physician should examine your gland by touch to check for swelling, nodules, or other abnormalities. Here is another way to test thyroid function: Does your foot bounce when someone taps the tendon at the back of your ankle? This is a good indication that you do not have a sluggish thyroid.[7] If your reflex is slow, keep testing it throughout therapy. Your foot should begin to bounce nicely.

THYROID BLOOD TESTS

Because the TSH is not a reliable blood test, and because you won't be able to get thyroid medication easily unless blood tests reveal a problem, you can—and should—insist that the following five tests also be performed: free T_4; free T_3; reverse T_3; and antithyroglobulin and antimicrosomal antibodies.

Free T_4. T_4 (short for the amino acid tyrosine plus four iodine molecules) is a primary hormone manufactured by the thyroid gland. Although T_4

may be the most plentiful thyroid hormone, it is not the most potent. Sixteen percent of T_4 is used directly by the cells. The rest is converted by them into its sister hormone, T_3, which is ten times more dynamic. T_3 is the thyroid hormone that has the greatest effect on the body's metabolic function. Actually, it must be present on the nucleus of every cell in the body to properly activate our DNA.

Reverse T_3 (RT_3). This test measures a substance, called RT_3, that blocks T_3 receptors in your cells. You may have quite a bit of it blocking your T_3. RT_3 increases with stress, particularly the stress of undereating or anorexia. When RT_3 is high, the use of T_3 medications (like Cytomel) is often more beneficial than that of any of the T_4-containing medications.

Thyroid Antibody Tests. These two tests measure the number of immune system terminators created specifically to do battle against the thyroid. There are two types of these antibodies, and so two tests are needed: for antithyroglobulin and for antimicrosomal. This is the test that helps identify whether you have thyroiditis, an allergy to your own thyroid. This autoimmune condition is quite common and shares many of the symptoms of "low" thyroid. See more on page 68.

TEST RESULTS: LOW, LOW-NORMAL, OR NORMAL

Note: In more than twenty-five years, our clinic has seen only two people with *over*active thyroid test results. But many of our clients' mothers or grandmothers have been hyperthyroid and had their glands irradiated or removed.

Many people seem to get false-negative results on their thyroid tests, particularly on TSH. There are lots of people who score in the low-normal range. They almost always have plenty of symptoms to indicate some kind of foul-up involving their thyroids. But sure enough, their doctors don't attend seriously to their symptoms and refuse to give thyroid medication a try. The patient gets worse, but again is admonished and sent away with a low-calorie diet. (I hope that you know by now that low-calorie diets make things even worse.) Yet a standard medical textbook advises that "patients with subclinical hypothyroidism [low-normal test results] may benefit from therapy even though their symptoms are not obvious."[8]

Fortunately, there are doctors who interpret the test scores differently. According to their interpretations, your low-normal score could be considered *sub*normal. These practitioners will usually be glad to give you a monitored trial on thyroid medication. (See page 175 for assistance finding these doctors.) Remember that blood tests for thyroid function are relatively recent. Up until the 1940s, doctors treated thyroid problems by looking carefully for certain symptoms rather than relying solely on a blood-test number!

If your test results are outside of the normal range, or if they indicate low-normal thyroid function, your physician will have recommendations to make. Bring this book with you to the visit in which you review the test results that have come in and the treatment options described in chapter twelve.

If your first results are negative—in other words, no thyroid (or adrenal) problems are reflected by them—you and your physician will have to look carefully at your symptoms and history again, and then decide whether a trial of medication is in order if you have already tried the nutritional strategies in chapter twelve.

Most of my clients with many symptoms of low thyroid have found that test results have confirmed a problem. But almost 25 percent have had no confirming blood-test results. In most of those cases, a trial of thyroid medication has been very successful.

ARE YOU ALLERGIC TO YOUR OWN THYROID?

Another common cause of low-thyroid symptoms is thyroiditis, which means that you are actually allergic to your own thyroid. If your body's immune system is mistakenly trying to destroy your thyroid gland and its hormones, you will, at some point, suffer many of the symptoms in the questionnaire. Some thyroid experts now believe that *most* low-thyroid symptoms are caused by thyroiditis.

Our clinic's experience is that about 25 percent of our clients with thyroid problems have had thyroiditis identified by blood antibody tests and by certain unique symptoms. They have all improved from various treatments that are described in chapter twelve, but recovery can be complex.

Stephen Langer, M.D., in his *How to Win at Weight Loss*, gives this excellent summary of thyroiditis symptoms:

In descending order of frequency [they] are: (1) profound fatigue, (2) memory loss, (3) depression, (4) nervousness, (5) allergies, (6) heartbeat irregularity, (7) muscle and joint pain, (8) sleep disturbances, (9) reduced sex drive, (10) menstrual problems, (11) suicidal tendencies, (12) digestive disorders, (13) headaches and ear pain, (14) lump in the throat, and (15) problems swallowing.

Nervousness ranges from mild anxiety to full-blown panic attacks, of which some are true psychiatric emergencies. These are as puzzling to the patients as to their physicians, who, in desperation, recommend psychotherapy and powerful tranquilizers.

As with anxiety and panic attacks, patients tell me, "I feel so depressed, but I have no reason to feel that way. I have a loving husband, a good job, and caring friends."

... [D]eep fatigue and psychological problems are the most prevalent complaints of patients with HAIT [Hashimoto's autoimmune thyroiditis].[9]

When your thyroid is under attack from your own immune system, you may experience flat, apathetic, low-thyroid depression; plus an agitated, distraught, even panicky depression. One of our nutritionists, who suffered from (and conquered) this difficult condition, calls it "tired and wired." You may not have a weight problem or even a low body temperature with thyroiditis. Malfunctioning adrenals can be a big part of this problem.

Whether you have simple low thyroid (hypothyroidism) or thyroid allergy (thyroiditis), you will find that changing your diet and adding nutritional supplements can help. Many of you, however, will have to get further help from thyroid medicine. In chapter twelve, you will learn all about the many tests for evaluating thyroid function and how to maximize your thyroid's health.

FIVE

Food Addictions and Allergic* Reactions

In this chapter, you'll discover whether or not you are actually allergic to the foods you are crazy about. I explained in chapter one that the brain is the site of our addiction to foods. But not just any foods can hook the brain. Sugar is the most addictive of all, but you may not realize that it can also set off potent allergic reactions. Many of us are both addicted *and* allergic to sugar.

There are two other foods that you're likely to be addicted and possibly allergic to. These two foods have a reputation for being much healthier than sugar, and they really are loaded with nutrients. Unfortunately, among those nutrients lurk two proteins that can be very destructive allergens. Remarkably, they can also stimulate heroin-like reactions in the brain, providing all the comfort in comfort foods. The two foods I'm talking about are, along with sugar, the most popular foods in America: flour products and milk products. The "opiate" allergen in milk products is a protein called casein. In products made from wheat, rye, oats, or barley, the protein is gluten. Both trigger the release of exorphins (similar to endorphins, but a slightly different molecule) that can fit right into our brains' opiate receptors: instant comfort and pleasure.[1] Think cereal and milk, bread and cheese, ice cream and cookies! Right. When combined with sugar or chocolate, they become triply addictive. But even without sweetness, we have irresistible macaroni and cheese and pizza.

---

*   I'm using the word *allergic* to broadly define any adverse effects that result from ingesting particular foods.

How do you know if allergy-addictors are a problem for you? (1) You consistently eat too much of them, and you are horrified at the idea of losing them; (2) you have uncomfortable, even dangerous allergy symptoms that you may never have associated with your diet; and (3) when you totally eliminate these foods, these symptoms disappear.

We aren't going to be talking here about immediate, obvious kinds of allergic reactions to foods. After all, no one gets addicted to foods that close the throat! We're talking about "delayed" food reactions that you are so used to that you may just consider them normal, like bloating, stomachaches, gas, constipation, low energy, joint pain, headaches, earaches, postnasal drip, and ADHD. These are some common symptoms of food intolerance or allergy. Ironically, the most "intolerable" foods, the ones most likely to cause these symptoms, are often our very *favorite* foods.

It is possible to have allergic reactions to any number of foods, but there are only a few foods that can also cause addiction.

HAVE YOU EVER BEEN ON AN ALLERGY-FREE DIET, BUT DIDN'T KNOW IT?

Think back to your "best" diets. When (if ever) did you really feel good on a diet? I don't mean feeling good because you were losing weight—try to remember how you felt physically and what your mood was like as you were losing the weight. Of course, cravings and starvation eventually kicked in and you had to quit every diet you ever tried. But before you reached that point, did you ever feel really good?

The diets that reduce carbohydrates and emphasize proteins, fats, and vegetables are usually the ones our clients have felt the best on. The Atkins diet is one that people often remember feeling good on. But if these diets worked so well, why did you, and most other dieters, continue to have weight problems? Why were you unable to "stay on maintenance"? Many of my clients felt that Dr. Atkins's diet was too fatty and low in vegetables and other healthy carbohydrates for a permanent plan but that most other diet plans were far too low in calories. Low-cal dieters can't maintain their energy, their sense of well-being, or their weight loss for long, because the low calories trigger the starvation response: a rebound increase in food cravings and a decrease in the ability to burn calories. Fasting programs can make some people feel great. But fasting is not a permanent maintenance possibility!

If only the diet despots understood better. Some of them almost have it right. They have diets that initially pretty much eliminate the big-three allergy-addictors. It isn't the calories; it is the *kind* of calories that they eliminate that make certain weight loss diets more "successful" than others.

Most diets actually create a second insurmountable obstacle to long-term success, besides being too low-cal: *none excludes all three allergy-addictors entirely*—the grains wheat, rye, oats, and barley; cow's milk products; and sweets—or even suggest it as an option. To maintain weight loss, Atkins advises against most refined sweets and starches, but allows wheat and dairy products. The Zone Diet's Dr. Barry Sears puts sugar and chocolate in his bars, and he is adamant about the importance of oats and cottage cheese. He also allows moderate amounts of pasta, bread, and the other gluten-containing grains, as does vegetarian diet guru Dean Ornish, M.D. Most diets do suggest that sugar and flour be kept at low levels, but *any* amount of these foods can overcome even the most Herculean willpower in many people by triggering allergy-addiction. All three also advocate the use of soy, a known thyroid inhibitor.

What about the other leading diet plans, like Weight Watchers and Jenny Craig? Besides being too low cal, they also recommend small or moderate amounts of all the allergy-addictive three. At least in the maintenance phase, *all* diets that I know of allow at least two of the three prime allergy-addictors.

When you are allergy-addicted, following these diets is like attending Alcoholics Anonymous meetings and being served small glasses of beer. The low-fat vegetarian diets may be the worst. They allow too little fat, escalating fat cravings by starving us of good fats, and they promote excessive consumption of starchy carbs made from the highly addictive and nutritionally feeble allergen wheat (and its cousins rye, oats, and barley).

Overeaters Anonymous, in its wisdom, bans all foods made from sugar or flour for everyone (and any other food that a particular person cannot stop overeating). That's the kind of "diet" I support!

GRAINS, MILK PRODUCTS, AND SUGAR

It is obvious to the food industry that many people crave wheat products, milk products, and sugar, so, not surprisingly, the three can be found everywhere, "conveniently" combined as cheesecake, milk chocolate brownies, and cookie dough ice cream. Other common but somewhat less addictive allergens, like peanuts and almonds, may be added to further enhance the effect. I include chocolate in this category since it's a semi-common allergen and a heavyweight addictor, especially when combined with any or all of the big three.

So what makes the big three so irresistibly comforting? They can set off powerful drug reactions in your brain. Sugar consumption can trigger a brain release of your powerful natural painkillers, the endorphins; and a release of antidepressant serotonin all at the same time![2] Casein, a protein in cow's milk, and gluten, a protein found in the grains wheat, rye, oats, and barley, stimulate the production of exorphins, opiate chemicals very similar to endorphins.[3] Over time, these pleasurable brain surges can become heavily addicting. If you don't have your bagel and cream cheese with your sweet latte, you won't get that feeling that you like so much.

In fact, going without one or more of the big-three allergy foods could land you in an unbearable withdrawal state, causing your body to start screaming like any addict's body does without its drugs. You probably already know how hard it can be to "withdraw," especially if you are addicted to more than one of these three allergy foods. Even one allergy-addiction can easily become a nightmare of cravings, overeating, weight gain, mood swings, and guilt.

Reba is a good example of someone who had troubles caused by allergy-addictors. A graduate student in psychology, Reba came from a large Italian family and loved pasta, bread, and sweets. For years she'd had frequent digestive trouble: bloating, constipation, gas, and joint pain. Over the prior six years she had gained twenty extra pounds that she could not shed. She had been aware that her heavy consumption of sugar was certainly part of the reason she was gaining weight, but she also suspected that wheat was a problem. Bread and pasta made her feel blocked and drowsy, with a heavy feeling, but she ate them anyway because they tasted so good to her.

I suggested that she try going off of wheat and sugar and recommended some supplements that would stop her sweet-dough craving and improve her mood. Reba suffered no withdrawal discomfort. Just a few days later, she said she had begun to feel "lighter," physically and mentally. After a week, her clothes became loose and her energy increased. Although she was eating plenty of food, in one month she had dropped fifteen pounds and her digestive problem was gone, along with her joint pain.

Moreover, Reba found it easier to concentrate and produce at school, yet she felt calm and peaceful, which amazed her. And best of all, she said, was that she "didn't miss the pasta and bread that, being Italian, I never thought I would be able to go without." She found she enjoyed rice pasta and loved polenta-crust pizza.

Because food allergies often have a genetic basis, they may have caused problems from birth for you as well as for other family members. Allergy-addiction can impair your digestion and the absorption of anything you eat, creating general malnutrition. Food allergies can also seriously affect your immune system by diverting it from its other jobs, such as protecting you from viruses, bacteria, and airborne irritants like pollen. As a rule, allergy-food addicts usually feel low and run down. They have often had inhalant allergies, to pollens and other plants, for years—allergies that disappear when their allergy foods are withdrawn. This is because by eliminating allergy foods, they free up their immune system to take care of all their other health needs, and it begins to do a much better job.

ALLERGY-ADDICTOR 1: A FAMILY OF GRAINS

The family of grains that is made up of wheat, rye, barley, and oats is actually a family of hybridized grasses. Grasses are high on the list of the most common causes of inhalant allergies. It makes sense that eating grasses is apt to cause problems as well! The proteins in these four grassy grains contain a substance called gluten (think "glue"), which is very hard to digest. Gluten can actually inflame and even damage your digestive lining rather easily. It can, and has, killed infants by damaging their tiny digestive tracts (many of our gluten-intolerant clients report having been colicky infants).

The most severe kind of reaction to gluten-containing grains has a special name: celiac disease (CD). One in every four persons is genetically vulnerable to CD, especially if they have northern European ancestors.[4] CD is closely associated with both diabetes and colon cancer, as well as mental conditions such as depression and mania. Anemia, osteoporosis, thyroiditis, and a blistery skin condition called dermatitis herpetiformis are also associated with celiac disease.

You might have this most severe celiac reaction to the four gluten-containing grains, but you are much more likely to have a somewhat milder form of the problem: gluten intolerance. Because these grains are universally so hard to digest, I don't recommend that anyone eat them often, even if there are no obvious adverse reactions to them. They also contain phytic acid, which blocks the absorption of calcium. And they are not particularly nutritious foods anyway.

In general, wheat is far and away the most problematic of all these gluten-containing grains. Some people can actually digest gluten in small amounts, as it appears in oats, barley or rye, and spelt and kamut (old forms of wheat that have less gluten than the hybridized form that we eat today). After you have carefully investigated all of the possible gluten-containing grains, you'll discover which causes your problems.

Eating foods made from these four grassy grains, particularly wheat, may have many surprising consequences. Routinely I read the food diaries that my incoming clients have written. Many people who love bread and pasta describe feeling heavy and tired after eating them. Others say, "I want a nap right after I have a sandwich every day at lunch." Low energy is a very common symptom of gluten intolerance, and it can lead to excessive need for stimulating caffeine and chocolate. Some of my clients also often complain that they continue to feel hungry even after eating big meals, and they just keep on eating. They never feel full, because their gluten-damaged intestines aren't absorbing food very well. Often they crave and eat sweets soon after they eat a meal that contains bread or pasta, because sugar *will* get into their systems, like a drug, no matter how damaged their digestive tract is, and give them a brief lift.

After eating even small meals that contain wheat or gluten, many people complain of bloating and gas, or say, "I feel too full after I eat." Some even want to—or do—throw up after their heavy, gluten-containing meals. When they bring in their initial food diaries, it is clear that after meals in which the only carbs consumed are rice, corn, or potatoes, these same people feel light and energetic. They tend not to crave or binge on these carbs the way they do bread and baked goods, like croissants, pretzels, and crackers. Yet all these foods are equally starchy carbs with identical calorie contents. The crucial difference turns out to be what kind of carbs they are—whether they contain gluten or are gluten-free.

Another reason for weight gain, besides the overeating of baked goods, is that the allergic reaction includes water retention. Our clients tend to lose five to ten pounds in their first week off these foods; water weight is very easy to lose.

Because gluten-containing foods interfere so much with digestion, they set up some people to have problems with other foods that also tend to be hard to digest, like dairy and soy products and the grains buckwheat, millet, amaranth, and quinoa. Only a first-class small intestine can handle these foods well. Because of intestinal inflammation caused by wheat, the digestive tube can eventually have trouble digesting anything at all. Many of my clients avoid food all day, then eat a lot at night and just sleep off their allergic reactions, sometimes waking up feeling hungover. If you tend to get through the morning with a cup of coffee and juice, and keep going on coffee or diet soda and some candy, it may be because common foods such as cereal and sandwiches don't agree with you.

The wife of one of my colleagues suspected she was gluten intolerant, so we told her to eliminate the suspicious grains for a week and then try eating some wheat to see how she felt. She felt less bloated and more energetic right away. But on her test day, as we'd suggested, she took a nice big piece of homemade bread to work with her. She had her bread with a cup of tea at her ten A.M. break. Fifteen minutes later she woke up, startled by her unexpected nap. Her experience was the most extreme we've seen, but drowsiness is the most common symptom we hear about from gluten "testers." Bloating, gas, bowel trouble, and general tiredness are common, too. Another grain-allergy clue is not being "regular." As soon as I see a dough junkie who tends to have bowel problems (constipation, diarrhea, or both), low energy after eating, and a distended abdomen, I propose seven to fourteen days off gluten-containing grains. Of course, I also propose amino acids and other nutrients to stop grain cravings and make it easy to give up the dough. Typically the characteristic problems, often lifelong, disappear for good in the first few days off these grains.

One of the problems with having a wheat allergy is that wheat can show up in lots of unusual places, from gravies and sauces to ketchup. (See pages 195–196 for a list of hidden sources of gluten.)

ALLERGY-ADDICTOR 2: MILK PRODUCTS

Unlike human breast milk, and even goat's or sheep's milk (which are often fairly easily digested by human beings), cow's milk can cause big problems. One of the least known of them is addiction. Do you drink lots of milk, or overeat cheese, ice cream, or frozen yogurt? If you crave foods full of milk, you are likely to be intolerant of them. More understandably, if you hate (or ever hated) any of these foods, you are also likely to be intolerant of them. Did you need special formula as a baby because you couldn't tolerate milk? Ask your parents if you or anyone else in the family have ever had problems with any dairy products. Do you have respiratory problems? Many of our clients have had everything from runny noses to asthma and chronic earaches since they were children, due to a milk allergy. Respiratory congestion is a classic symptom of intolerance of milk products, though it can be symptomatic of other food or inhalant allergies, too. (Antibiotic and cortisone treatment for childhood milk-allergy symptoms, like earaches and asthma, often set off major addiction to sweets and starches by encouraging yeast overgrowth, as I discuss in chapter seven.)

The other part of your body that cow's milk products can typically affect is your digestive tract. Stomachaches, gas, bloating, belching, cramping, and diarrhea are typical allergic reactions to cow's milk products. The good news is that even the most severe symptoms can be cured overnight by eliminating milk, cheese, ice cream, and other milk products from your diet. If you are addicted to milk-based foods, you are probably having a reaction not only to milk sugar (lactose), but to milk protein, or casein. It can trigger the release of powerful pleasure chemicals in the brain, keeping you hooked. According to allergist Doris Rapp, M.D., digestive problems are most likely caused by a reaction to lactose, while respiratory problems are most likely to be caused by other ingredients in milk, such as casein.[5]

If you can't digest milk sugar, you can use lactose-free milk and take a supplemental enzyme, lactase (brand name Lactaid), which helps you break down the lactose. Thirty to 90 percent of us are not naturally equipped with our own lactase, depending on our genetic background. In fact, according to the National Institute of Diabetes and Digestive and Kidney Diseases, of the National Institutes of Health, 12 percent of American Caucasians, 75 percent of African Americans, and 90 percent of Asian Americans and Native Americans are lactose intolerant.[6]

Lydia, a dynamic Middle Eastern mother, had been having food problems all her life. She'd been a picky eater as a child (a red flag for food allergy) and had been force-fed by her nanny. By age 20 she'd developed an ulcer and was living on Tagamet, a liquid antacid. Whenever she got upset, she would vomit. By 34 she was having alternating constipation and diarrhea, constantly taking Zantac, another potent antacid, and sometimes having stomach cramps after meals. At 44 she came to the clinic and reluctantly agreed to try going off all foods made from cow's milk, including milk chocolate, which she loved.

Lydia used amino acid supplements to stop her chocolate, milk, and cheese cravings, but she only needed them for eight weeks. After that, she was able to stay away from her old dairy favorites with no struggle. Some people who have problems with wheat (or other gluten-containing grains) and milk can tolerate milk products more easily after cutting wheat and other gluten-containing grains out of their diets for a while. Grains can damage the digestive lining and make many foods difficult to digest, especially foods, like milk products, that are already troublesome. So after you've been off of wheat, rye, oats, and barley for three months, you could try milk, yogurt, or cheese again to see if you can better tolerate them. Worldwide research indicates that milk consumption, especially in childhood, can lead to serious problems: diabetes, heart disease, infant anemia,

Crohn's disease, multiple sclerosis, infertility, and asthma. There are several good reasons for all of us to minimize the use of milk products, whether we can "stomach" them or not. Unless they are organic, milk products are laced with the antibiotics and hormones that are regularly used to treat dairy herds. In any case, because they are homogenized and pasteurized they are even harder to digest, so they're *not* the best source of calcium, which is one reason why osteoporosis is still so common among milk-drinking women.

OTHER ALLERGY-ADDICTORS

Dr. Ellen Cutler, author of several books on allergy elimination, reports that 80 percent of her patients have significant allergic reactions to sugar. That doesn't surprise me, but the worst common reactions we've seen are joint pain, headaches, and hyperactivity. Other symptoms are very much like the ones that sugar's cousin alcohol can produce: mood and energy swings, hangovers, headaches, agitation, and irritability. A sugar addiction might be caused by any of the imbalances that are described in this book, but if sweets literally make you feel high and then sick (with a headachy, groggy, heavy feeling), you are probably having an allergic reaction.

Sugar is a drug that can be extracted from many foods—corn, barley, sugar beets, sugarcane—and it is called by many names. It's important that you recognize sugar on food labels; it is often a hidden ingredient going by a different name (such as dextrose). A list of "sugar" words to help when you're reading labels is included on page 198.

Other addictive and nonaddictive foods and additives can also cause negative reactions, of course. I'm addicted to peanuts, which give me stomachaches. Many studies have confirmed that pediatrician Benjamin Feingold's elimination diet can quickly cure ADHD in children. It has similar benefits for adults who are sensitive to certain additives or foods. Mood and attention problems can clear up overnight when food coloring or an allergy food such as apples (because of their high salicylate content) are removed from the menus of sensitive people. Amino acids and other supplements can make avoiding any allergy-addictors easy, but any experimental return to them will usually trigger a reappearance of the original allergy symptoms. Doris Rapp, M.D., a pediatric allergist, has produced fascinating videos of children before and after exposure to sugar and other allergy foods. Their allergic reactions of restlessness, tears, rage, violence, or exhaustion are immediate and obvious. So is the relief when the reactions are reversed with a neutralizing treatment.

Some allergy-addictors are harder to give up than others. If you are allergic to sugar or chocolate, you'll have to say good-bye to these sweet drugs. You may experience a few days of druglike detox, but you've probably been through that many times before. This can be your last farewell to them, partly because you understand more about why you can't tolerate them, but mostly because your supplements and new way of eating will silence your sweet cravings—*permanently*.

The Blood Type Clues to Possible Allergies

Your blood type may give you a clue about food allergies. Two generations of naturopathic physicians and authors, John and Peter D'Adamo, have researched this possibility. Son Peter's *Eat Right for Your Type* asserts that all four blood types—O, A, B, and AB—have trouble with the gluten-containing grains, especially in terms of weight gain, but that B and AB blood types can tolerate milk products. (More on this in chapter eighteen.)

TESTING FOR FOOD INTOLERANCES

Allergist Theron Randolph paved the way in the 1970s for a broader definition of *allergy* by describing case after case of patients with severe physical and mental reactions that could be turned off overnight by removing a single food, then turned back on instantly by reintroducing that food.[7] Psychiatrists such as William Philpott, coauthor of *Brain Allergies*, and pioneering biochemists such as Carl Pfeiffer, author of *Nutrition and Mental Illness*, developed exciting nutritional techniques to clear up unbalanced emotional states by identifying and removing allergy foods.[8] The trick is how to identify them. The addictive allergens are easy to spot, but if removing them does not relieve all allergy symptoms, there are tests that can help, though none is foolproof.

Most doctors still insist that food allergies are very rare. This may have a lot to do with the unreliability of the testing methods available. Neither the conventional blood test for allergies (RAST) nor the skin-prick testing pick up food allergies anywhere near as reliably as they do inhalant allergies. Perhaps because of this, many doctors refuse to test for food allergies at all. Some testing does a good job of identifying allergies to gluten and milk protein, but not to lactose. At Recovery Systems, we recommend blood testing if our clients' symptoms continue even after they eliminate the big-three allergens (see chapter thirteen).

THE HOME TEST FOR HIDDEN ALLERGIES

Home testing for food intolerance is called "elimination and challenge" and is the most commonly accepted and accurate way of identifying problem foods. When you are ready, eliminate the suspected allergens—gluten-containing grains or milk—one at a time for seven days each, then reintroduce them for one day. (See chapter thirteen for specific instructions on how to perform a home test for allergies.)

Please note that there are special problems with testing for severe gluten intolerance (i.e., celiac disease). If you have extensive intestinal damage from gluten, you have CD. Once you start religiously avoiding gluten, this damage will heal. If you "test-try" gluten after a few months of healing, you may not get the old symptoms right away. It may take a few weeks of re-damaging your gut before you notice them again.

There is also the problem of delayed reaction. Some people get arthritic or muscular pains days after the allergy food is eaten, making it extremely difficult to connect the symptoms to the food eaten two or three days before. But if you eliminate the foods again and these symptoms go away, you have your answer.

As for determining whether you are allergic to sugar, I feel it's not worth testing. Do you think you might be allergic to the poison strychnine? You could try it and see. . . . . That's the way I feel about suggesting that you try sugar once you've gotten off of it. After fifteen years of seeing how much damage sugar can do, I would much rather *everyone* stay off it. But if you want to find out for sure whether your addiction to sugar is associated with an allergic reaction, you'll get a quick answer after you've been off of it for seven to fourteen days, by reintroducing sugar on *one* day at both breakfast and lunch.

Don't just suddenly decide to reintroduce because you're at someone's birthday party and getting pressure to try the cake. Do it in a situation in which you can watch your reactions carefully, not in a social situation, in which it might be hard to keep close track of any emerging symptoms. Your old adverse symptoms should return within forty-eight hours.

From the allergy testing we describe in chapter thirteen, you might be able to find out which types of sugar are worse for you. For instance, you may be allergic to corn syrup but not beet sugar. This might give you more freedom in your food choices, but, again, freedom to use sugar is not a goal that I would encourage. Sugar in any form will cause problems, even if they aren't allergic problems.

For milk intolerance, if you eliminate milk products from your diet for a week or two, then you reintroduce them and find that your nasal congestion and bowel problems come back along with your cravings, first try raw milk products, which can be more easily digested by many than pasteurized and homogenized milk products. Then try eating only lactose-free milk products or taking lactase supplements, like Lactaid. You may find that cottage cheese, aged cheese, buttermilk, and yogurt are easier to digest, because they are already partially digested by cultures. If you still have problems, it's time to move on to milk derived from just goats or sheep instead of cows. If you react to those foods, too, then forget about trying to consume any milk products.

Saliva, Stool, Blood, or Biopsy for Testing Severe Gluten Intolerance or Celiac Disease

Saliva testing is not very accurate, because the salivary antibodies (SIgA) are destroyed by gluten. Stool tests (e.g., EnteroLab) are very sensitive. Blood testing for IgG antibodies and transglutaminase vary in reliability. (These blood tests measure antibodies.) Biopsy of the small intestine used to be the gold standard for diagnosing celiac disease, but its accuracy is now in question. (See chapter thirteen for specifics on these test procedures.)

ARE YOU AFRAID OF FEELING RESTRICTED OR DEPRIVED?

If giving up bread or milk makes you feel deprived, I sympathize. You've probably been tortured by food restricting—that is, dieting—much too often already. Believe me, I would not propose these restrictions if I knew any guaranteed way around them.

Remember, though, that this time you will *not* be restricting *calories*. I know, too, that many of you will feel socially awkward having to refuse foods that you are allergic to. But I also know from years of experience that if you are very upset about giving up these foods, this in itself is a strong clue that you are allergy-addicted. Would you have the same feelings if I suggested that you might need to give up celery or cabbage for life?

What you probably won't believe, until you experience it, is that the amino acids and other supplements that you'll be taking from day one will stop the cravings that are causing you to panic. They will minimize your withdrawal symptoms, too. So this will be totally unlike any food eliminating you've ever done before! I promise. And the outcome will be thrilling: your energy will rise, your digestion and bowels will normalize, your mood will elevate, your extra weight will fall off, and your health prospects for the future will be greatly improved.

Now that you have an idea of whether or not you are allergy-addicted to wheat, milk, or sugar (or other foods), it's time to learn how to avoid these trouble foods. Turn to chapter thirteen for details on testing you can do to turn off your cravings and on what tasty substitutes you can use.

SIX

Hormonal Havoc

PMS, Menopause, and
the Food-Mood Connection*

After more than twenty-five years of helping people with food addictions of all kinds, I know that nothing matches the ferocity of hormone-driven cravings. Premenstrual chocolate cravings have brought more women to Recovery Systems' door than any other single problem. Fortunately, it's an easy problem to correct. If you erupt in premenstrual sweet cravings every month, or have developed permanent cravings and unnecessary weight gain (among other woes) in menopause, you will find solid answers here. Most of our menstruating clients lose all of their hormonal cravings and other, more debilitating symptoms of PMS, such as irritability and cramping, within two months. The same is true of many of our menopausal clients, who have suffered from hot flashes, night sweats, and insomnia. Relief from these symptoms is a result of a significant improvement in their diets, combined with the amino acids that correct their brains' appetite and mood chemistry (detailed in chapters one and nine).

But sometimes more help is needed. This chapter will introduce you to the world of hormone imbalance and point you toward the rebalancing solutions in chapter fourteen.

---

* Men, please turn the page.

The Male Box

Men should be aware that two common things can eventually result in consistently lower testosterone levels (that is, male menopause):

1. Eating too many high-carbohydrate foods (sweets and starches) for too long.
2. Too much stress wears out the adrenals, major testosterone-producing glands, especially as you age.

If you are past age 40 and are overeating carbs, gaining weight, and becoming moody, check the symptoms of low testosterone below. If you then feel it is indicated, test your levels of free and total testosterone, DHEA, estrogens, sex hormone binding globulin (SHBG), dihydrotestosterone, cortisol, and others, like PSA, that your physician may recommend.

DHEA (available over-the-counter) converts to both testosterone and estrogen (too much or too little of either can cause problems). It also shores up your adrenal stress response. Bioidentical testosterone is available by prescription. (Don't get methyltestosterone, which may cause cancer and is very hard on the liver.) Your holistic physician can help prevent the conversion of DHEA and testosterone into estrogen.

See the solutions to excessive stress on pages 163–174.

Eating more protein and low-carbohydrate vegetables and less sugar and starch and repairing adrenal stress will naturally raise your DHEA/testosterone levels. To eliminate carbohydrate cravings, use the introductory questionnaire to identify which imbalances are causing them and follow the recommendations in the pertinent chapters.

Symptoms of low testosterone in males:

 ✦ reduced muscle mass
 ✦ reduced sense of well-being
 ✦ reduced energy, vitality
 ✦ reduced sex drive
 ✦ moodiness, lack of motivation
 ✦ apathy; reduced purpose, courage, direction

✦ increased insulin and blood glucose
✦ increased abdominal fat and carbohydrate consumption
✦ coronary clogging
✦ increased total and LDL (bad) cholesterol
✦ bone loss, hip fractures[1]

(Mellowing and compassion may also result!)

ESTROGEN AND PROGESTERONE IN PMS AND MENOPAUSE

Normally, your estrogen level should peak when you ovulate, in the middle of your menstrual cycle. Then it should subside until after menstruation, gradually rising again to its ovulation peak. Once you have peaked, your estrogen levels deflate, but your progesterone levels quickly begin to swell dramatically. Progesterone supports pregnancy (think "pro-gestation"), and if you become pregnant your levels of it will remain elevated for the duration of the pregnancy. When your body is sure you aren't pregnant, your progesterone levels deflate. Then around menstruation its levels become as low as estrogen's, the only time in the month that the two hormones are at equal levels.

Estrogen stimulates many of your brain's mood sites, leading to the production of serotonin (your natural Prozac) as well as catecholamines (your natural caffeine) and endorphins (your natural painkillers and pleasure enhancers). If estrogen levels drop too low, during PMS or menopause, your mood can drop with them. This is one way that hormonal food cravings get triggered: sweets and starches briefly lift your mood by indirectly increasing all three key pleasure enhancers in your brain.

Here are other ways that mood and eating are affected: Progesterone can increase your levels of GABA, a brain chemical similar to Valium. If progesterone levels don't rise high enough, you might be tense, wired, and sleepless. If progesterone levels are high, they can either destress and relax you or make you tired, or both. They can also make you want to eat more, yet they keep your metabolism high enough, usually, to burn off the excess calories (as in PMS). If you, like so many of us, are already deficient in your mood-enhancing chemicals (see chapters one and nine), you are likely to have even more mood and craving problems if you have deficits in estrogen or progesterone. If your testosterone levels are also too low, more depression can result, as can low libido (and muscle and bone loss). When testosterone dominates, PCOS (polycystic ovary syndrome) can also result. See sympotoms of PCOS on page 93.

Signs and Symptoms of Premenstrual Syndrome

- ✦ Craving for sweets
- ✦ Nervous tension
- ✦ Increased appetite
- ✦ Mood swings
- ✦ Irritability
- ✦ Mild to severe personality change
- ✦ Fatigue, lethargy
- ✦ Forgetfulness
- ✦ Confusion
- ✦ Weight gain
- ✦ Uterine cramping
- ✦ Diarrhea and/or constipation
- ✦ Abdominal bloating
- ✦ Heart pounding
- ✦ Oily skin
- ✦ Anxiety
- ✦ Heightened or diminished sex drive
- ✦ Depression
- ✦ Crying
- ✦ Insomnia
- ✦ Swelling fingers and ankles
- ✦ Backache
- ✦ Breast tenderness and swelling
- ✦ Headache
- ✦ Dizziness or fainting
- ✦ Acne[2]

After age 35 your ovaries gradually make less of both estrogen and progesterone, until they run so low that your adrenals (and abdominal fat stores) have to start extra production to compensate. Menstrual cramping can become more painful and bleeding heavier.

These are among the most common signs that premenopausal changes (perimenopause) are underway. If you are in perimenopause or have already reached menopause, think back to what your periods were like before age 30, and if they changed over time. Are you having any of the clearly menopausal symptoms, such as hot flashes, night sweats, memory loss, or more intense food cravings?

Pre-Perimenopausal and Menopausal Symptoms

- Menstrual irregularity
- Hot flashes and/or flushes; night sweats
- Dry vagina
- Memory problems
- Insomnia and/or weird dreams
- Sudden, intense food cravings
- Sensory disturbances (vision, smell, alterations to taste)
- Waking in the early hours of the morning
- Lower back pain (crushing of vertebrae)
- Fluctuations in sexual desire and sexual response
- Onset of new allergies or sensitivities
- Sudden bouts of bloat (waistline increases by two to three inches for an hour or two)
- Annoying itching of the vulva (area around the vagina)
- Indigestion, flatulence, gas pains
- Chills or periods of extreme warmth
- Overnight appearance of long, fine facial hairs
- Rogue chin whiskers
- Crying for no reason
- Bouts of rapid heartbeat
- Waking up with sore heels
- Graying scalp and pubic hair
- Aching ankles, knees, wrists, or shoulders
- Thinning scalp and underarm hair
- Frequent urination
- Mysterious appearance of bruises
- Prickly or tingly hands with swollen veins
- Nausea
- Light-headedness, dizzy spells, or vertigo
- Urinary leakage (when coughing or sneezing, or during orgasm)
- Weight gain, especially in unusual parts of the body
- Sudden and inappropriate bursts of anger
- Sensitivity to being touched by others
- Inexplicable panic attacks
- Tendency to cystitis (inflammation of the bladder)
- Vaginal or urethral infections

✦ Anxiety and loss of self-confidence
✦ Depression that cannot be shaken off
✦ Painful intercourse
✦ Migraine headaches
✦ Easily wounded feelings
✦ Crawly skin[3]

A WOMAN WHO HAD IT ALL

Farrell was a redhead with a big laugh. She was a clothing artist who came to Recovery Systems originally at age 40 because she had food cravings that were completely out of control during the ten days before her period. She put a quick stop to her PMS cravings with a good multi–amino acid supplement, a multivitamin/multimineral, and a low-carbohydrate diet that daily included eight cups of vegetables and eighteen ounces of animal protein (she was a meat-eating, O-blood type); she ate no refined carbohydrates. She also began to attend Overeaters Anonymous meetings. Her weight normalized as her cravings disappeared, and Farrell quit bingeing and vomiting. All of her PMS symptoms, including chocolate cravings, were gone in two months.

Eight years later, at 48, Farrell suddenly began craving carbohydrates again, even though she had continued to eat very well, take her supplements, and attend therapy and OA. Her problem? Menopause. It had sent her into exhaustion and deep depression as well as back into compulsive overeating, night sweats, weeping, nausea, and insomnia. Before returning to see us, she had checked with her doctor. He had tried her on the hormonal drugs Premarin and Provera. Her energy had improved, but her cravings worsened, her weight gain sped up, and she became bloated, depressed, and full of rage. Finally, Farrell quit both drugs and came back to see us and our holistic medical consultant, hoping for a more natural and effective solution to her hormonal imbalance. She got it: we gave her L-glutamine, 5-HTP, and DLPA. Her cravings disappeared and she began to eat well again, increasing her protein and vegetable intake. Her new holistic M.D. evaluated her thyroid function, which had always been borderline. Indeed, her thyroid test results showed that she needed thyroid hormone medication. Her energy increased and her sleep improved. To rebalance her estrogen and progesterone, she was given natural progesterone pellets and a Climara skin patch that administered 17 beta-estradiol (which is exactly like human estradiol and not implicated in the adverse effects found in studies that used Premarin). This combination eliminated her night sweats, nausea, and rages.

Why did Farrell have so many hormonal problems in the first place? Her biggest problem was that she lived in the USA.

WHAT IS HORMONALLY HAZARDOUS ABOUT THE USA?

It is unnatural and unnecessary to have uncomfortable hormonal symptoms. Women in healthier, less developed countries, like Indonesia, don't experience hot flashes (they don't even have a word for them!). They often love menopause because they're so happy to stop dealing with their periods and pregnancies. PMS is not a common problem for them, either. The American diet is responsible for much of the PMS and other hormonal problems that so many American women suffer. For example, women in Japan traditionally have much lower breast cancer rates than do women in the United States. However, once Japanese women start eating an "American" diet, their breast cancer rates shoot up.

Several studies have shown that America's poorest immigrants are healthier than most Americans raised here are, but that after they've been on our diet for a few years, their health deteriorates dramatically. This is why the nutritional suggestions that you will find in this book are so vital. They can help you back to a "primitive" nutritional state that can protect you from some of the discomforts and the dangers of modern hormonal imbalances.

Poor countries tend to be much richer nutritionally because they don't have as much junk food. It seems the more supermarkets and fast-food outlets a country has, the more its women suffer from PMS and menopausal troubles. Caffeine can be a big contributor to PMS, too. Too many sweets, refined starches, and junk fats (e.g., fried foods) and too much soy, chocolate, and alcohol raise estrogen levels too high. Too much estrogen relative to progesterone seems to be a common cause of PMS and menopausal discomfort as well as more serious hormone-related problems, such as breast cancer.

YOUR HORMONAL HISTORY

UNBALANCED BY GENETIC FACTORS?

What are the hormonal patterns and trends among the women in your family? When did each of you begin menstruating? Did you develop breasts and hips quickly or slowly? Has pregnancy, miscarriage, or childbirth affected your appetite, mood, or weight long-term? Do you all crave and craze premenstrually? Have you had more difficult periods as you've moved into your forties? Have you all gone into menopause at a particular age?

Does low thyroid function run in your family? Chapter four explained the thyroid's tendency to falter at hormonal milestones such as the start of menstruation and menopause or after a pregnancy, slowing down metabolism, thereby reducing the ability to maintain comfortable energy or weight. Be sure to review the symptoms of low thyroid on pages 56–58 as you consider your own and your family's hormonal history. Unusually early or late onset of menstruation (13 is the average age), heavy menstrual bleeding, permanent weight gain after childbirth, and infertility can all be examples of thyroid-related problems. If your thyroid is a culprit, chapter twelve will help you check it out and get it functioning properly again, helping your thyroid-related PMS and menopause symptoms to disappear.

HOW ELSE CAN YOU UPSET YOUR ESTROGEN/ PROGESTERONE/TESTOSTERONE BALANCE?

Undereating. The foods we *don't* eat can cause even more problems. Do you avoid fresh vegetables and fruits and high-protein foods such as fish and eggs because you want to cut your calories to make up for eating junk food? Do you skip breakfast? Do you try to subsist on coffee, cigarettes, and diet soda instead of food as much as possible? If so, your hormones can be stressed and starved into imbalance and depletion. Have your periods become irregular or stopped as a result of undereating? Are you bulimic or anorexic?

Too little body fat can also reduce your sex hormones. Fat is hormonally vital. In fact, all of your reproductive and stress-fighting hormones are made from the much maligned fatlike substance called cholesterol! In menopause, the fat on your abdomen can actually produce estrogen when you run low, as your ovaries start making less estrogen. This is a good thing. Because dieting encourages slowed metabolism and weight gain, it hampers your ability to maintain a good weight in menopause, when your metabolism is already naturally slower from naturally lowered thyroid and progesterone, as well as aging factors.[4]

Alcohol, Drugs, and Drug Foods. I already cautioned that certain foods— caffeine, chocolate, sugar, refined starches, soy, and fried foods—can alter estrogen-progesterone balance. Tobacco, with its high sugar content (up to 90 percent!), can interfere, too. So can alcohol, which reliably increases the risk of breast cancer. Another way that alcohol and drugs can distort hormone levels is by impairing your liver function. Your liver removes hormonal excesses if it is functioning well.

Chemical Hormones. The pesticide residues in nonorganic meats, dairy products, and produce supply fake estrogens that can raise your estrogen levels too high. Also, drug estrogens such as DES are fed to cattle and poultry to fatten them; then, when we eat their fat, we ingest the estrogen. That's why you should eat pasture-fed or organic meat and poultry, and leaner meats.

Petrochemical products such as plastic containers (and, sorry, even water bottles) are now known to emit estrogen impostors as well, particularly when exposed to heat. These are all factors in a surge of estrogen-related problems, such as migraines, breast cancer, and low sperm count.[5]

Another cause of hormonal imbalance for many women is *the birth control pill.* Sixteen-year-old Maria had a steady boyfriend and an allergic reaction to condoms, so she decided to start taking the pill. She stayed on it for eight years and loved the regular, light periods and sense of safety. But she gained twenty pounds, and when she quit the pill, she developed a huge fibroid tumor in the lining of her uterus and suffered miserable PMS and heavy periods. The pill, with its estradiol and progestins (artificial progesterone), had kept the levels of her natural estrogen and progesterone (which can protect against fibroid tumor growth) unbalanced.

Taking the birth control pill can add to or create a hormonal imbalance—even years after going off the pill. Staying on the pill for more than ten years (especially with the higher-dose versions) can raise your risk of breast cancer.

HORMONE IMBALANCES

The following are lists of adverse symptoms associated with either too much or too little estrogen, progesterone, and testosterone. (Remember: estrogen is made out of testosterone!) If you experience any of these symptoms, you should test your hormone levels. Then make sure your test results conform with your symptoms. Finally, if both processes indicate a hormone imbalance, you might try low-dose hormone balancing to correct it. Monitor carefully. It sometimes takes a while to find the perfect dose. And be sure to retest regularly to prevent over- or underdosing. (More on this in chapter fourteen.)

Symptoms of Possible Progesterone Imbalance

+ Sweet cravings
+ Tiredness
+ Bloating
+ Sleeplessness
+ Bone loss
+ Constipation
+ Depression
+ Lower sex drive[6]
+ Breast tenderness
+ Acne[7]

Symptoms Indicating Possible Estrogen Imbalance

+ Irritability, negativity
+ Weight gain
+ Increased blood pressure[8]
+ Sleeplessness (low melatonin)
+ Diarrhea
+ More sensitive to emotional pain (weepy)
+ Tension, anxiety
+ Increased weight around the abdomen
+ Hot flashes
+ Headaches[9]
+ Racing heart
+ Incontinence
+ Reduced memory or concentration[10]
+ Tearfulness
+ Vaginal dryness (low estriol)
+ Gallstones

Symptoms of Testosterone Imbalance in Women

Too Little
+ Low energy
+ Loss of sex drive
+ Depressed
+ Thin, fine hair
+ Dry, thin skin
+ Fewer dreams
+ Osteoporosis
+ Muscle loss
+ Cognitive decline

Too Much
+ Hyper feelings
+ Increased libido
+ "Scattered" thoughts
+ Irritable, anxious
+ PCOS (polycystic ovary syndrome): Facial or body hair, acne, endometriosis, ovarian cysts, insulin resistance
+ Intense dreaming
+ Aggressive dreams
+ Violent dreams[11]

HOW ADRENAL STRESS AFFECTS YOUR HORMONAL BALANCE

The adrenal glands and the ovaries make your reproductive hormones. The adrenals actually produce at least 50 percent of your sex hormones as well as all of the hormones that assist you in responding to stress. These stress-coping hormones—adrenaline, cortisol, and DHEA—are deployed at the first sign of emotional upset or physical danger. Levels of cortisol and DHEA continue to be high during prolonged stress, such as illness, and can remain on the job for years, helping you to cope. The adrenal glands are also forced into overdrive by dieting. Their mission is to organize the cannibalizing of muscle and bone to salvage the proteins and minerals that the body must have circulating at all times in the bloodstream. And if you are overexercising to keep the weight off, as so many Americans do, your adrenals regard that as stressful, too, and have to march out more troops.

All of this keeps the attention of your adrenals firmly off your reproductive needs. Your levels of estrogen, progesterone, and testosterone can all begin to falter as a result. In fact, adrenal exhaustion from too much stress is a major factor in sex hormone imbalance. See chapters three and eleven for more on adrenal exhaustion and how to treat it. It is particularly implicated in perimenopause and menopause, during which accumulated stress can accelerate naturally diminishing hormone levels to cause severe hormonal deficiencies.

MENOPAUSE AND
HORMONE REPLACEMENT THERAPY

Are you perimenopausal or menopausal, or for any other reasons do you take Provera (progestin, an inexact, or nonbioidentical, copy of human progesterone) or Premarin (made with estrogen derived from pregnant mares' urine), as hormone replacement therapy (HRT)? Sometimes we see someone who is really happy and satisfied with these drugs. They report the disappearance of memory loss, hot flashes, and mood swings. More often our clients, like Farrell, have found that they have not only not eliminated the problem symptoms, but the drugs have caused serious new problems. You might not be aware of these problems until you begin to see signs of breast cancer, cardiovascular disease, or cancer of the uterine lining (endometrial cancer). These or other problems can occur because your own hormonal levels are unbalanced to begin with, or because you're using unnatural HRT such as Prempro or too little of any HRT. Such factors can increase your risk of developing these cancers by 50 to 75 percent or more, depending on which drug or combination of drugs you use, especially without first testing to check your own symptoms and blood or saliva levels. I hope that the following information will clarify the actual risks involved.

The Shocking Results of the First Large Study of the Effects of the Hormone Replacement Drugs Premarin and Provera Among 122,000 Nurses

Their Increased Risk of Breast Cancer When Taking:

Premarin (estrogen) alone   36%

Premarin plus Provera (progestin)   50%

Premarin and testosterone   78%

Provera alone   240%

Plus a doubled risk of gallbladder disease and lupus from hormone therapy (mainly Premarin).[12]

Other Possible Unwanted Effects of the Estrogen Premarin Used Alone, Without Either Bioidentical Progesterone or the Nonbioidentical Progesterone Mimic Progestin (e.g., Provera)

✦ Breast tenderness
✦ Blood clots
✦ High blood pressure
✦ Nausea and vomiting
✦ Fluid retention
✦ Impaired glucose tolerance
✦ Headaches
✦ Leg cramps
✦ Gallstones
✦ Worsened uterine fibroids and endometriosis
✦ Vaginal bleeding
✦ Increased risk of endometrial cancer and breast cancer (but less breast cancer with a hysterectomy)[13]

Other Possible Unwanted Effects of Progestin Alone

✦ Depression
✦ Bloating
✦ Menstrual bleeding resumes
✦ Increased heart disease risk
✦ Increase in the risk of breast cancer by 240 percent
✦ Cancers become more invasive

More Prempro Scandal

Another large National Institutes of Health (NIH) study, the Women's Health Initiative (2002 to 2010), was halted early when researchers discovered that the widespread use of Prempro had created a health crisis affecting up to 40 percent of the menopausal women in America. The study showed that those on Prempro had:

✦ A 41 percent increase in strokes
✦ A 29 percent increase in heart attacks
✦ A doubling of rates of blood clots
✦ A 22 percent increase in cardiovascular disease
✦ A 26 percent increase in breast cancer
✦ A 50 percent increase in dementia

A 2010 *JAMA* follow-up study on the Women's Health Initiative (WHI) found that those taking Prempro in 2002 had:

+ Twice the incidence of breast cancer
+ Twice the incidence of death from breast cancer

NEW INSIGHTS INTO HRT

Since 2002, the percentage of U.S. women taking Prempro (most of whom are menopausal) has dropped from 40 to 15 percent. Many women have, understandably, been too afraid to use any supplemental hormones, even low-dose bioidentical ones—none of which the WHI Prempro study included—guided by testing. Fortunately, numerous studies have identified the Prempro culprit: progestin, the inexact, nonbioidentical, synthetic progesterone-like drug called medroxyprogesterone acetate. (This drug is also found under other names and in birth control pills.) Fortunately, many studies using *bioidentical* progesterone have found that it does *not* cause the problems associated with nonbioidentical progestins such as Provera. Premarin or more bioidentical forms of estrogen, estradiol, taken with progestins or alone, could be dangerous. Taken along with bioidentical progesterone, they appeared to be quite safe as well as beneficial. Natural, bioidentical progesterone actually has many protective effects, including against cardiovascular problems and breast cancer.[14] Conventional doctors and pharmacies carry the bioidentical forms of both progesterone (e.g., Prometrium) and estradiol (e.g., Vivelle patches). Compounders have many other forms.

In chapter fourteen, you'll learn how to test for hormonal imbalances and how to get your hormones back in balance using diet, supplements, herbs, and acupuncture. Finally, you'll learn about the use, when necessary, of low-dose, bioidentical, symptom- and test-based hormone replacement therapies.

SEVEN

Yeast Overgrowth

A Hidden Cause of
Food Cravings

Years ago at Recovery Systems, although we were having spectacular success eliminating food cravings, we were troubled by the occasional client who did not respond as expected. Typically we'd hear that cravings had subsided considerably but were reappearing every three or four days. Often we would hear, "It doesn't even feel like it's me wanting this stuff." It turned out that our clients were right. It *wasn't* them; it was an organism called yeast.

This yeast, called *Candida albicans*, is in some ways similar to bread-raising yeast. Much like bread-making yeast, it gobbles up the sugar and starch in the gut, making a big, puffy, gassy stew. And that's essentially the way our yeast-afflicted clients usually feel: bloated, puffy, gurgly, and distended, especially after sweets, starchy foods, or alcohol. Some have also had chronic vaginal yeast infections or sinus infections, both reliable tip-offs that something beyond depleted brain chemistry or allergies is at work. Other common symptoms are a history of antibiotic use, mental fog or spaciness, nail fungus, and athlete's foot.

Check your own symptoms on the following questionnaire to see if too many yeasts could be contributing to your cravings.

Identifying Yeast Overgrowth

Section A. General Indicators
Choose the score that fits your symptom best and circle it. Scoring:
No Symptom = 0; Mild = 4; Moderate = 8; Severe = 12

Mental/Emotional Functioning
0 4 8 12   Depression
0 4 8 12   Feel spacey, light-headed, or disoriented
0 4 8 12   Poor memory
0 4 8 12   Inability to make decisions and to concentrate

Digestive Symptoms
0 4 8 12   Bloating, distension, or gas
0 4 8 12   Abdominal pain

Reproductive System
0 4 8 12   Loss of sexual interest or ability
0 4 8 12   Troublesome vaginal burning, itching, or
               discharge
0 4 8 12   Premenstrual tension or cramps

Muscles and Joints
0 4 8 12   Cold hands or feet or physical chilliness
0 4 8 12   Pain or swelling in joints

The Most Indicative Symptoms
Scoring: No Symptom = 0; Mild = 3; Moderate = 6; Severe = 9
0 3 6 9   Chronic eczema, rashes, or itching (e.g., anal,
              under breasts)
0 3 6 9   Body odor or bad breath not relieved by
              washing/brushing
0 3 6 9   Chronic sore throat, laryngitis, cough, or tender
              glands
0 3 6 9   Urinary frequency, burning, or urgency
0 3 6 9   Pain or tightness in chest, wheezing, or short-
              ness of breath
0 3 6 9   Recurrent ear infections, fluid in ears
0 3 6 9   Chronic sinus infections
0 3 6 9   Food sensitivity or intolerance

_____ Total, Section A

Section B. Major Influences–Personal History
Scoring: Yes = Number Indicated; No = 0

Antibiotics and Drugs as Factors
35   Have you taken tetracycline or other antibiotics for one month or longer?

35   Have you taken frequent short courses of other broad-spectrum antibiotics?

15   Have you taken prednisone or other cortisone-type drugs for one month or more?

10   Have you taken birth control pills for more than a year?

Key Symptoms
25   Have you had persistent yeast infections, prostatitis, vaginitis, or other reproductive problems?

20   Have you been frequently exposed to high-mold environments and seemed to have a sensitivity to mold?

20   Have you had severe athlete's foot, nail or skin fungus, ringworm, or other chronic fungus?

10   Have you been treated for internal parasites?

Cravings
10   Do you crave or consume lots of sweets?

10   Do you crave or consume lots of starches, such as pasta or bread?

10   Do you crave or consume lots of alcoholic beverages?

_____ **Total, Section B**

_____ **Grand Total, Sections A and B**

A score over 100 suggests the possibility of a yeast overgrowth; over 175 indicates a high probability.

Adapted from *Inner Health*, © 1997, J. Anderson, N. Faass, T. Kuss, J. Ross, and J. Stine.

There is a lot of skepticism in the medical community about just how common or problematic yeast overgrowth really is. Actually, we used to be skeptical, too. But now we're believers, having seen so many clients who finally lost their bloat and cravings only after their yeast problem was addressed. We are also located in the San Francisco Bay Area, where opportunistic infections (i.e., yeasts) kill AIDS victims every day. We know how real and damaging yeast overgrowth can be.

WHAT IS *CANDIDA* AND HOW DOES IT CAUSE CRAVINGS?

Candida albicans is the most well known of the problematic yeasts, but it is just one of many different types of yeasts that are commonly found in human bodies, in bread, and even in the air. From the time we are born, we have some *candida* and other yeasts living in our intestinal tracts. Normally, *candida* and other yeasts live in harmony with us. It is only when they overgrow their normal boundaries that yeasts such as *candida* pose a problem.

When you have too much yeast in your system, it's called a "yeast infection," or yeast overgrowth. Since yeasts love warm, wet places, yeast infections show up in places such as your intestines, your vagina, or your mouth (where it is called "thrush"). When enough of these yeasts overgrow in your body, they can become quite troublesome. They also have the chameleonlike ability to change to fungi as they overgrow, producing long rootlike structures that are invasive and can penetrate the lining of your intestine. A fungus can release toxins and incompletely digested food and fecal matter into your bloodstream. This damages the digestive tract and causes food sensitivities, allergies, and other problems.

THE EMERGENCE OF YEAST AS A MAJOR CAUSE OF FOOD CRAVINGS

Yeast infections are fairly common. Researchers estimate that 25 to 35 percent of the population suffers from yeast and related fungal conditions. Many more women than men are affected.[1]

Yeast infections became a much greater health risk in the second half of the twentieth century than ever before. Modern medicine's introduction of the wonder drugs known as antibiotics started yeast on its rise to prominence. Antibiotics kill all bacteria, regardless of type. This means that they also destroy good bacteria, mainstays of our immune defenses. The "friendly" bacteria—such as *Lactobacillus acidophilus* and *Lactobacillus bifidus*—are killed off by antibiotic therapy. Opportunistic yeasts quickly overgrow, stepping in to fill the void left behind after antibiotic therapy kills off the helpful bacteria that used to line the intestinal tract. Birth control pills and steroids also directly contribute to yeast overgrowth.

When you swallow sweets and starchy carbs, you feed the yeasts, which starts a fermentation process, hence the gurgle and bloat. Of all the food groups, undigested and unabsorbed carbohydrates (sweets, starches, and alcohol) most directly feed the growth of these intestinal microbes. Good digestion absorbs the carbs that you eat quickly into your body, but if you have been eating too many sweets and starches, you may have overwhelmed your gut's ability to digest and absorb them. As the yeast feeds on excess carbs, it multiplies and spreads, and its feeding frenzy is felt as the overwhelming cravings for carbohydrates that so many people now suffer from.

WHO GETS YEAST INFECTIONS?

Exposure to antibiotics is the cause of most yeast overgrowth. Many women are afflicted with vaginal yeast infections, specifically because of earlier illness (e.g., childhood earaches) treated with antibiotics. The most typical symptoms are a white vaginal discharge and itching of the genital area, irritation, swelling, and redness; discomfort during sex; and painful urination. Recurrent yeast infections are an indication that a yeast overgrowth may be affecting your whole system. But many of our yeast-ridden clients don't get them. Males can contract yeast infections yet be without obvious genital symptoms (e.g., jock itch), but they can reinfect their partners if they're not tested and treated along with them.

HOW DO YEASTS MULTIPLY AND TAKE OVER?

Antibiotics. These wonder drugs kill off the good along with the bad, wiping out lots of beneficial bacteria that normally keep yeasts in check.

The Pill. The hormones in birth control pills encourage yeast overgrowth. They also increase levels of glycogen (sugar) present in vaginal secretions, promoting further yeast growth.

Spermicidal Creams and Foams. The active ingredient in these creams, nonoxynol-9, fosters the growth of both *candida* and *E. coli* (a bacterium

that causes cystitis). Nonoxynol-9 also destroys vagina-friendly lactoba-
cilli bacteria, which are part of the body's natural defense system against
yeast.[2]

Cortisone, Prednisone, and Similar Steroids. Use of these medicines
encourages yeast growth because they suppress the immune system.

Nutritional Deficiencies. Deficiencies of *Lactobacillus acidophilus* (helpful bacteria) and the B vitamins (such as biotin) allow opportunistic
yeasts to spread.

Poor Digestion. Poor digestion and malabsorption set the stage for yeast
overgrowth. If you don't have enough digestive juices (hydrochloric
acid) in your stomach, yeast is more likely to overgrow. If you have
enough, the yeast gets burned up as you digest. Eating foods you are allergic to, such as dairy and gluten-containing grains (especially wheat),
can slow down, irritate, and damage your gastrointestinal tract, allowing
yeasts more feeding time and more defenseless tissue to invade.

Poor Diet. The lack of nutrients in fast food and junk food directly lowers immunity, allowing yeasts an easy takeover.

Excessive Carbohydrate and Sugar Intake. Of all the food groups, these
foods most directly fuel yeast overgrowth.[3]

Antibiotic Residues in Commercial Meat. Most commercial meats contain small amounts of residual antibiotics. Eat antibiotic- and hormone-
free meats instead (see chapter twenty).

Weakened Immune Function. Are you highly stressed? Do you have
frequent colds and flus? Yeasts thrive when your immune response is impaired or debilitated. AIDS patients are typically killed by yeast that
takes over as they grow weaker.

Use of Recreational Drugs. Alcohol, marijuana, tobacco, and other recreational drugs stress the liver, adrenals, and immune system, further depleting the body and its resistance to yeasts.

Operations, Catheterization, Radiation, Anticancer Drugs. Opportunistic yeast thrives after these traumas to the body.

PREVENTING YEAST OVERGROWTH

When the following three conditions are met, the yeast in your body usually remains harmless:

1. You have a stable population of friendly, beneficial bacteria in your intestines.
2. Your immune system is strong and intact.
3. Your diet is balanced with adequate protein, vegetables, and essential fats, and you're not overeating carbohydrates (particularly sugar, refined carbohydrates, and grains).

HOW YEAST SPREADS

When yeast spreads in the GI tract, you'll know it's there, mostly from the gas and bloating. You'll definitely get major cravings for sugar and starches—the foods that yeasts prefer. The more you feed the yeast, the more it proliferates, releasing toxins and interfering with your digestion as it expands.

Eventually the yeast may enter your bloodstream and spread through your body. At this point, your immune system really can begin to be overwhelmed and falter. A frail, sluggish immune response is an open invitation for yeast to overgrow, as yeasts are far more aggressive even than viruses.[4]

As the yeast spreads, your symptoms may grow more diffuse and convoluted: depression, lethargy, mental fog, mood swings, PMS, confused thyroid function, susceptibility to infections (sinus, respiratory, bladder, gums, etc.), sensitivity to pollutants and fumes (which can become full-blown "environmental" illness), achy muscles and/or joints, and skin and nail fungus.

TESTING FOR YEAST OVERGROWTH

If you believe you might have a yeast infection, given the symptoms listed in the Quick Symptom Questionnaire and the more complete questionnaire here, you might have some stool testing done to be sure. Either way, you can start a three-month anti-yeast food and supplement plan, which usually stops yeast-related symptoms very quickly, even in the first week. Effective yeast-eradicating medications are also available.

A diagnostic stool analysis at a specialty lab (see page 362, for listings) is one fairly good method of diagnosis. We tend to get the best results from the Genova Diagnostics Microbiology Analysis. Any health professional can order this or other similar analyses, and some labs will let you order these tests yourself. Another route would be to take a yeast-antibody blood test. If your yeast-antibody presence is above 100, you probably have a yeast overgrowth. Yeasts and fungal organisms are hard to test for, as are parasites. But testing is important, because some of you will want to be treated with the more potent and simpler anti-yeast medications, which require a prescription. Without test results showing the presence of excessive yeasts, it's hard for a physician to justify the use of such meds. See the end of chapter fifteen for more testing information.

In chapter fifteen, you'll also learn about how to effectively kill off these unwelcome diners with or without medications and start feeling better and eating better than you've been able to for quite a while.

The Problem with Parasites

This year we had two clients whose cravings did not stop until we found and killed certain parasites. Like yeasts, microscopic parasites are aggressive organisms that can cause cravings, bloating, and many other problems. Some people with parasites such as giardia may have no noticeable symptoms, but others will manifest severe symptoms. Parasites usually affect already weakened systems. For example, if you have a predisposition to weakness in the lungs because you are asthmatic or have had pneumonia in the past, you might develop wheezing, shortness of breath, or respiratory symptoms.

Parasites are surprisingly common due to world travel, which spreads them around so that even non-travelers get them. They can be extremely difficult to kill off, and they can be quite destructive, so if you suspect you have parasites, please work with a health professional to test for and eradicate them. You or your health professional can send for a protocol like the one that we use at our clinic, from our supplier, Infinity Health in Denver: (800) 733-9293, Monday–Friday, 9:00 A.M.–5:00 P.M. MST. But frequently, antiparasitic meds are required.

A stool test (see chapter twenty-one) can help identify both parasites and yeast overgrowth. The presence of yeast progressively suppresses immune function, which may lead to a parasite invasion, and vice versa. If it turns out that you have both a yeast infection and a parasite infection, you should start an anti-parasite program first, *before* tackling the yeast. At Recovery Systems, we tried to do it the other way around and failed a number of times before we learned this valuable lesson. Fortunately this dual infestation has not been a common problem.

Parasite Questionnaire
Please circle the appropriate number next to each question.
A = Symptom never occurs/never exhibit this behavior
B = Symptom/behavior occurs occasionally
C = Symptom/behavior occurs often
D = Symptom/behavior occurs most of the time

	A	B	C	D
1. Chronic fatigue for no apparent reason	0	1	2	3
2. Swollen or achy joints	0	1	2	3
3. Increased appetite, hungry after meals	0	1	2	3
4. Eat out at restaurants	0	1	2	3
5. Nervous or irritable	0	1	2	3
6. Restless sleep/teeth grinding during sleep	0	1	2	3
7. Night sweats	0	1	2	3
8. Blurry, unclear vision	0	1	2	3
9. Fevers of unknown origin	0	1	2	3
10. Frequent colds, flu, sore throats	0	1	2	3
11. Constipation	0	1	2	3
12. Diarrhea alternating with constipation	0	1	2	3
13. Thinning or loss of hair	0	1	2	3
14. Elevated A.M. cortisol (on saliva tests)	0	2	4	6

	A	B	C	D
15. Irritable bowel	0	2	4	6
16. Rectal or anal itching	0	2	4	6
17. Bloating or gas	0	2	4	6
18. Abdominal or liver pain/cramps	0	2	4	6
19. Mucus in nose that is moist or encrusted	0	2	3	4
20. Dark circles under eyes	0	2	3	4
21. Bowel urgency	0	2	3	4
22. Skin problems, rashes, hives, itchy skin	0	2	3	4
23. Vertical wrinkles around mouth	0	2	3	4
24. Kiss pets, allow pets to lick your face	0	2	3	4
25. Go barefoot outside the home	0	2	3	4
26. Travel in Third World countries	0	2	3	4
27. Eat lightly cooked pork/salmon products	0	2	3	4
28. Eat sushi, sashimi	0	2	3	4
29. Swim in creeks, rivers, lakes	0	2	3	4
30. History of parasitic infection	0	2	3	4
31. Loose stools or diarrhea	0	2	3	4
32. Pale, anemic, or yellowish skin	0	2	3	4
33. Foul-smelling stools	0	2	3	4
34. Low-back or kidney pain	0	2	3	4
35. Indigestion, malabsorption	0	2	3	4

Total _____

Scoring Index:
0–19   Possible parasitic presence
20–29   Likely parasitic infection
30–39   A stronger possibility of parasitic infection
40 or more   Odds are quite strong that parasites are present

Note: If your score is 15 or higher, there is some likelihood that parasites are affecting your health. Consult your health care practitioner for further discussion and laboratory testing. Questionnaire was mutually developed by Timothy Kuss and Dr. Jack Tips, of Apple-A-Day Clinic in Austin, Texas. © 1996 Timothy Kuss, Infinity Health, 1519 Contra Costa Boulevard, Pleasant Hill, CA 94523, (925) 676-8982.

EIGHT

Fatty Acid Deficiency

Why You Can't Stop Eating
Chips, Cheese, and Fries

Are you someone who doesn't care too much about bread or pota-toes unless they are drenched in butter or cheese, or deep-fried? If you like sweets at all, do you only lose control with peanut butter cups or ice cream? Do you love potato or corn chips, but not the baked kind? If this sounds like you, you're addicted to fat. In this chapter, you'll dis-cover why. Then in chapter sixteen you'll discover painless ways to ex-tract your "fat tooth."

We see a few pure-fat addicts every month. But usually fat cravers are also carbohydrate lovers who are stuck with uncontrollable cravings for both, much like 32-year-old Bronnie, a typical fat-and-carbohydrate ad-dict. She had a fascinating, high-energy lifestyle, working as a producer of dance exhibitions all over the country. She had lots of friends, whom she loved to entertain with lingering candlelight dinners. But those dinners, and all of the other food that she ate, tended to be overly rich. Bronnie had always craved cheese, chips, olives, salami, nuts, ice cream, popcorn with lots of butter, and creamy sauces. By age 18, she was a hundred pounds overweight. She weighed 285 pounds when she came to our clinic for help. We started out by eliminating her sweet cravings with 5-HTP, chro-mium, and L-glutamine. Then we went after her fat cravings.

Bronnie had mixed northern European ancestry that included some Scandinavian forebears. Her family history also contained depression, anxiety, alcoholism, fatigue, PMS, and winter depression, all signs of fatty acid deficiency. With the right nutrients to treat her cravings, she was able to begin the changes in eating habits that had been so impossible for her to adopt before.

FAT IS NOT THE ENEMY

Like Bronnie, most of the fat-cravers we work with lose their interest in fats in a few days. The secret? Foods that contain very particular fats!

The fact is that human beings actually need lots of high-quality fat in their diets and on their bodies. Here are just a few of the reasons why:

+ For the production of all hormones
+ To protect their internal organs and insulate them from cold
+ To burn for energy when carbs are scarce
+ To cover every single body and brain cell
+ To make hair and skin lustrous
+ To keep sex drive from waning
+ To maintain mental stability and concentration
+ To prevent carbohydrate cravings
+ To keep bowels regular

The brain must be 60 percent fat (and 25 percent cholesterol) to function properly!

The complete list of the benefits of fats is actually much longer as is the list of health problems that occur when you are too low in certain essential fatty acids.

TOO MUCH AND TOO LITTLE FAT

Ironically, many people who overeat fatty foods today are deficient in healthy fats. Like most Americans, you are undoubtedly taking in far too many fragile and overprocessed vegetable oils and not enough of the traditional fats that kept us so healthy and weight-perfect up until the 1970s. What are the traditional, safe, nourishing fats? Saturated fats such as butter and coconut oil, extra virgin olive oil, nuts, seeds, avocadoes, fatty fish (especially wild and low in mercury), poultry (with skin), and meat (especially organic or free-range). These are the foods that, combined with plenty of protein and wholesome carbs, kept us fit and free of degenerative disease for millions of years. For example, we had *no* heart disease until after 1930, when margarine and hydrogenated shortening began to replace butter and lard.

If you are a fat addict, your real problem probably is not just that you are eating too much of certain unhealthy fats; it's that you aren't eating enough of the healthy fats. You may be so deficient, in fact, that your body continually calls for oily, creamy foods, hoping that you will eventually swallow the particular kind of fat that it really needs. And you are not alone. For example, according to Artemis Simopoulos, M.D., distinguished researcher and author of *The Omega Diet*, we are getting one tenth of the essential omega-3 fats we need, and 20 percent of us have levels so low "as to be undetectable."[1]

Actually, U.S. women have been trying to restrict all fat intake since the 1970s. Partly because they lost pleasure, calories, and nutritional satisfaction when they quit eating adequate healthy fat, their intake of sweets and starches has increased from 30 percent to 50 percent of their total dietary intake. But some low-fat dieters have rebounded out of low-fat dieting into fat obsession. To find your fat balance you need better information, here and in chapter twenty-one.

FAT REEDUCATION

FAT IS RICH IN MANY WAYS

It turns out that fats are fascinating and complex as well as essential to our health and well-being. There are many kinds of fats (or fatty acids), each fulfilling a special need in the body. Butter, for example, contains at least five hundred different fatty elements. The many types of fat in beef (in grass-fed beef, especially) include vitamin D and both the essential omega-3 and omega-6 fats.

Instead of taking in the traditional, safer oils, you may be getting too much soy or canola oil, fried food, or hydrogenated fat, which prevent the absorption of the good fats. The traditional fats are very stable and protective of our tissues. Their high saturated fat content is actually beneficial! In the 1990s, the same studies that proved that hydrogenated vegetable oils (i.e., shortening and margarine) caused heart disease concluded that "there was no association between the intake of saturated fat and coronary death."[2]

Coconut oil, butter, and cocoa butter are types of saturated fats. Eaten moderately, they cause no harm and can actually help lower the levels of damaging triglycerides. Fats high in medium-chain fats (MCFs), especially coconut oil, can also raise metabolic rates and promote weight loss. MCFs are saturated fats whose metabolism-enhancing properties have been well researched; they are used extensively by bodybuilders and athletes to enhance fat-burning and stamina.[3] When we ate lots more of them, before 1970, our weight was generally ideal.

Saturated fats keep our cell walls firm, while the unsaturated vegetable and fish oils make them flexible. We need both kinds of fat to stay in balance. Red meat actually includes many beneficial fats, as well as the critically important minerals iron and zinc. Unfortunately, animal and milk fat also harbor pesticides, hormones, and antibiotics. Buy the organic or range-fed versions whenever you can. Remember: animal fat is only junk fat if you consume it in excess. But you will not be doing that, because you're going to start eating balanced fats that will stop your excess fat cravings.

As for cholesterol, most of it we make ourselves from carbs and proteins as well as fats. Cows make it from grass. Low-carb diets reduce cholesterol, while diets low in saturated fat don't—as the studies on Dr. Atkins's diet have proved. *Cholesterol* is a word, like *fat*, that we have learned to fear. But guess what is made from the cholesterol in our bodies? Estrogen, testosterone, adrenaline, and all of our other sex and stress-coping hormones. Fats such as butter, cheese, coconut, and the fats in shellfish, meat, and poultry contain cholesterol, but 70 percent of us are not adversely affected by it. Our bodies know how to both make and dispose of unneeded cholesterol. Actually, only cholesterol levels over 260 are associated with adverse health consequences (and so are levels under 170).[4] Only a small percentage of us are born with a tendency to make too much cholesterol, and those people have a genetic problem, not a dietary one, so a low-cholesterol (low saturated fat) diet does not help much.

The omega-6 and -3 fats are called the "essential fats," because our bodies can't make them out of other fats. It's essential that we get them directly from foods, though only in relatively small amounts. The omega-3 fats are sometimes called vitamin F_2, because, like vitamins, they are essential to life. (*Vita* means "life.") Without them, we cannot protect ourselves from hormonal imbalances, dry skin and hair, immune system weakness, and adverse effects on the brain, eyes, and arteries, among other things. Both omega-6 and -3 fats must be consumed in balance with each other on a regular basis.

Hundreds of studies have convinced us of the extraordinary benefits of these two essential oils in preserving our health, but we need only small amounts of them; a serving of high omega-3 fish and a handful of nuts and seeds for our omega-6 needs a few times a week will sustain us. Remember that the fat in milk products, meats, and poultry also contains omega-6 fats. Most important for fat-cravers, their ratio should be 1:1, not 25:1 as it is now, with dangerous excesses of omega-6 oils that can set off cravings for the balancing (but harder-to-find) omega-3 fats. Too much omega-6 fat contributes to cardiovascular disease, rheumatoid arthritis, asthma, Crohn's disease, osteoporosis, cancer, and Alzheimer's disease. These frightening effects are partly a result of omega-6 oils being so out of ratio with omega-3 oils. But another shocking factor is that most of our common vegetable oils, *except* extra virgin olive oil and coconut or palm oil, are so fragile and so overprocessed that they are dangerously rancid before they're even bottled. Because they are deodorized, we can't smell the rancidity, but our bodies can tell.

Whether you've been eating junk food or healthy food, you are probably getting too much omega-6 fat and you probably aren't getting enough omega-3 fat. You'll see some quick improvements as well as long-term health benefits when you put your fat habits into reverse.

THE OMEGAS AND WEIGHT

Studies have shown that adding fish oil to the diets of lab animals causes their weights to drop, even when they continue to eat the vegetable fats that had originally caused them to gain weight.[5] Our clients, too, experience a drop in weight when they add fish or flax oil to their menus, even though they also eat nuts, seeds, and other kinds of fats in their full-calorie diets. Why? One reason is that omega-3 fats raise our metabolic rate so that we burn calories more briskly. They also act as diuretics, helping the kidneys to flush out excess water from our tissues. Omega-3 fats also help energize us, allowing us to exercise more easily. Getting these benefits requires that half of your essential-fat calories come from omega-3 fats—rich fish and fats from cold water fish; the other half should come from high omega-6 fats like vegetable oils, preferably directly from nuts and seeds. Together they should total just 4 to 8 percent of your calories for the day.[6] Note: There are concerns about the processing and purity of fish oil supplements. Cod liver oil is less processed and also contains vitamins D and A, but delivers less O-3, as it must be used in limited doses to avoid too much vitamin A. More on this in chapter sixteen.

One omega-6 fat offers anti-inflammatory benefits similar to those of omega-3. It is called GLA. Like fish oil supplements, GLA supplements have been shown to reduce weight by stimulating more active burning of fat by the body, and by stimulating the thyroid gland to raise metabolic rates. It can reduce PMS discomforts dramatically as well. The best source of GLA is oil from the evening primrose plant or black currant seeds. My clients with PMS use it, along with fish oil and/or flax oil, but at half the dose (that is, one GLA per two fish oil capsules).

DO YOU HAVE FAT-LOVING GENES?

There are certain groups of people, from specific genetic stock, who we know have very special needs for the omega-3 fats, the fatty nutrients found only in cold-water fish such as sardines and salmon. Did you descend from them? Even a distant ancestor could have passed the genetic need for fish fat to you, though you are most likely to have the problem if your ancestry includes 25 percent from one of these specific genetic stocks:

+ Scandinavians
+ North American coastal
+ Native Celtic Irish (native to Ireland, not England; these people are or were usually Catholic, not Protestant), Scottish, or Welsh

If you are descended from any of these genetic groups, or possibly other island or coastal people, you may crave fats because your ancestors relied heavily on fish for as long as twenty thousand years.[7] Your genetic code adapted itself to a fish-based diet. Your body design may still require lots of fish fat, and it may not be able to substitute the fats from other animals or vegetables.

What's so special about the fat found in fish? It is a particularly rich kind of fat. For example, fatty nutrients in fish provide DHA, one of the most activating brain foods and the highest source of Vitamin D—so crucial in these sun-deprived areas. Those of us who do not come from this coastal stock have bodies that can make these special fatty nutrients out of flaxseeds, walnuts, leafy greens, or any other food that contains the raw form of omega-3 fatty acids. But the descendants of fish-dependent peoples cannot. They need to eat fish regularly or take fish oil supplements or algae oil. See chapter 16 for information on testing for fatty acid levels.

Many of our clients come from alcoholic families that are Scandinavian, Irish, or Native American and suffer alcoholism and depression at unusually high rates. Depression and cravings for alcohol, as well as fat, can be relieved by the use of fish oil. Without the omega-3 fats in their food, these genetic types suffer depression as a brain fat deficiency symptom. They use alcohol to numb the depression, and/or overeat all kinds of fat, blindly searching for the right one—omega-3, which is hard to find in a standard American diet.

One researcher gave fish oil (or GLA-rich evening primrose) supplements to chronic alcoholics and found that their interest in alcohol disappeared. The depression that their alcohol use had relieved was eliminated by the supplements. These supplements also helped them to detox comfortably after they quit drinking, by preventing seizures.[8]

THE OTHER CAUSES OF FAT CRAVINGS

DO YOU HAVE ENOUGH PLEASURE-BOOSTING ENDORPHINS?

Fat consumption triggers the pleasure response—a release of endorphins, our natural pain killers. This built-in pleasure response to fatty foods has been used to addict us to commercial foods that carefully combine poor-quality fats, sweets, and starches with salt in an irresistible and lucrative health disaster. Chapter sixteen will explain how to raise your endorphin levels in minutes so that you won't need to keep using extra fat for a pleasure boost. Chapters five and thirteen will explain how all milk products, including fatty ones like ice cream and butter, can have an extreme effect on some people.

HAVE LOW-FAT DIETS DEPLETED YOU OF HEALTHY FATS?

Like so many of us, you are probably shocked by the idea that fat can be good, let alone essential for your health. The anti-fat movement has been very successful, though misguided, since the 1970s, when the Pritikin Institute's now-famous low-fat heart disease diet hit the headlines. What never got into print was important information from the institute's own former head nutritionist, Ann Louise Gittleman. As noted previously, in her book *Beyond Pritikin*, Gittleman reported that Pritikin clients who went very low fat (10 percent) for more than three months developed new health problems and regained unneeded weight. A big part of their new problems stemmed from the fact that they had lost the healthy fats along with the unhealthy ones. Gittleman helped us to see how vital some fats can be. She found that adding healthy fats back into the diet quickly helped return weight to ideal levels. Why? Because certain fats control how much fat is burned by our bodies and how fast it is burned. Recall that medium-chain triglycerides from saturated fats such as coconut oil are used by athletes and bodybuilders for metabolic enhancement. Gittleman described in *The Fat Flush Plan* how fatty acid supplements can help with weight loss. In fact, eating just 8 percent of your calories as balanced essential fatty acids (1:1 to 2:1 omega-6 to omega-3) will help keep your fat-burning capacity at its peak.[9] That's largely because the omega-3 fats are *activating* fats.

As you can see, although you want to quit *overeating* fat, you can't do it by cutting fat out of your life. Please stop trying to eat a super-low-fat diet. Even if you have been able to lose pounds on low-fat regimens such as Ornish's, you have probably rebounded out of them eventually and into the opposite extreme, overeating fats more than ever.

DO YOU DIGEST FAT WELL?

You may be eating plenty of healthy fats, but if you aren't an efficient fat-processor, you may not get the benefits from them. You may not be making enough of the enzymes that do your fat digesting. Or your liver and gallbladder, key players in fat digestion, may be in some kind of trouble. How do you know if you're digesting fat poorly? If you are, you will feel overly full, heavy, or nauseous after a high-fat meal or experience belching after eating fatty foods.

Lipase is part of the digestive brigade that breaks down fats so that your body can use them most beneficially. Lipase (*lipid* is another word for *fat*) meets up with your fat soon after you swallow it. So does bile, a powerful acid made by the liver and stored in the gallbladder. Bile breaks fat into little pieces so that lipase can easily dissolve it for your body to utilize rather than just store.

If you are having trouble digesting fats, try taking lipase supplements to help you break down the fats you eat. These supplements are exactly like your own digestive enzymes. You have many kinds of enzymes in your digestive tract, each one capable of digesting only one particular kind of carbohydrate, protein, or fat. If you don't have enough lipase, your body can't get the full nutritional value of the fats you eat.

Once you've improved your general eating and health over the next few months, you'll be making lots of your own lipase and you won't need lipase supplements anymore. That's because your pancreas, which produces digestive enzymes such as lipase, will no longer be stressed by a high-carbohydrate diet. Now it will be able to manufacture enough of the enzymes you need instead of working overtime to produce insulin to handle all those extra carbs.

Fat and the Liver and Gallbladder

The liver and its intimate partner, the gallbladder, process much of our incoming fats. If either is unable to do its job, our bodies may not receive the fats that they need, and they will put out the call for more fat. This can turn into a vicious cycle as the liver gets more inefficient because of an overload of fats to process, on top of whatever problems it had to begin with (for example, from drug, alcohol, or high fructose sugar use; hormones; or toxins such as pesticides).

Your liver is the gallbladder's boss in processing the fats that come into your body. It can get overworked and congested. It can even become diseased, especially now, with various forms of hepatitis becoming more and more common. Symptoms of liver problems include yellowing of the skin and eyes, intolerance of greasy foods, and unusual (especially pale) bowel movements and pain under the rib cage and in the big toe.

There are a number of nutritional supplements that can help your liver function better. You'll see in chapter sixteen why the herbs milk thistle (or silymarin) and artichoke can be so helpful, and what to do if you've lost your gallbladder (as 25 percent of low-calorie dieters have).

MICROBIAL PARASITES AND FAT CRAVINGS

Tiny intestinal invaders can increase your appetite for fatty foods. The parasite *Blastocystis hominis* ("blasto") actually feeds on the fat that you eat until it literally explodes. These and other parasites can invade the liver and affect the gallbladder, too. If you increase your omega-3 and saturated fats, reduce your high omega-6 vegetable oil intake, raise your endorphin levels, take lipase, and improve your liver and gallbladder function, and you still have strong cravings for fats, then take the Parasite Questionnaire, on page 105, and if your score is high, explore testing and treatment.

Whatever the cause of your fat cravings, you don't have to be enslaved by them anymore. When you get the correct fat balance for your body, you won't miss the fats you don't need. Turn to chapter sixteen for liberating nutritional solutions.

Part II

Correcting Your Imbalances

NINE

Refueling Your Brain with Amino Acids

This may be the most exciting chapter in *The Diet Cure*, because it will teach you how to use amino acid supplements to correct the brain chemistry deficiencies that are forcing you to the chocolate chip cookies. Soon you'll be free of food cravings and the depression, irritability, anxiety, and overstress that trigger them. The Amino Acid Therapy Chart, on pages 122–123, will help you to spot which aminos you'll need, at what dosages, and when to take them.

As part of your Master Plan, you'll of course be taking the Basic Supplements (see chapter seventeen). And while amino acids and the Basic Supplements will do wonders for your brain chemistry, certain foods are also fundamental to your brain-refurbishing project. So once you have chosen your amino acid supplements here, you'll read the general supplement- and food-related chapters in Part III.

Finally, I'll give you some guidance in this chapter on when you can stop taking your amino acid supplements and simply continue with your basic supplements and Master Eating Plan, happily (and permanently) in control of your own appetite.

Precautions: Not all amino acids and supplements are safe for all people. See chapter seventeen, page 257. If you are pregnant or nursing, the complete free-form blend, Total Amino Solution, by

Genesa, is preferable to individual aminos. (It's also great for vegans to add to their individual aminos.) For even more on the amazing aminos and their uses, see my second book, *The Mood Cure*.

USING THE AMINO ACID THERAPY CHART: RESTORING YOUR DEPLETED BRAIN CHEMISTRY

The following chart will help you determine what amino acids you should take, in what amounts, and when, to stop your food cravings and negative moods. Let's start at the top of the chart.

Column A, Deficiency Symptoms. This tells you how you might feel if you did not have enough of each natural mood booster. Check off the symptoms that apply to you.

Column B, Addictive Substances Craved. Here is a list of the drugs or druglike foods you will be drawn to if you don't have enough natural mood boosters. Check off each one that applies to you.

Column C, Natural Solution: Amino Acids. This lists the amino acids that correct the deficiencies. Look first at the boxes you checked off in columns A and B. These are the areas of your brain chemistry that need the most mood food (amino acids). Column C then tells you which specific aminos you will need.

Column D, Neurotransmitter or Brain-Fuel Promoters. These are the natural brain boosters, or neurotransmitters, that are made from the amino acids you will be taking. This column indicates what benefits will result from building up these neurotransmitters.

Now let's look at each of the five horizontal sections, starting at the top of the chart on pages 122–123.

Section I, Relieving Hypoglycemic Cravings for Sweets, Starches, and Alcohol. If your cravings are triggered by a drop in blood sugar (hypoglycemia), the L-glutamine should alleviate them in just a day. Two 500-milligram capsules three times a day between meals is usually sufficient. For fast, emergency relief of carbohydrate cravings (and/or alcohol cravings), take 500 milligrams of L-glutamine or more, if needed, by opening a capsule under your tongue. As L-glutamine stabilizes your brain's blood sugar level, your mood will stabilize as well.

Section II, Curing the Lack of Energy and Focus That Drives You to Caffeinated Drinks and Chocolate. For low energy and poor concentration, take 500 to 1,500 milligrams of L-tyrosine up to three times per day (before breakfast, midmorning, and midafternoon). L-tyrosine is an energizing and stimulating amino acid. If it is too stimulating (for example, if it interferes with sleep), eliminate it or reduce the dose, particularly the midafternoon dose.

If you look for a "lift" or better concentration from foods or drugs such as lattes, chocolate, nicotine, or Skittles, you probably need to overhaul your brain's natural energy system. I usually recommend L-tyrosine first. If the tyrosine makes you feel wired or jittery, try a similar but somewhat less stimulating amino acid, L-phenylalanine. Work with these two aminos until you get your own natural energy and concentration back. If they don't do the job, your master energy glands—the adrenals and the thyroid—probably need help. We cover them in chapters three and four.

Section III, Enhancing Your Ability to Relax and Stop Stress Eating. If you have checked off several of the symptoms and substances in this section in columns A and B, try adding 100 to 500 milligrams of GABA (gamma-aminobutyric acid) to your daily regimen of amino acids whenever you need extra help relaxing. Taking GABA for the first time early in the day may not be a good idea, because you might get too relaxed to drive. If so, take less next time. Several popular formulas combine GABA with two other relaxing amino acids, taurine and glycine, 300 to 500 milligrams each. This combination can be even more calming for some people than GABA alone. GABA Calm, by Source Naturals, a fast-acting, chewable product, contains 100 milligrams of GABA and 25 milligrams of tyrosine (to prevent you from getting too relaxed). Another,

AMINO ACID THERAPY CHART

Sec. No.	A. Deficiency Symptoms	B. Substances Craved	C. Natural Solutions	D. Neurotransmitter Promoters
I	☐ frequent cravings for sugar, starch, or alcohol ☐ irritable, stressed, shaky if meals are delayed	☐ sweets ☐ starches ☐ alcohol	L-glutamine 500–1,500 mg x 2–3 early morning, midmorning, midafternoon	**Back-up fuel source for entire brain** makes us feel stable, calm, and balanced
II	☐ crave pick-me-ups from substances in column B ☐ apathetic depression ☐ lack of energy ☐ lack of drive ☐ lack of focus, concentration ☐ attention deficit disorder ☐ easily bored	☐ caffeine ☐ sweets ☐ starches ☐ chocolate ☐ aspartame ☐ diet pills ☐ cocaine ☐ meth ☐ tobacco ☐ marijuana	L-tyrosine 500–1,500 mg early morning, midmorning	**Catecholamines** arousal energy mental focus drive
III	☐ overstressed ☐ stiff and tense muscles ☐ hard to relax/loosen up, get to sleep ☐ overwhelmed and burned out ☐ eat to relieve stress	☐ sweets ☐ starches ☐ tobacco ☐ marijuana ☐ Valium, Xanax ☐ alcohol	GABA 100–500 mg as often as needed (add relaxing taurine or theanine, if needed)	**GABA** calmness relaxation sleep muscle pain relief

AMINO ACID THERAPY CHART

Sec. No.	A. Deficiency Symptoms	B. Substances Craved	C. Natural Solutions	D. Neurotransmitter Promoters
IV	☐ very sensitive to emotional (or physical) pain ☐ tear up, cry easily ☐ crave treats for comfort, enjoyment, reward, or numbing ☐ "love" or get a high from foods in column B, drugs, or behaviors such as over exercise, infatuation, self-harm, starving, purging	☐ sweets ☐ starches ☐ chocolate ☐ exercise ☐ heroin ☐ oxycontin ☐ marijuana ☐ alcohol ☐ flour or milk products ☐ fats	DL-phenylalanine (or D-phenylalanine) 500–1,500 mg midmorning, midafternoon	**Endorphins** emotional and physical pain relief pleasure reward loving feelings numbness
V	☐ afternoon or evening cravings ☐ negativity, depression ☐ worry, anxiety, low self-esteem ☐ obsessive thoughts/behaviors ☐ winter blues ☐ PMS ☐ irritability, rage ☐ panic, phobias ☐ fibromyalgia, TMJ ☐ night-owl, hard to get to sleep ☐ insomnia, disturbed sleep ☐ hyperactivity ☐ benefit from SSRIs	☐ sweets ☐ starches ☐ alcohol ☐ marijuana ☐ Ecstasy	5-HTP 50–150 mg midafternoon and, if needed, for sleep (by 10 P.M.); or L-tryptophan 500–1,500 mg midafternoon and, if needed, for sleep (by 10 P.M.) Melatonin 0.5–5 mg for sleep at bedtime (by 10 P.M.)	**Serotonin** emotional flexibility self-confidence optimism sense of humor **Melatonin** (made from serotonin) good sleep

True Calm, by NOW Foods, has 200 milligrams of GABA and higher doses of taurine and glycine. Try 500 milligrams of GABA only if you need even more relaxation. (*Note:* If these aminos do not relieve your stress, you may be suffering from adrenal exhaustion. See chapter three.)

Section IV, Eliminating the Need for Comfort Foods. Which amino acids can free a food junkie? D-phenylalanine is the single most helpful amino acid for building up optimal amounts of our natural painkillers. Many studies have confirmed its usefulness in increasing pain tolerance by keeping our pleasure-promoting endorphin levels high.

Most supplement formulations combine D-phenylalanine with equal amounts of L-phenylalanine, its mildly stimulating twin. This combination, DLPA (DL-phenylalanine), usually works well, especially if energy is needed. If DLPA makes you feel too stimulated, the D-form can be taken alone, though it's harder to find. If you overeat, try DLPA on arising, midmorning, and midafternoon for a "treat" or to help deal with emotional pain. You will also need to consume lots of high-protein food and, perhaps, add a complete blend of amino acids, because endorphin building requires many more amino acids than are needed to construct any of the other three key neurotransmitters.

Section V, Raising Serotonin, Our Natural Prozac. The deficiency symptoms in column A of the last section of the Amino Acid Therapy Chart make it clear that depleted brain serotonin can cause some of the most extensive suffering and overeating of all.

Taking Your Aminos

If you're in a hurry for relief, taking an amino acid (or any other nutrient) sublingually—that is, opening the capsule and pouring the contents under your tongue—speeds its effect. (Though only L-glutamine tastes good.) Try to take your aminos at least twenty minutes before or ninety minutes after a meal in which you eat protein; otherwise, the protein in your food will compete with the amino acid and less of the amino will get into your brain. If you are still having cravings or other deficiency symptoms in column A an hour after taking a 500-milligram capsule (the smallest dose usually available), go up to 1,000 to 2,000 milligrams, gradually increasing 500 milligrams at a time. *Stop if you have any adverse reactions such as shortness of breath or agitation.* Keep going up only if benefits increase at higher doses.

Note: GABA doses start at 100 milligrams and go up to 500 milligrams max per dose.

For children and sensitive adults: try small (e.g., ¼–½) doses at first. Raise as tolerated.

If you have low serotonin levels, try a 500- to 1,000-milligram dose of tryptophan midmorning, midafternoon, and two hours after dinner (or at bedtime, if sleep is a problem, because, as explained in chapter one, tryptophan converts to serotonin, which can create melatonin, which helps you sleep).

Since tryptophan is somewhat less readily available, there is another, more easily accessed supplement that you can take to boost serotonin: 5-HTP (hydroxytryptophan). It is widely available in health food stores and some drugstores, as well as Walmart. Our clients find that they often benefit from 50 to 150 milligrams two to three times a day.

Serotonin fuel in either form, as tryptophan or as 5-HTP, usually works best when it is taken thirty or more minutes before rival amino acids (tyrosine or phenylalanine), caffeine, or protein foods. Too much tryptophan can make some people sleepy, even when it's taken in the daytime. If you have this problem, eliminate morning doses, experiment with smaller amounts, or take tryptophan with meals. You may need to vary your dose quite a bit according to your response to tryptophan, as different individuals respond differently to this amino acid (more so than to any of the other aminos). 5-HTP is more stimulating; avoid it at bedtime if insomnia is a major problem and try tryptophan instead. Tryptophan is a famous sleep promoter. Be sure to take the multiple vitamins and minerals in your Basic Supplement Plan while you are taking either form of tryptophan, as you should with any amino acid. Vitamin B_6 and zinc are particularly important because they help the brain to manufacture its neurochemicals out of the amino acids. Vitamin B_3 (niacin) is also important, because your body makes it out of tryptophan, and you want your limited store of tryptophan making serotonin, not niacin.

Eat serotonin-promoting foods. Emphasize the following protein sources of tryptophan and serotonin, along with moderate amounts of carbohydrates at meals.

Most foods that are high in protein, though they are the only concentrated source of tryptophan, contain much less tryptophan than they do the other amino acids. Here are some foods that have higher amounts of tryptophan:

+ Pork
+ Beef
+ Wild game
+ Shrimp
+ Chicken
+ Turkey
+ Duck
+ Milk products, especially cottage cheese (if you are not intolerant)
+ Seeds (pumpkin, sunflower, and sesame)
+ Filberts and almonds

Try St. John's wort. *Wort* means "herb," and this one increases serotonin activity. Studies from Europe and the United States find that it is as effective as Prozac, without as many side effects. Some people do best taking St. John's wort in combination with L-tryptophan or 5-HTP; some do better on St. John's wort alone. Try taking 300 milligrams of St. John's wort (which includes 0.3 percent of the active ingredient hypericin) three times a day. Start with the tryptophan or 5-HTP, and then add St. John's wort (which is more likely to cause a negative side effect, such as sensitivity to sunlight) if you need it (most people don't).

Be sure to get enough exercise. Moderate levels of exercise can temporarily raise serotonin levels. That's why many of us feel so good after even moderate physical activity. The exercising muscles pull all of the competing amino acids out of the bloodstream, allowing L-tryptophan to pass freely through to the brain. *Caution:* When exercise is the only tool used to raise serotonin, exercise addiction can result. (See chapter twenty-one for more on exercise.)

Expose yourself to enough natural light. If you tend to get depressed and/or overeat in winter or in the evening, it is probably because you are not getting enough light to produce enough serotonin. In the late summer, your brain registers a decrease in light levels and begins to reduce serotonin levels in favor of melatonin—your "hibernation" or sleep chemical. As fall and winter set in, your serotonin levels can drop too low. This is called SAD, or seasonal affective disorder. Specially designed SAD lamps, over three thousand lux, help trick your brain into raising serotonin to summer levels. Three thousand lux is about ten times brighter than normal office lighting (one lux represents the brightness of one candle; ten thousand lux is as bright as a sunny day at noon); to get that intensity with regular lightbulbs you would expose yourself to far too much infrared light, which would hurt your retinas, so the key is either sunlight or cool fluorescent lighting. Visits to tanning booths in winter have likewise lifted the moods of many of our clients suffering from winter depression. Tanning has other benefits, including activating the synthesis of vitamin D, and is strictly monitored for skin safety. (For sources of high-lux, full-spectrum lamps, see Resources on page 133.)

Consider taking SSRIs (selective serotonin reuptake inhibitors). As I mentioned in chapter one, raising serotonin can make the difference between life and death if you are severely depressed, anorexic, or bulimic. Since the effects of tryptophan and 5-HTP can be felt in a day or two, try them first. If they don't make a vast and rapid improvement in how you feel, I suggest you consult a medical doctor, preferably a psychiatrist, and ask about possibly taking an SSRI or similar drug. Unfortunately, these drugs improve but do not eliminate all symptoms of low serotonin. Even worse, you may experience mild or severe side effects such as suicidal depression, inability to achieve orgasm, insomnia, or weight gain. Lastly, SSRI withdrawal can be very uncomfortable, and any benefits are not usually sustained after discontinuation. Fortunately, my clients almost never need SSRIs long-term. Why? Because the aminos usually work or we direct clients to physicians who help them with their low thyroid function, which is the most common reason we've found for tryptophan or 5-HTP not to work better than an SSRI.

To ease withdrawal from medication, consider combining 5-HTP or tryptophan with one SSRI. Do this in consultation with your prescribing physician. In *The Mood Cure*, I cite studies documenting L-tryptophan's successful coadministration with SSRIs, and I include a whole chapter on natural alternatives to SSRIs. Though most had no problems, a few patients in initial studies on Prozac experienced agitation, restlessness, and mild digestive distress when they took Prozac and 5-HTP or L-tryptophan together. Many of the psychiatrists whom we work with are happy to combine the two, and the results have been excellent as long as the aminos are taken at least five hours away from the SSRI and only one type of SSRI is being taken per day.

If the combination of medication and tryptophan is successful, you might (in the spring or summer, preferably) try reducing your medication. At our clinic, we have often collaborated with M.D.s or D.O.s (Doctor of Osteopathy, an M.D. equivalent with specialty in skeletal adjustment) to get clients off of their Prozac or similar medications with a trial of L-tryptophan or 5-HTP, which often worked better than the SSRI alone right away.

Melatonin: More Help for Nighttime Overeaters

Your brain begins to make its own sleeping pill, melatonin, out of serotonin as the sun gets lower in the sky each afternoon. If it can't produce enough, you don't sleep well. The food that your brain needs as raw material to manufacture melatonin is the amino acid tryptophan. In the afternoon and evening, you need extra supplies of serotonin because your brain begins to convert it into melatonin. As serotonin levels decline in this daily cycle, if you are low in serotonin to begin with, you will start to crave carbohydrates, which can give you a temporary lift of serotonin (especially if they are simple carbohydrates, like sugar). Your midafternoon cravings may get worse as the evening wears on. Unable to sleep, you eat more sweets and starches, usually along with milk products. Ice cream and cereal are common favorites.

Because too much melatonin can cause grogginess and troubling dreams, as well as add to depression for someone already deeply depressed, I recommend melatonin for relieving late-night cravings only when L-tryptophan or 5-HTP does not normalize sleep. Taking 500 to 1,500 milligrams of L-tryptophan (or 100 to 150 milligrams of 5-HTP) at bedtime is usually effective for insomnia and night-owl syndrome. If you still wake up after 2 A.M. and can't get back to sleep, try a 1–3-milligram time-release capsule of melatonin at 9:30 P.M. This is also a good strategy if you are trying to adjust to a change in time zones because of traveling. If none of the above helps, read the sleep chapter in my book *The Mood Cure*.

If you need to take L-tyrosine or DLPA and tryptophan. Remember that L-tyrosine and DL-phenylalanine (DLPA) compete with tryptophan, so either take them at different times of the day or take L-tryptophan or 5-HTP thirty minutes or more before either of the other two amino acids. If you take them together they will still help, but not as effectively.

We often will only recommend L-tyrosine and DLPA for early morning (AM) and midmorning (MM) use, and 5-HTP or L-tryptophan only for midafternoon (MA), evening (predinner), and bedtime (BT) use, when all are needed.

Finding DPA. A few companies carry D-phenylalanine (DPA) via the Web, but not in stores. If emotional or physical pain is a real problem for you, it can be well worth ordering it. (See Resources at the end of the chapter.)

Amino Acid Supplementation

With a pencil, check off the amino acids and other supplements listed below that you should be taking, as indicated by your responses on the Amino Acid Therapy Chart and the other information in this chapter. You should photocopy the supplementation chart to make clean copies for future use, because your amino plan is likely to change as you begin using the supplements; by your reactions to them you may find that you need more or fewer. Where a range of doses is listed, start with the lower amount to see how it affects you.

Note: It is important that you also take the vitamins, minerals, and other nutrients in the Basic Supplement Plan in chapter seventeen to optimize the effects of your amino acids on your appetite and mood.

	AM	B	MM	L	MA	D	BT*
❏ L-glutamine, 500 mg (to stop sweet, starch, and alcohol cravings and enhance relaxation)	1–3	—	1–3	—	1–3	—	—
❏ GABA, 100–500 mg; or GABA with taurine† (to destress and relax muscles)	—	—	1	—	1	—	1
❏ L-tyrosine, 500 mg (to energize and focus)	1–3	—	1–3	—	1–3	—	—
❏ DLPA, 500 mg; or DPA, 500 mg (to enhance feelings of comfort and pleasure and to reduce pain)	1–2	—	1–2	—	1–2	—	—

	AM	B	MM	L	MA	D	BT*
❏ L-tryptophan, 500 mg (to improve mood, sleep, and P.M. cravings) *or*	—	—	1–2	—	1–2	—	2–3
❏ 5-HTP, 50 mg *or*	—	—	1–2	—	1–2	—	2–3
❏ St. John's wort, 300 mg, with 900 mcg (0.3%) hypericin (to help raise serotonin levels)	—	—	1	—	1	—	1
❏ Complete essential amino acids, 500 mg	1–4	—	1–4	—	1–4	—	—

*AM = on arising; B = with breakfast; MM = midmorning; L= lunch;
MA = midafternoon; D = with dinner; BT = at bedtime.
†GABA Calm, by Source Naturals, and True Calm, by NOW, combine
GABA with taurine.

Note: Add the complete free-form amino acid blend if:

1) You are unable to eat enough protein-containing foods at first or are a vegan.
2) You have been severely malnourished (e.g., after major surgery, anorexia, or alcoholism).
3) Your endorphins seem to be very depleted. (See section IV of the Amino Acid Therapy Chart on page 123.)
4) You are pregnant or nursing (take it instead of any individual aminos).

Caution: Find an amino blend that contains at least the nine essential amino acids, in the free form (e.g., Total Amino Solution, by Genesa, which includes tryptophan):

Lysine
Phenylalanine
Leucine
Threonine
Isoleucine
Tryptophan
Methionine
Histidine
Valine

AMINO FOODS

Protein is the only food source of amino acids. Mature adults should be sure to have at least 20 grams of protein at each of their three meals. You must build adequate protein into your diet in order to be able to stop using the amino acid supplements in three to twelve months. Chapter eighteen, "Your Master Eating Plan—The Best Foods for Your Diet Cure," will help you determine how much protein you will need and detail more about your Master Eating Plan, including what kinds of carbohydrates and fats will work best with your protein. But don't forget, muscle and brain power can be built *only* from protein.

SHOULD YOU TEST FOR AMINO ACID OR NEUROTRANSMITTER LEVELS?

If you would feel more comfortable getting tested to confirm your need for amino acids, you can ask your doctor for a blood plasma test for amino acid and neurotransmitter levels, both before and three months after you start taking amino acids. The initial test may show you have adequate neurotransmitters or amino acids, but your symptoms might indicate that you need more. The tests are only rough guides as levels in your plasma change very quickly. The real proof is in how the aminos make you feel. The most accurate testing, blood platelet testing, is hard to find. We know of only one commercial lab that offers it: Health Diagnostics and Research Institute in New Jersey. We discourage the use of urine testing for evaluating nuerotransmiter status because it is so unreliable. (For more information, see my article at moodcure.com/articles.)

Note: We recommend all pregnant or nursing women get all of these tests before trying the aminos.

WHEN IS IT TIME TO STOP YOUR AMINOS?

Unlike the basic supplements, your amino acid supplements will be needed only temporarily. But how will you know when you no longer need them?

 ✦ You start to get adverse symptoms, like headaches, tiredness, or jitteriness.

✦ You stop taking them (one by one) to see if your cravings or mood symptoms return, and they don't.

When should you start tapering off your aminos to see whether they are still needed? After one to three months, start consciously skipping your amino doses to see what happens. Experiment with one amino at a time; don't drop all of them at once. If you still need your aminos, try eliminating them again monthly until you are ready to do without them. But keep them on hand for short-term use during any future brain slumps.

Note: If you try to taper off after, say, six months and your symptoms return, you should return to your strongest dose. If your symptoms are long-standing, or severe, or run in your family, it might take a year on the aminos before you can do well without them.

ACTION STEPS

1. Study the deficiency symptoms on the Amino Acid Therapy Chart in this chapter and the Amino Acid Precautions (pages 257–258).
2. Try the supplements indicated by your symptoms as directed, along with your basic supplements, detailed in chapter seventeen.
3. Eat plenty of protein as suggested in chapter eighteen.
4. If you continue to have symptoms of low serotonin:
   ✦ try using a full-spectrum lamp
   ✦ exercise regularly
   ✦ consult your doctor about using SSRI drugs
5. Especially if you are pregnant or nursing, consider, with your physician, testing your amino acid and neurotransmitter levels before and three months after you start taking aminos to verify that you have a deficiency that both you and the baby need amino help with.
6. Cut down, then eliminate, your amino acids over the next three to twelve months, as you no longer need them.

Further Reading

Eric R. Braverman, M.D., et al., *The Healing Nutrients Within* (Laguna Beach, CA: Basic Health Publications, 2003).

Robert Erdmann, Ph.D., with Meirion Jones, *The Amino Revolution* (New York: Fireside, 1989).

Joan Mathews Larson, Ph.D., with Keith W. Sehnert, M.D., *Seven Weeks to Sobriety: The Proven Program to Fight Alcoholism Through Nutrition* (New York: Ballantine Books, 1997). *Depression-Free Naturally* (New York: Ballantine Books, 2000).

Michael J. Norden, M.D., *Beyond Prozac: Brain-Toxic Lifestyles, Natural Antidotes and New Generation Antidepressants* (New York: ReganBooks, 1996).

Julia Ross, M.A., *The Mood Cure* (New York: Penguin Books, 2003).

Priscilla Slagle, M.D., *The Way Up from Down* (New York: St. Martin's Press, 1994).

Resources

Most amino acids can be purchased from health food stores, drugstores, websites, supplement catalogs, or our clinic's website. Visit dietcure.com or call 800-733-9293.

DPA (D-phenylalanine) and the most pure L-tryptophan are available only through a few companies on the Web (e.g., Bios Biochemicals, Montiff, or dietcure.com).

Theraputic lamps: 3,000 to 10,000 lux lamps are easy to find. We prefer full spectrum lamps with radiation shielding and flexible necks that can be used as desk lamps. The Ultralux 55-watt desk lamp by Full Spectrum Solutions (fullspectrumsolutions.com or 888-574-7014) is an excellent lamp.

TEN

Nutritional Rehab for the Chronic Dieter

Whenever I see someone with signs of any of the eight physical imbalances described in this book, I immediately look for the role of low-calorie dieting. In addition to all the damage it can do by itself, it can set off several of the other imbalances as well.

Some dieters can recover on their own by making a decision to stop dieting forever. But you may need more education and deprogramming in order to return to wholesome, non-diet eating, which can then restore optimal appetite, energy, and mood, often very quickly. With the help of nutritional supplementation, you will eliminate your anxiety and food cravings, which will dissolve your fears about weight gain. Then you will be able to start enjoying healthy eating and recover from the many adverse effects of low-calorie malnutrition. It will help, too, for you to see the results of research on the benefits of Atkins-type diets, lower in carb and adequate in fat and calories, to weight and overall health. (See pages 138–140.)

In this chapter, you'll get more suggestions about how to break out of the dieting mentality. I'll also provide nutritional supplement protocols designed for soon-to-be ex-dieters, including bulimics and anorexics, whose profound nutritional needs are, oddly, seldom addressed. Finally, I'll suggest some resources, books, CDs, DVDs, magazines, and supportive organizations and professionals that can help keep you safe from dieting.

DEFECTING FROM THE DIET CULT

One young woman came to Recovery Systems after years of intermittent dieting and ten- to twenty-pound weight shifts. She was eating candy bars in the afternoons and, too often, lots of ice cream after dinner. When I went over her diet diary with her, I immediately pinpointed the culprit: she was always skipping breakfast. This particular client did not even seem to need any special nutrient supplements to help get her back on track. As soon as she began to eat a protein-rich breakfast daily, her afternoon and evening junk-food cravings just disappeared. Soon she was eating three well-balanced meals per day and finding her weight stable for the first time in years.

By returning to eating three meals a day you, too, will be able to eliminate overeating and weight gain. Unfortunately, many of you are too afraid of putting on pounds to try eating normal amounts of food again, but you don't have to be, as you will learn in this chapter.

YOUR "IDEAL" WEIGHT

When I wrote the first edition of this book, the obesity epidemic had just begun. Since then, while bulimia and anorexia still rage on, overeating and overweight have become a totally unprecedented phenomenon. Why? The amazingly and increasingly addictive nature of fructose-based sodas and sweets, doughy starches, and fried foods. Since dieting has proved to be useless in the face of this menace, more and more often we are just giving up. Unable to protect ourselves from our cravings for these increasingly addictive foods, we are gaining weight and becoming diabetic at a tremendous rate. We should be enraged that the food industry fattens us while the media makes us think we should be super skinny. What we are left with is fear and self-hate. While you use this book to fight free of these addictive weight- and health-destabilizing foods, use chapter two and this chapter to win back your self-respect along with a healthier relationship with food.

Unfortunately, too many of us have looked to the media to get a sense of what we "should" look like. Entire books have been written on the effect of our culture's distorted image of women's bodies. Try some of the following exercises to resist the media hype and the self-hate it generates:

1. Stop weighing yourself. Toss out your bathroom scale. Even at the doctor's office, do not allow yourself to be weighed (unless you are underweight) or insulted about your weight.
2. Pick one day a week to totally avoid any conversation about anyone's weight, especially yours! Expand this to seven days a week as soon as possible.

3. Check the body shapes of people on your family tree. If you don't know what your grandparents, great-grandparents, or great-aunts or -uncles looked like when they were young, before they ever dieted, get photos and study them. Go as far back into pre-dieting (pre-1970) family history as you can. You'll probably find your genetic double, who will be the healthy ideal weight that you should be. Remember, the further back you go the healthier the diet, and the more realistic the weight standards. I found that my body was almost identical to my paternal grandmother's and to no one else's on either side of my family. You may wish that you had your aunt's green eyes or your uncle's long eyelashes, but you know it's impossible. Remember, the rest of your body is inherited, too.

4. Question your family messages about weight. Did you grow up hearing things like, "I hope you don't get my thighs," or "Don't eat so much or you'll end up looking like your uncle Benjamin"? It's sad to think that these inherited body types are held up as something you should, or even could, try to avoid developing. If only we all grew up hearing messages like, "I think you'll be built just like your wonderful aunt Jane," with no negative baggage attached to any particular body type.

5. Look at old photographs and great artwork of the past. Take a trip to the flea market, a store that sells old magazines or prints, a museum or art-reproduction shop, or view some old movies. Look at the bodies of models, actors and actresses, and ordinary people of the past. You may be astonished to see the beefy thighs and arms on 1940s pinups or on women in paintings (such as those of Rubens, Michelangelo, and Botticelli), or the fleshy legs on 1920s bathing beauties. Notice the thick middles of some of the most dashing male movie stars of the past. Remember, Marilyn Monroe varied from a size 10 to size 14, and the full-figured Mae West was considered quite the sex symbol. You may want to get copies of these old photographs or artworks to hang on your wall as a reminder that the "ideal" body has changed drastically over time for no good reason.

6. Stop reading fashion magazines and watching soaps and sitcoms with emaciated actresses and super-buff actors. Women and gay men will have an especially hard time avoiding unrealistic body images in magazines and media aimed at them. Keep in mind that television, magazines, movies, and even newspapers rarely show images of average-shaped bodies. Moreover, print images are often drastically altered by computer to "fix" every possible flaw. You can try reading

magazines that feature larger-size models and realistic body shapes, but if they still make you hate your body they will have to go, too. Hating your body, like any hate or other strong negative emotion, contributes to unneeded weight gain by triggering junk-food binges.

7. Keep in mind the following eye-opening facts:

   ✦ Only 5 percent of us have "skinny" genes.

   ✦ In healthy 20- to 50-year-old women worldwide, 28 percent body fat is ideal.

   ✦ Eskimos traditionally consumed a 75 percent fat diet. This kept their bodies healthy, fat, and warm.

   ✦ If Barbie were a real person, she would have so little body fat that she would be unable to menstruate, not to mention she'd fall over.

   ✦ Among elderly women, the thinnest have a death rate 50 percent higher than average-weight women.

   ✦ In a study of seventeen thousand Harvard alumni published in *The New England Journal of Medicine*, the men who had the best chance of living the longest were those who gained the most weight (twenty-five pounds or more) but stayed physically active.[1]

While it's true that with serious obesity we can have health problems, modest weight loss will get rid of them. Weight loss, even in those cases in which excess weight is causing real health problems, has to be approached very cautiously. Many studies worldwide have confirmed that weight loss in both men and women correlates with a shortened life span. For example, the famous forty-year Framingham Heart Study found that those whose weight fluctuated frequently, or by many pounds, had a 50 percent higher risk of heart disease.[2]

Bypass the Bypass

The increasingly common gastric bypass and other bariatric surgeries are often unsuccessful because of continuing or increasing food cravings, malnutrition, and adverse "complications" (including death) for at least 40 percent. As an alternative (or as post-operation support), the Diet Cure is a must.

Sadly, many of my clients look back at the weight that prompted their first diets and tell me, "That was a great weight. I'd love to be that weight again, even though I wasn't skinny." Quite often that was their "ideal" weight and they never needed to diet in the first place. They were strong, full of energy, and emotionally positive. It was dieting that sapped their energy, disturbed their moods and appetites, and caused them to forfeit their true weight. If you have dieted, you've probably been yo-yoing above and below your true weight for years. Often, inherited low thyroid function prevents you from finding your true weight. (Dieting, of course, just slows your thyroid even more.)

Fortunately, whatever the reason you lost track of it, your body can often find its own natural weight again, if it is allowed to. Just as your natural voice reappears after a bad cold, your natural weight can reappear after the yo-yo years.

YOUR NEW IDEAL MEAL: HOW MUCH PROTEIN, FAT, AND CARBS?

In chapters eighteen, nineteen, and twenty, you'll find lots of ideas for creating healthy meals that will enhance your particular biochemistry and get you on the road to health. To eat healthfully, you will have to reeducate yourself about what a meal should look like.

To start, try to forget about counting calories or fat grams. Focus on new ways of viewing food. What is a healthy portion of chicken for you? Six ounces? Three ounces? What constitutes a "balanced" meal? After reading chapter twenty, you will, I hope, have a different idea of what you should be eating.

THE TRUTH ABOUT DR. ATKINS'S LOW-CARB CRUSADE

In his famous diet, Dr. Atkins did not restrict saturated (or other) fat consumption because he knew, as a cardiologist, that carbs were the real problem. The Harvard School of Public Health concurred. Its study "found no association between low-carbohydrate diets and increased cardiovascular risk, even when these diets were high in saturated animal fats."[3]

Other studies have confirmed the superiority of Atkins-type diets' positive impact on blood pressure and on the lowering of cholesterol, triglycerides, glucose, insulin, and A1C levels.[4] These last three are diabetes markers. Several studies on diabetes document the benefits of lowering carbs and including fat in the diet. To quote one such study's author, "When we took away the carbohydrates, the patients spontaneously reduced their daily energy consumption by 1,000 calories a day. Although they could have, they did not compensate by eating more proteins and fats and they weren't bored with the food choices. In fact, they loved the diet. The carbohydrates were clearly stimulating their excessive appetites."[5]

A one-year study published in the *Journal of the American Medical Association* comparing the Atkins diet with the Ornish (high-carb), Zone (low-carb, low-cal) and LEARN (low-fat, high-carb) diets found that "overweight and obese women assigned to follow the Atkins diet, which had the lowest carbohydrate intake, lost more weight and experienced more favorable overall metabolic effects at 12 months than women assigned to follow the Zone, Ornish, or LEARN diets."[6]

All this without restricting fat and rarely even discussing calories!

So, with all his practical and well-tolerated dietary advice and his sophisticated knowledge of nutritional medicine and the use of supplementation, where did Atkins's system fall short? Why do Atkins dieters quit and regain the weight, just like higher-carb, lower-calorie dieters do?

Missing Link One: Dr. Atkins did not know that carbs could be more addictive than cocaine. Since his death, researchers at Princeton[7] and the University of Bordeaux,[8] among others, have documented this phenomenon (already so obvious to most Americans!). More important, he did not know about the extraordinary effectiveness of individual amino acid supplements (except for L-glutamine) in completely turning off the carb cravings that never quite leave too many of his followers. The high protein content of his diet helped a lot, because protein is made up of twenty-two amino acids, but there is often not quite enough of any single amino acid to completely turn off the craving signals in the brain. The use of individual amino acid concentrates, used briefly, solves this problem beautifully. (I explain this in chapters one and nine.)

Missing Link Two: Dr. Atkins specifically did not recognize the addictive power of certain common grains, particularly wheat, and milk products for many people. Instead he included small amounts of both in his menus. For too many, this perpetuated the addictions to doughy and creamy foods that eventually erupted into pizza and pasta relapse. As I explain in chapters five and thirteen, both should have been totally excluded for those who overate them (as sugar was), and amino acids used to stop the cravings for them, allowing people to abstain without feeling deprived. I am happy to be able to introduce these missing links into the lifesaving system Dr. Atkins so heroically pioneered.

VEGETARIANISM

Are you a strong, vigorous, healthy vegetarian with rosy cheeks? Or are you tired a lot and a bit pale? Are you in between? Vegetarian dieters can be extra deficient in certain nutrients, because they not only cut calories; they often eliminate whole groups of foods from their diets, notably protein. The other nutrients that are most commonly deficient in vegetarian diets are the minerals iron and zinc, vitamin B_{12}, and the amino acid L-carnitine. (These are all easy to find in red meats.) Supplements for vegans can be found in chapter seventeen. If you are a vegetarian or vegan, get your iron and ferritin levels tested, and check your blood count (CBC) for signs of anemia. Get professional suggestions for B_{12}, iron, and/or folic acid supplementation if you are anemic. Monitor your levels by retesting regularly.

GOOD-BYE TO DIET SWEETENERS

Many dieters have become dependent on aspartame, also known as NutraSweet or Equal. You may find it surprisingly hard to do without your sweetened diet drinks and foods and your pink packets. Rather than search for another sweetener (I don't know of any that are problem-free), I'd like you to eliminate the drinks and foods that you've felt the need to sweeten. Think instead about why you crave those beverages. Do some nutritional investigation and repair work. If you like diet sodas only with caffeine, take some tyrosine (500 to 1,500 milligrams) at the times you'd usually drink your caffeine (before or between meals is best). You should lose interest in caffeine very quickly. Ditto decaf coffees or lattes, which still contain some caffeine. If you like only (or mostly) non-caffeinated beverages sweetened with aspartame, try DL-phenylalanine (500 to 1,000 milligrams) when you'd usually have your diet drink. You should not miss it. If you decide that you miss both caffeinated and NutraSweetened foods, you can try L-tyrosine (500 milligrams) and DL-phenylalanine (500 milligrams) together first thing in the morning and between meals.

You won't need these extra amino acid supplements for long. If they begin to make you a little jittery, or if you've been free of cravings for a month, go off of them. If your yearning for aspartame or caffeine comes back, take a dose for another month or so, then try going off again. Repeat until you're permanently free of cravings. You might think about your old drug favorites, but if you don't actually crave them, you're fine.

What should you drink instead? Warm beverages are a good idea, especially in the morning, when you're at your coldest after eight hours of inactivity and no food, especially in cold weather. Think hibiscus, rooibos, or lemon verbena tea.

Pure or mineral water with a squeeze of lemon, lime, or grapefruit juice is delicious.

RESPECT YOUR RED FLAGS

If at any point after you start the Diet Cure you find yourself regularly wanting a cup of coffee, a diet soda, or some chocolate, that is an important red flag that can alert you to nutritional problems that need attention. Keep a food-mood log (see page 369) so that if you experience cravings you can spot any problems that might account for them. You'll usually find that you've skipped meals or supplements, or eaten foods that make you tired, or not eaten enough for your unique nutritional needs.

You might also discover that you'll need to review the Quick Symptom Questionnaire again. Even if your total score in a particular section was not very high, a few significant symptoms might indicate a real imbalance. For example, if you tend to have cold hands and feet, and you've never taken your temperature in the morning but assume it's normal, take your morning temperature as instructed in chapter twelve, and explore the possibility that you have a sluggish thyroid.

HOW TO UNDIET

1. **Do not skip meals.** Eat three substantial, balanced meals (containing protein, fat, and carbohydrates) per day. Skipping breakfast automatically slows metabolism and induces afternoon and evening food cravings and overeating.
2. **Eat at least 25 percent of the day's calories at breakfast.** Breakfast is the only meal that speeds up calorie burning. You may be able to stop all compulsive eating simply by adding a solid breakfast that emphasizes protein (at least 20 grams).
3. **Do not undereat.** Dr. Wayne Calloway, an expert in Third World malnutrition as well as eating disorders, describes patients who had dieted so often that they were gaining weight on 700 calories per day. When he raised their intake above 1,500 calories (with 25 percent taken in at breakfast), they finally began to lose weight and gain energy.

4. **Start your meals with plenty of protein** (like fish, chicken, beef, turkey, and eggs, among other foods). Twenty grams or more of protein will reduce your interest in empty carbohydrates and make you alert and strong.
5. **Eat unlimited amounts of green vegetables with your protein. Eat some red and yellow ones, too.**
6. **For snacking, eat fruit or vegetables with proteins** (for example, apple and cheese), not sweets or starches (like bagels or pretzels).
7. **Be sure to include some good fats in each meal** for optimal health and to trigger your appetite to turn off. Eat butter, nuts, seeds, olive oil, and avocados.
8. **Stop counting calories and fat grams.** If you are eating according to the guidelines of *The Diet Cure*, you don't have to worry about crunching numbers to be healthy.
9. **Turn to chapters eighteen, nineteen, and twenty for detailed guidance on using food to recover from dieting,** including a list (on page 270) of how much protein common foods contain.

SUPPLEMENTS FOR EATING DISORDERS

You will need to take the basic vitamin, mineral, and other nutrient supplements recommended in chapter seventeen. If, however, you have an eating disorder, you will need some extra nutritional help.

HELP FOR BULIMIA

Please combine the following nutritional suggestions with visits to expert counselors and health professionals. I urge you to work with a physician who can monitor your progress and your health. I'm particularly concerned that you get your heart and your electrolyte levels checked regularly. You must also confer with a doctor about adding the serotonin-increasing nutrients 5-HTP or tryptophan to whatever prescribed SSRI (such as Prozac or Paxil) you may be taking. Taking them together is sometimes necessary in the first few months of recovery to effectively relieve you of your compulsion and your mood swings. Be sure to take your 5-HTP or tryptophan at least six hours away from the SSRIs.

If you've been bulimic for less than ten years, you should respond immediately to this program. If you have a more severe problem that has gone on for more than ten years, be patient. It won't be long. You are on the right track. One long-term bulimic who purged fifty times a day had cut down to twice a night within two weeks. It took her a few months, but she was even able to escape those last evening episodes.

The supplements that will stop food cravings and binge eating overnight are amino acids (see chapters one and nine). To heal the digestive tract, include aloe vera juice, which repairs your damaged gut lining and gets your bowels moving; chromium and glutamine to decrease your sugar cravings by stabilizing your blood sugar; and calcium, magnesium, and potassium to support your heart (plus extra magnesium if you have constipation). GABA, vitamin C, and B complex lower stress. L-tyrosine will decrease caffeine cravings and increase your energy. DLPA (or DPA) stops cravings for chocolate and other comfort foods, and replaces the high of the binge (or purge) with a natural sense of well-being. Fish oil capsules will help stop fat cravings and help with PMS symptoms. 5-HTP or L-tryptophan will raise your serotonin levels, eliminating obsessive thinking, negativity, irritability, and insomnia. (Check with your doctor if you are taking antidepressants, and see page 258 on mixing these supplements with your medication.)

Eating soft or pureed food for a while and taking digestive enzymes and aloe juice should help enormously in getting rid of that awful "too full" feeling that makes you want to throw up even when you've "been good." If not, get a chiropractor or other expert bodyworker to adjust the sphincters that won't close or open properly (as they do with hiatal hernias). Delayed gastric (stomach) emptying is a double problem. Because it takes so long for you to get the benefit of the foods you eat, it can trigger severe low blood sugar cravings in addition to the bloated feeling that makes you want to throw up. Bulimics share this problem with many diabetics; you'll find great advice that can help get your stomach moving in the right direction in *Dr. Bernstein's Diabetes Solution*, by Richard K. Bernstein, M.D.

RELIEVING THE SPECIAL STRESSES OF BULIMIA

Bingeing, purging by vomiting or with laxatives or diuretics, fasting/restricting, and overexercising are extremely hard on your adrenal glands, which have to take care of all your ordinary stresses, too. Your adrenals can malfunction badly after a while. That knocks your other hormones (like estrogen, progesterone, and testosterone) out of balance and contributes to anorexic amenorrhea and to the particularly vicious PMS that many bulimics suffer. It also makes you too easily stressed and overwhelmed in general.

Of course the first step in bulimic recovery is to turn off the cravings, which can happen overnight on the amino acids (chapters one and nine). But I recommend that you also have your adrenal cortisol levels checked with easy, accurate, and readily available saliva testing. (See chapters three and eleven.) Many of you will continue to produce abnormal levels of the adrenal hormone cortisol, even in recovery. This can keep you anxious, stressed, tired, and sleepless.

Testing for your reproductive hormone levels is also helpful if you continue to have severe PMS in recovery (otherwise, you'll be thrown off every month, back into demoralizing bursts of bulimia) or have stopped menstruating. Once you find out how your reproductive hormones are out of balance, you and your doctor can act effectively to get them rebalanced. (See chapters six and fourteen.)

Antidepressants to the Rescue?

The serotonin-activating antidepressants, which can be quite beneficial for bulimics, typically fail with anorexia. Yet both eating disorders display low-serotonin symptoms. The difference? Most bulimics actually keep some food down. They are better nourished and at safer weights, so that, though always low, their serotonin function is closer to normal. This gives the SSRIs more to work with. The anorexics we see are typically able to expand their shrunken serotonin levels using tryptophan (not 5-HTP). This helps them respond better to SSRIs as needed.

Because of side effects, bulimics often want to get off their SSRIs and do, quite successfully, by substituting 5-HTP or tryptophan. They first inform their prescriber that they'd like to add 5-HTP or tryptophan (six hours away from the SSRI) for a week or two to see if the amino provides significant benefits. If so, they ask for suggestions about tapering off their meds at an agreed-upon time. See *The Mood Cure* and moodcure.com for more on alternatives to antidepressants.

HELP FOR ANOREXIA

Anorexia note: You must work with a medical specialist. Do not try to follow the Diet Cure suggestions by yourself. See suggestions for holistic inpatient and other help on page 152.

Starvation is one of the techniques that researchers use to study stress reactions in lab animals. Forced exercise is another. You've proba-bly been suffering from both if you are anorexic. Anorexics' adrenals typically produce too much cortisol—but it has a purpose: to pull nutri-ents out of what is left of your bones and flesh to keep you alive. Test your cortisol levels, as per chapter eleven, but do *not* try to lower your cortisol with the indicated supplements until you are eating and out of crisis. It may normalize on its own. Retest and see. Taking the basic supplements will help relieve your overworked adrenal glands gently to renew your ability to handle stress. Vitamin B_1 along with your B complex and vita-min C (with electrolytes), will be especially helpful.

The way back from anorexia is unique to each person. The deadly biochemical—*not* psychological—phenomenon of "the voice" is tena-cious. Even animals who have been inadvertently underfed can take a long time to tolerate normal feeding. Your immediate enemy, of course, is your mind. Your survival depends on changing it. Fortunately, the amino acids can help. Tryptophan (*not* 5-HTP, which can further raise cortisol levels) is your best friend. It can help turn off the obsession. Ad-just your dose as needed. (One ballerina took 10 grams of tryptophan be-fore "the voice" was silenced.) Others need to add St. John's wort or an SSRI five hours away from tryptophan. Zinc helps restore taste and ap-petite. Drink a bottle a day of diluted zinc until it begins to taste awful, signifying that you've absorbed enough. (Or use 50–100 milligrams in capsules instead of the liquid.) Then taste-test the liquid zinc once a week to be sure that it still tastes awful. Finally, taste-test once a month. Take extra zinc again as needed. You'll of course also need to take the basic multivitamin/multimineral, extra B complex, and vitamin C (e.g., Emergen-C Lite, with electrolytes, though you may well need more po-tassium or sodium, as per testing). If you are constipated, drinking aloe vera juice and/or taking an extra 200–600 milligrams of magnesium will help. GABA will reduce your stress (share with your worried loved ones!);* L-tyrosine will bring back your energy and sparkle by stimulat-ing your brain and thyroid function (without caffeine or diet pills). Your basic fish and flax oil will help your dry skin and hair and your heart and brain. DL-phenylalanine (DLPA) will help you wean yourself off Nutra-Sweet, if you're addicted to diet gum, soda, etc. If it is too stimulating, try D-phenylalanine (DPA—without the L form). Anorexia stimulates en-dorphin release, but you can build up these natural pleasure chemicals

---

* GABA Calm, by Source Naturals, is a good 125-mg GABA formula. Stronger (250–500 mg) versions are also available. (Watch for low blood pressure.) Available through stores and at dietcure.com.

with DLPA or DPA instead, so that you won't need to starve to get the high. A complete free-form amino acid blend will help restore vital protein to your heart, muscles, and brain, and support other vital functions as you increase your ability to eat.

George's aloe vera juice is wonderful for anorexics who vomit or use laxatives. It heals and stimulates the digestive tract. Complete digestive enzymes (with HCl) will help you to break down and utilize your food efficiently. This is particularly important if you have been vomiting. Remember: supplements contain almost no calories, so don't fear them, but begin eating more as soon as possible; you cannot rely on these nutrients to substitute for food.

Another reason that anorexics often respond so well to zinc and B vitamin supplementation is that they sometimes suffer from a genetic condition called *pyroluria*, which results in a deficiency of zinc and B_6. Zinc is essential for a healthy appetite (among many other things), while B_6 allows mood-regulating neurotransmitters, like serotonin, to be produced and is the substrate of hydrochloric acid, which allows for comfortable digestion. (See *Depression-Free, Naturally* by Joan Matthews-Larson for more pyroluria information, a symptom questionnaire, and a supplement protocol.)

COULD YOU BE PYROLURIC?

Pyroluria is a relatively unusual genetic (and stress-exacerbated) condition in the general population (11%) but higher in some groups that tend to have quite stubborn mood problems. Dieting can radically exacerbate symptoms, which include a lifelong tendency to feel shy and left out, having few friends, always avoiding breakfast and usually high protein foods, and not remembering your dreams. It can weaken stress-tolerance and increases anxiety and serotonin deficiency symptoms generally (see chart on page 123), preventing full response to amino acid therapy until it is addressed.

To address: Try zinc capsules (30-50 mg/day) until the zinc tally tastes unpleasant. Retest weekly. Take B_6 (200-600 mg/day) or P5P (50 mg 3 times/day) until dream recall returns. Urinary testing may be helpful but is not always accurate. (See *The Mood Cure* for the complete pyroluria questionnaire and more suggestions.)

Supplements to Support Recovery from Bulimia or Anorexia

Chose the nutrients you seem to need after reading pages 139–141, and try them, along with the basic nutrients covered in chapter seventeen.

	AM	B	MM	L	MA	D	BT*
❏ L-tryptophan, 500 mg	__	__	1–4	__	1–4		1–4
❏ or 5-HTP, 50 mg		__	1–4	__	1–4		1–4
❏ and/or St. John's wort, 300 mg (if not on SSRIs)	__	1	__	1	__	1	__
❏ Liquid zinc, 40 mg (Ethical Nutrients' Zinc Test, Biotics Research's Aqueous Zinc, or Metagenics' Zinc Tally)	__	1/3 bottle	__	1/3 bottle	__	1/3 bottle	__
or Zinc capsules, 50 mg	__	1–2	__	1–2	__	1–2	—
❏ George's aloe juice, 4–8 oz	1	__	__	__	__	__	1
❏ L-glutamine, 500 mg, for cravings and blood sugar drops	1–2	__	1–2	__	1–2	__	__
❏ Vitamin B₆, 100 mg, for mood, PMS, digestion	__	__	1	__	1	__	__
❏ Vitamin B₁ (thiamine), 200 mg, for stress and appetite	__	1	__	__	__	1	__
❏ Emergen-C Lite packets (1,000 mg vitamin C with electrolytes)	1	__	1	__	1	__	__
❏ Extra potassium, or other electrolytes as per M.D./testing	__	__	__	__	__	__	__

	AM	B	MM	L	MA	D	BT*
❏ DLPA, 500 mg (or DPA 500 mg), for pleasure and energy without aspartame or the binge, purge, starvation high	1–2	_	1–2	_	_	_	_
❏ GABA, 100–500 mg, to reduce stress	_	_	1	_	1	_	1
❏ Tyrosine, 500 mg, for energy and caffeine cravings; do not use with caffeine	1–2	_	1–2	_	_	_	_
❏ Digestive Enzymes with HCl	_	1–2	_	1–2	_	1–2	_
❏ Total Amino Solution, 750 mg (Genesa), especially for anorexia, bulimia, vegans	_	1–2	_	1–2	_	1–2	_

*AM = on arising; B = with breakfast; MM = midmorning; L = with lunch; MA = midafternoon; D = with dinner; BT = at bedtime.

GETTING HEALTHY PROFESSIONAL SUPPORT

1. See chapter twenty-one for guidance in finding holistic help, especially if you have an eating disorder. Remember that all health professionals have their own biases and most do not understand the dangers of undereating.

2. If you need help with your Diet Cure, find a holistic nutritionist knowledgeable in the traditional-foods (Weston A. Price) approach. Most dietitians are not holistic.

3. Do not allow any health professionals to prescribe fasts, low-calorie or low-fat diets, or surgery, unless you are very ill and this book does not help.

4. Do not allow yourself to be weighed (unless you are underweight) or insulted about your weight by any health professional.

5. Join a support group to get in touch with your inner image, adjust your body image, and get it all into positive perspective.

6. Explore Overeaters Anonymous (see Resources at the end of this chapter). Stick to the Diet Cure food plan. Don't get obsessed with "goal weight."

7. For individual counseling: Before committing to a counselor, check his or her stance on weight, body image, and diet issues. A women's issues or an eating disorders specialist might be your best bet. Find one who is open to holistic nutritional care.

Note about anorexia: Holistic nutritionists who are anorexia specialists are rare. So are good holistic inpatient treatment programs. (See Resources at the end of this chapter.)

ACTION STEPS

1. **Deprogram yourself about dieting.** Stop weighing yourself and counting fat grams, carbs, and calories (unless it's to make sure you're getting enough!).

2. **Reject unhealthy messages about body image and fat.** Use some of the suggestions in this chapter to do this.

3. **Be sure to eat**
   + 3 meals *minimum* per day;
   + 4 cups *or more* per day of colored low-carb veggies, mostly green;
   + 20 grams protein *or more* per meal;
   + at least one quarter of your day's total calories at breakfast (600 calories or more);
   + other whole-food carbs—beans, corn—as needed after you've eaten your vegetables, protein, and fat;
   + extra virgin olive oil in your salad dressings and coconut oil in your sautéed dishes.

4. **Keep a food-mood log** of what you eat (or don't eat) and how you feel (strong, energetic, free of cravings, or the opposite). See chapter twenty-two for information on how to set it up.

5. **Use the amino acids, basic supplements, and special supplements** listed here to eliminate food cravings, dieters' malnutrition, and the obsessions of eating disorders.

6. **Consult with a health professional and an individual counselor** as needed if you have an eating disorder.

Resources

Explore these materials on the food and dieting industries, body image, self-acceptance, and eating disorders.

FURTHER READING

Frances M. Berg, *Health Risks of Weight Loss* (Hettinger, ND: *Healthy Weight Journal*, 1995). And many other priceless books on weight sanity.

Carolyn Costin, LMFT, M.A, M.Ed., *100 Questions and Answers About Eating Disorders* (Sudbury, MA: Jones and Bartlett, 2007).

Glenn A. Gaesser, Ph.D., *Big Fat Lies: The Truth About Your Weight and Your Health* (Carlsbad, CA: Gürze Books, 2002). One of my favorites. This exercise physiology professor reviews the research on healthy body weight with surprising results.

James M. Greenblatt, M.D., *Answers to Anorexia: A Breakthrough Nutritional Treatment That Is Saving Lives* (North Branch, MN: Sunrise River Press, 2010). A lifesaving approach including hopeful treatment resources.

Gürze Books catalog of books, CDs, DVDs, and more. Order a free catalog: bulimia.com; (760) 434-7533. Gürze focuses on body image and eating disorders, and also publishes a bimonthly newsletter, *Eating Disorders Review*, summarizing relevant research on physiology, treatment, and other aspects.

Lydia Hanich, *Honey, Does This Make My Butt Look Big?: A Couple's Guide to Food and Body Talk* (Carlsbad, CA: Gürze Books, 2005).

Gregory L. Jantz, Ph.D., with Ann McMurray, *Hope, Help, and Healing from Eating Disorders: A Whole-Person Approach to Treatment of Anorexia, Bulimia, and Disordered Eating* (Colorado Springs: WaterBrook Press, 2010). By the founder of the premier holistic treatment program in the United States, the Center for Counseling and Health Resources, in Edmonds, Washington.

David A. Kessler, M.D., *The End of Overeating: Taking Control of the Insatiable American Appetite* (New York: Rodale Books, 2009). The ex-FDA chief reveals how the food industry made us a nation of food addicts.

Gina Kolata, *Rethinking Thin: The New Science of Weight Loss—and the Myths and Realities of Dieting* (New York: Picador, 2008). The latest word on dieting, including research comparing low-carb with other approaches.

Margo Maine, Ph.D., and Joe Kelly, *The Body Myth: Adult Women and the Pressure to be Perfect* (Hoboken, NJ: Wiley, 2005). Among many fine works by this insightful, weight-sane clinician.

Jenni Schaefer with Thom Rutledge, *Life Without Ed: How One Woman Declared Independence from Her Eating Disorder and You Can Too* (New York: McGraw-Hill, 2003). Help with the central anorexic struggle to escape the weight-obsessed "voice."

Naomi Wolf, *The Beauty Myth: How Images of Beauty Are Used Against Women* (New York: Anchor Books, 1992). A classic.

DVDS

Jean Kilbourne (jeankilbourne.com). A terrific resource for DVDs on body image and advertising.

America the Beautiful: Is America Obsessed With Beauty? directed by Darryl Roberts (El Segundo, CA: Gravitas Ventures, 2008). A marvelous film available at americathebeautifuldoc.com.

ONLINE SUPPORT

About-Face (about-face.org). Created and blogged by the inspired Kathy Bruin, who has led successful national campaigns against emaciated models in Calvin Klein ads.

Body Positive (bodypositive.com). Boosting body image at any weight: "Remember, your body hears everything you think."

Healthy Weight Network (www.healthyweightnetwork.com). Research and information on the truth about weight and dieting.

Kay Sheppard (kaysheppard.com). Find this pioneering food-addiction expert's books, consultations, workshops, the Food Plan, the Loop (e-mail mailing list), online OA meetings, articles, and more.

National Eating Disorders Association (nationaleatingdisorders.org). NEDA supports individuals and families affected by eating disorders. Call toll-free for information and NEDA's helpline: (800) 931-2237.

National Eating Disorder Information Centre (nedic.ca). NEDIC provides information and resources on eating disorders and weight preoccupation. (The marvelous Margo Maine is a central contributor.) Call toll-free: (866) NEDIC-20 (633-4220).

Overeaters Anonymous (oa.org). Look up local numbers for meetings in each county. (I would suggest OA over other twelve-step food-addiction programs because of food restriction and sponsorship problems in some of the offshoots of OA.) In the United States, call: (505) 891-2664.

Something Fishy (something-fishy.org). Loaded with information and support, this site is maintained by a very creative recovering anorexic but is not limited to anorexia and bulimia.

Resources Especially for Girls and Parents

READING

Joan Jacobs Brumberg, *The Body Project: An Intimate History of American Girls* (New York: Vintage, 1998).

Kaz Cooke, *Real Gorgeous: The Truth About Body and Beauty* (New York: W. W. Norton, 1996).

Dr. Barbara Mackoff, *Growing a Girl: Seven Strategies for Raising a Strong, Spirited Daughter* (New York: Dell, 1996).

New Moon Girls (Duluth, MN: New Moon Girl Media). A sweet magazine for girls and their dreams, available at newmoon.com or (218) 728-5507.

Kathleen Odean, *Great Books for Girls: More Than 600 Books to Inspire Today's Girls and Tomorrow's Women* (New York: Ballantine Books, 2002). Created by Odean, a librarian, this invaluable resource for parents is a guide to hundreds of books with positive female characters.

Debra Waterhouse, M.P.H., R.D., *Like Mother, Like Daughter: How Women are Influenced by Their Mothers' Relationship with Food—and How to Break the Pattern* (New York: Hyperion, 1998).

HOLISTIC OPTIONS FOR EATING DISORDER TREATMENT

For inpatient treatment, I used to rely on twelve-step (OA-oriented) programs, but now it's hard to find ones like Rader Eating Disorder Programs, in Oxnard, California (raderprograms.com). These programs remove sugar and white flour from the "abstinent" recovery food served. It is unfortunate that there are so few still open, because most conventional programs require the consumption of pizza, pasta, and chocolate chip cookies, and see the desire for healthy food strictly as a symptom of obsessiveness (which it can sometimes also be). An excellent program in the Seattle area that is truly holistic-health oriented is called the Center for Counseling and Health Resources (aplaceof hope.com). Another holistic program, called Mirasol, in Arizona, can provide care for moderate to mild cases, but, in my experience, not for the depth and breadth of severity that the above programs can handle.

As more inpatient options open up or there are changes in the preceding programs, I will post them on the eating disorders treatment page at dietcure.com.

NOTE ABOUT ANOREXIA TREATMENT

If you are at a dangerously low weight and unable to eat, you'll need more intensive care for a while. Any approach that can get more food into you will help revive your authentic self. Even if the food quality is mediocre (as it is in all but the holistic and twelve-step programs), it will help. After completing any inpatient program that prevents your use of Diet Cure supplement or food suggestions, use them immediately upon discharge.

See dietcure.com also for an updated list of specialized outpatient practitioners and programs. Many of those listed will have been trained by me through the NeuroNutrient Therapy Institute.

ELEVEN

Balancing Your Blood Sugar and Reviving Your Adrenals

I hope that you now understand how dangerous sweets and starches can be to your health and mood. You may already have known this but been fighting a losing battle with these carbs for years anyway. Fear not: you are about to receive some new weapons that will help you win the war, as they have for so many of my clinic's clients.

Most of you have been struggling with chronic low blood sugar; that is, hypoglycemia. Rather than continue to rely on candy bars or coffee to perk you up in a hypoglycemic slump, you can learn to regulate your own blood sugar levels. Others of you may be diabetic or borderline diabetic. The truth is that most Americans now fall into two of these three categories because of what we eat and the way we eat it: skipping meals, especially breakfast; substituting caffeine for food; and when we do eat, filling up with fatally addictive high-fructose sweets and empty starches. Regardless of type, you can eliminate these problems through key changes in your eating habits made possible by very special nutritional supplementation.

In this chapter, you'll learn how to use one spectacular amino acid and a few other marvelous nutrients to get rid of hypoglycemic carb cravings, keep your blood sugar stable, and get your adrenals overhauled. These supplements will make it much easier for you to stick to a blood sugar stabilizing diet, which focuses on increasing protein and fat, reducing carbohydrates, and adding plenty of low-carb vegetables.

Special Note to Diabetics

Before you even think about using any of the techniques laid out in this chapter, be aware that they will lower your blood sugar, so you must be ready to use your glucometer throughout the day to be sure you don't drop dangerously low. Also, consult with your doctor as soon as possible, so you will be ready with a medication-reduction plan to keep you from getting into trouble as your diet and blood sugar improve.

One of our diabetic clients, addicted to both sugar and alcohol, really had not believed that she'd be able to quit both so easily. When suddenly she really did lose her interest in them, she found that she had not prepared for the consequences. The next thing she knew, she was being hauled out of her office on a stretcher by paramedics. She had gone into hypoglycemic shock. Now she measures her blood sugar frequently and has worked out an insulin-decrease plan with her M.D.

In addition, I highly recommend *Dr. Bernstein's Diabetes Solution*. Dr. Bernstein's approach is remarkably effective. At Recovery Systems we have seen even severe diabetics follow this high-protein, high-fat, very low-carb plan and find their blood sugars stabilize as never before, on less medication!

TESTING FOR BLOOD SUGAR PROBLEMS

The standard three- to six-hour glucose-tolerance test is guaranteed to make you feel worse than you do already—dizzy, headachy, nervous—because you can only have sugar water during the test period. We typically request one fasting A.M. test each for glucose and insulin and one postprandial test (after a high-carb breakfast) plus a glycohemoglobin A1C test. But you may get more extensive testing through your M.D., N.D. (naturopathic doctor), or D.O. (doctor of osteopathy) or other practicitioner.

USING NUTRITIONAL SUPPLEMENTS TO REGULATE BLOOD SUGAR

The following information will open the door that you've been banging on for years. It will allow you to choose what you are going to feed yourself and to really enjoy foods that are not overly sweet or starchy. You're going to be able to easily eliminate foods containing sugar and white flour, which actually have less than no nutritional value, stripping you of whatever nutrients you take in from other, more nutritious foods. The B vitamins, vitamin C, and the mineral chromium are among the vital lost nutrients that you must replace immediately.

CHROMIUM AND OTHER PRIME BLOOD SUGAR REGULATORS

The United States is distinguished by being perhaps the most chromium-deficient country in the world. At least 90 percent of us don't have enough.[1] Chromium is crucial for keeping blood sugar stable, and it directly prevents carbohydrate cravings. Ironically, too much sugar, white flour, and alcohol deplete us of the chromium that would stop the yo-yo blood sugar and the carb cravings. One of our clients who tried chromium supplements had been eating 8 to 10 cups of vegetables a day, plenty of good fat, and 4 to 8 ounces of protein at each meal. She avoided all grains and other high-carb foods. In most ways she felt and looked wonderful, but she still got some mild low blood sugar cravings and daily headaches. The problem was that prior to getting on this food plan, she'd been a longtime junk-food binger, which had seriously depleted her of this key mineral. By taking 200 micrograms of chromium three times a day, she was able to bring her level back up and was completely craving- and headache-free from the first day on.

If any of us become too deficient in a nutrient, food alone may not give us enough of that nutrient to restore adequate levels. But supplements can replenish our supplies and quickly make a dramatic difference in how we feel. Most of our clients who elect to try chromium find that it helps stop their sugar cravings and all of their other low blood sugar symptoms. In fact, many studies have confirmed chromium's effectiveness in normalizing blood sugar levels in both hypoglycemics and type 2 diabetics.[2] Chromium also helps build muscle, promotes the burning of unneeded body fat, and helps normalize our cholesterol levels.[3] We prefer the amino acid chelate form, as in GTF (glucose tolerance factor) chromium.

Several years ago we began recommending that our hypoglycemic and diabetic clients use True Balance, by NOW Foods, or GlucoBalance, by Biotics, multiple vitamin and mineral formulations designed specifically to stabilize blood sugar. They have turned out to be the most useful multiple vitamin–mineral formulas that we have ever found. Two or three mealtime doses (of two caps per meal) provide 800–1,000 micrograms of the mineral chromium. They also provide 3,000 micrograms of the B vitamin biotin. Research has shown that biotin helps stabilize blood sugar and eliminate carbohydrate cravings in people with both low and high blood sugar. One of our advisers, William Timmons, N.D., found it more effective even than chromium for some people with low blood sugar.

A B complex is also crucial for blood sugar regulation, cellular energy, and protection from stress. True Balance and GlucoBalance contain the complete B complex at generous levels.

Diabetics, Biotin, Chromium, and Glutamine

A study of diabetics taking the B vitamin biotin found that high-dose biotin treatment for types 1 and 2 diabetics dropped blood sugar very fast.[4] The same is true for those taking chromium and the amino acid L-glutamine. So before you start taking them, be sure to work closely with your M.D. on medication adjustment.

L-GLUTAMINE: THE AMINO ANSWER

Don't leave the house without our other stellar blood sugar stabilizer, the amino acid L-glutamine. It can stop cravings for sweets, starches, and alcohol instantly (as I mention in chapters one and nine), by preventing the brain from dropping into the low blood sugar, code red, must-eat-candy-or-have-a-beer-or-hit-someone state. How? When the brain is low in glucose (blood sugar), it can burn glutamine instead. L-glutamine was first synthesized by a biochemist who quickly discovered how remarkable it was in eliminating alcoholics' cravings for alcohol. It can have the same miraculous effect on cravings for sweets and starches. It has many other health benefits as well. It works fastest when used as a powder. (Open a capsule in your mouth. It's great tasting.)

THE OTHER NUTRIENT HELPERS

The following nutrients, all vigorous blood sugar regulators, are included in the Basic Supplement Plan, laid out for you in chapter seventeen. Zinc supplementation helps restore the appetite for real food and is involved in the entire blood sugar regulation process. Zinc, like chromium, is stripped by sugar use and is particularly low in diabetics. It is also vital to blood sugar stabilization that your extra B complex contains niacin and thiamine. Vitamin B_5 (pantothenic acid) is famous for reviving adrenals exhausted by too much sugar. Vitamin E improves insulin's effectiveness. The mineral magnesium is notably deficient in diabetics (and is low in the general population, too). Omega-3 fat (naturally found in fish such as salmon as well as flaxseeds) raises your metabolic rate, regulates fat burning, and supports your insulin function to keep your blood sugar stable. In a study of obese diabetics and prediabetics, just adding omega-3 fish oil as a supplement brought both weight and insulin levels down. (The group fed a low-fat, high-carbohydrate diet got worse!)[5]

SUPPLEMENT	AM	B	MM	L	MA	D	BT*
❏ L-glutamine, 500 mg	1–3	—	1–3	—	1–3	—	1–3
❏ Biotin†, 1,000 mcg	—	1	—	1	—	1	—
❏ Chromium, 200 mcg	1	—	1	—	1	—	1

*AM = on arising; B = with breakfast; MM = midmorning; L = with lunch; MA = midafternoon; D = with dinner; BT = at bedtime.

†If you take True Balance or GlucoBalance multivitamins, you won't need this extra biotin or chromium or any of the nutrients listed above.

Help in Detoxing from a High-Carb Diet

For the first three or four days off sweets and white flour products, you may feel tired and headachy. These detox symptoms are caused by your system becoming too acidic. There are a few tricks to making it easier: Minerals in vegetables and fruits can neutralize that acidity, and your supplemental minerals will help speed up the antacid detox project. You can also use Alka-Seltzer Gold or 1,000 milligrams of powdered vitamin C (ascorbate). Try warm baths with four cups of Epsom salts, too. (For more on detox, see chapter twenty-two.)

THE FOOD SOLUTIONS

When the special nutrients have freed you from your cravings for sweets and starches, you can start eating foods that will keep you craving-free permanently. By that I mean you'll eat delicious low-carbohydrate foods along with as many wholesome carbs as you need and can tolerate. For example, if you rush around in the morning and don't have time for breakfast, you can try a high-protein coconut milk breakfast smoothie or cottage cheese with chopped tomatoes and cucumber. But you could also have eggs and healthy sausage with or without potatoes, or a feta cheese scramble with avocado and salsa, with or without beans.

You won't miss the doughnut. I promise.

Diabetics note: You may need to reduce or eliminate fruit and other whole-food carbs along with the junk carbs because for you they may be too destabilizing. At least for a while, concentrate exclusively on lots of protein, low-carb veggies, and good fats.

I recommend that you try to eat neither according to the guidelines of the USDA's Food Guide Pyramid nor to its similarly high-carb 2011 successor, MyPlate. The pyramid diet consists of more than 60 percent carbohydrates, with protein and fat deemphasized. When it first came out, it sounded hopeful, but it turned out that even whole grain starchy carbs are too much like sweet ones. Soon after a serving of bread or pasta enters your mouth, your blood sugar spikes, then dives. If these foods make up the bulk of your meals, you will most likely continue to crave carbs and experience the other consequences of blood sugar instability.

What has really made the difference for our hypoglycemic and diabetic clients is eating three to six times a day and avoiding too many high-carb foods. So what do they eat? Loads of salads and other low-carb vegetables, like asparagus, green beans, broccoli, red cabbage, and chard, topped with lemon and butter or extra virgin olive oil and garlic. (For a list of low-carb vegetables, see page 280.) They do not restrict fats, except deep-fried food, hydrogenated fats, and high-omega-6 vegetable oils (e.g., soy, corn, and canola). They eat generous portions of protein, like turkey and chicken, lamb chops, cracked crab, and salmon steaks, and smaller portions of whole high-carb foods such as squash, fruit, and beans. They enjoy these foods but don't overeat them or anything else, because they've quickly lost interest in their old high-carb standbys.

Over the years we've learned that some people, after an initial detox period, need to add more carbohydrates, particularly if they are very active physically. We help monitor our clients as they introduce more healthy carbs, like wild rice, winter squash, and potatoes. If these starchy foods trigger a return of sweet cravings or spike insulin, we recommend that they limit them further or cut them out altogether.

What Is Enough Protein in One Meal?

+ 3 eggs (24 grams of protein)
+ ½ to 1 can of salmon (22 to 45 grams of protein, roughly an 8-ounce can)
+ at least ⅓ of a 16-ounce carton (⅔ cup) of cottage cheese (20 grams of protein)
+ 4–6 ounces of meat, fish, or poultry, approximately the size of your palm (20–30 grams of protein)
+ 1–1½ cup of beans (15–24 grams of protein, but lots of carbs too)

PROTEIN HELPS KEEP BLOOD SUGAR STABLE

I would like you, too, to experiment until you find the balance of foods that makes you feel the best. Gradually you will learn how to eat to protect your hard-won blood sugar balance. You will find that one of the two foods that keep your blood sugar most stable turns out to be protein.

Foods high in protein trigger the release of glucagon, a hormone that helps provide balance when excess carbs trigger too much insulin. Glucagon stimulates fat burning instead of fat storage, shuts down cholesterol overproduction, and discourages water retention, among other things. Protein alone, or together with fat (most high-protein foods, like meat, eggs, and fish, contain fat as well as protein), stimulates glucagon activity. Carbohydrates trigger the release of insulin, which results in their conversion to fat and in low blood sugar cravings. But don't get glucagon-fixated. What you want is *level* blood sugar. When your insulin and glucagon are both normalized by adequate protein and fat, blood sugar stays level.

FAT IS EVEN MORE STABILIZING

Fat does not raise insulin; only carbohydrates do. Fat is also innocent when it comes to most weight gain. Fats can be converted into blood sugar if necessary—but slowly, not in bursts that overstimulate insulin release. And fat actually keeps the carbs in your meals from hitting you too hard. It also makes you feel satisfied so that you know when to stop eating, especially saturated fat, as you'll see here and in future chapters.

Convinced that a high-fat, low-carb diet will make you fat? Dr. Bernstein, the author of three books on the treatment of diabetes (and a fifty-year diabetic himself), describes a study published in the *Journal of the American Medical Association* in which two healthy men spent one year in a hospital eating 2,500 calories a day. Seventy-five percent of their calories came from fat and 25 percent from protein; none came from carbohydrates. By the end of the year, both men had lost six pounds and lowered their cholesterol. (One was a famous Arctic explorer, who had initiated the experiment after seeing Eskimos fare well on no-carb, high-fat fare.)

Eat some fat at every meal, because it helps stop carbohydrate cravings. The body yearns for fat and won't often stop eating until the fat arrives. You don't have to eat gobs of it—on the Diet Cure plan you will probably consume approximately 40 to 45 percent of your calories as fat (more if you're an insulin-dependant diabetic). A nutritious dressing of extra virgin olive oil and vinegar for a salad, guacamole with your sautéed shrimp and rice, and butter and lemon on your veggies will ensure that you enjoy your food and are satisfied by it, without harming your health.

Certain fats are better at keeping your blood sugar stable than any other food. They can be burned and provide energy, like carbs, but they burn longer and more steadily so that there are no spikes or slumps in your blood sugar level. These stabilizing fats are not the long-chain, unstable vegetable oils such as canola, corn, and soy oils; or even olive oils (the best of the vegetable oils). Instead, these fatty champs are saturated oils such as butter and coconut oil, the fats we ate lots of before 1970—when our weights were ideal and our diabetes rates insignificant!

If you've ever visited Thailand, you may have noticed how good you feel eating their native food, which is high in coconut fat. Eating these fats won't cause you to gain weight but will give you plenty of energy. The research backs up coconut oil as a powerful stress fighter, because its short- and medium-size fats burn steadily for long periods of time, preventing drops in blood sugar levels that drive you toward sweets for relief. Coconut oil is also stable enough to cook with. We find that clients who use full-fat coconut milk in their protein-fruit smoothies in the morning can go all day without a slump or a drop in blood sugar (of course, they eat a good lunch and dinner, too). These fats can boost metabolic rate by 50 percent, so weight gain is not a problem.[6]

So please relax, and don't worry; you're not going to become a fat addict. If you *already* crave and overeat fats (that is, you live for your next serving of french fries or cheese), you will need some help, so turn to chapter eight.

Watch your own reactions as you make changes in your protein, fat, and carbohydrate ratio. You'll know it's right if you feel energized and strong between meals. Unless you are diabetic, this kind of eating should work well for you right away. Diabetics often need fewer carbs and more fat.

VEGETABLES ARE VITAL

Along with protein and fat, vegetables are of primary importance. They should become your principal source of carbohydrates. Even low-carb, green veggies contain some slow-acting carbohydrates that won't spike insulin but will fill you up—if you eat enough of them. You'll need to make peace with vegetable preparation: washing, chopping, dressing, and cooking. Make vegetables your friends! Aim for 4 cups a day of colored veggies.

Veggies not only contain vitamins and fiber; they also contain crucial minerals and, particularly in the raw state, many digestive enzymes. If you've had low blood sugar for years, you are low on—or even out of—all four kinds of nutrients.

What Is 4 Cups of Vegetables a Day?

Enough to fill a 1-quart milk carton. Think green, red, purple, and yellow low-carb vegetables. Salad greens are so fluffy that they only count as half their volume, so one cup of lettuce contributes ½ cup to your daily minimum. (See chapter twenty for information on how to portion your vegetables for a meal.)

THE EATING ESSENTIALS

+ **Breakfast.** If you don't break the fast that has been going since you ate last night, your blood sugar will just keep dropping until you are so desperate that you will grab the first pastry that floats by. Break your night-long fast with protein—eggs, healthy sausage, a high-protein shake. Eat plenty of food—around 25 percent of your day's intake—within an hour after you wake up if you can (it gets easier quickly).

+ **Lunch.** If you can tolerate wheat, a sandwich loaded with protein (turkey, meat, or egg salad, for example) can be okay. Otherwise, try a large salad with chicken, beans, veggies, avocado, and dressing. Or a burrito without the flour tortilla wrap (ask for corn tortillas if you need them), with meat or chicken, beans, lettuce, salsa, and guacamole. Or a big bowl of chili and a mixed vegetable salad.

+ **Dinner.** Have fish or chicken, with sautéed butter-and-lemon veggies and a large salad with avocado. Or have a large shrimp-and-veggie stir-fry with peanut sauce and spicy red beans or a steak with a small buttered baked potato and piles of coleslaw.

+ **Don't skip meals.** Ever. If you do, I guarantee your blood sugar will crash. Then you'll eat cake.

+ **Snacks.** If your blood sugar has a great tendency to dip, you will need to shore yourself up with midmorning and midafternoon and maybe bedtime snacks that are strong on protein and good fat: peanut butter (unsweetened) and celery, an apple with cheese or almonds, salmon or turkey jerky, a between-meal protein smoothie (no juice, just whole fresh fruit; non-soy protein powder; and coconut milk, plain yogurt, or some raw nuts plus water).

+ **Legumes.** Try putting more legumes (beans, peas, lentils, and others) into your diet. If you can digest them easily (that is, without gas), I think you will like them as a carbohydrate source.* They are actually the highest-fiber food (which helps with blood sugar and bowels) and fairly high in protein and other nutrients. Have them in salads, chili, bean and pea soups, tacos, burrito fillings, and with rice, among other dishes.

---

* Sec chapter eighteen, page 281, for hints on reducing the gas-causing properties in beans and for a list of legumes you can try. They are actually the highest-fiber food, so they keep your digestive tract healthy, and beans are fairly high in protein and other nutrients. Remember, soybean products are hard to digest and produce many other health problems.

Diabetic note: Beans may not work for severe diabetics because of their relatively high carbohydrate content. Check your blood sugar.

✦ **Fruit.** Because it is the only food that we tend to eat uncooked, it retains its fragile vitamin and enzyme content (plus it's loaded with minerals and fiber). Remember, cooking destroys a good portion of the nutrients in your food (another reason we need supplements). But fruit is also loaded with fruit sugar, or fructose. You may find that fruit is too sweet for you, causing you to have a blood sugar dive up to two hours afterward. It does not tend to cause the immediate spike and dive of other sweet foods, but if you find yourself feeling tired and craving sweets after eating an apple as a snack, then next time be sure to eat it with nuts or cheese. Or avoid fruit for a while, until it does work for you. (For more meal and snack ideas, see chapters nineteen and twenty.) *Note:* diabetics may need to forgo fruit altogether.

✦ **Don't forget to take all of your supplements.** If you suddenly want a frozen yogurt, you can bet you have either forgotten a key blood sugar supporting supplement such as glutamine, or a meal!

✦ **Liquids.** Sweet juices and sodas (including diet sodas of any kind) are blood sugar monsters. Their high fructose corn syrup bypasses the usual blood sugar regulation processes, and we have no protection against these diabetes-provoking stealth bombs. Artificial sweeteners, notably aspartame, are also linked to diabetes. Drink filtered or spring water with a squeeze of fresh lemon, lime, or grapefruit. Try guava tea: in China, it is used to control and maintain proper blood sugar levels. Have mineral water or other low-phosphorus drinks such as carbonated Sodastream. The phosphorus in most sodas, especially any colas, leaches calcium.

I have already explained in chapter three that chronic blood sugar imbalance wears out the adrenal glands. In the final section of this chapter we will lay out what may be needed, beyond stabilizing blood sugar levels, to restore exhausted adrenals.

TESTING AND RESTORING YOUR ADRENALS

If you suspect that your adrenals are exhausted, as indicated by the symptoms listed in chapter three, I encourage you to get tested right away. It's time to find out exactly how worn down you and your adrenals are. It will take a week to get your results back, and in the meantime, you'll be getting some relief from your new foods and supplements. The test results will let you know if you need extra help. I strongly recommend that you use the following suggestions for testing and treatment in collaboration with a health professional.

BLOOD PRESSURE CAN INDICATE ADRENAL EXHAUSTION

Normally, systolic blood pressure (the first number in the measurement of blood pressure; for example, 120 in 120/80) is about ten points higher when you are standing up than when you are lying down. If the adrenal glands are not functioning well, however, this may not be true.

Have your health professional take and compare two blood pressure readings—one while lying down and one while standing up. First, lie down quietly for five minutes and have your blood pressure taken. Then stand up and immediately have your blood pressure taken again. If your blood pressure reading is lower after you stand up, suspect reduced adrenal gland function. The degree to which the blood pressure drops upon standing is often proportional to the degree of adrenal depletion.

BLOOD VS. SALIVA TESTING

Pregnenolone is the mother of all the adrenal hormones. Getting blood levels tested can be helpful. Blood cortisol levels rarely reflect actual deficiency, because they include bound (unusable) cortisol along with the free (usable) form. In contrast, saliva contains only the free (i.e., directly usable) form of cortisol. Saliva kits with four samples test your levels of both cortisol and DHEA—the adrenal glands' primary stress-coping hormones—throughout the day. (Ask for an extra vial if you typically wake up in the middle of the night.) Do not exercise or use caffeine, alcohol, or other drugs that day. Keep a log of sleep, food, activity, energy, and mood. If addicted to drugs such as Xanax, test just prior to taking the drug. Don't put yourself into withdrawal by trying to go off. You can have a holistic practitioner order this testing for you or order it yourself on the Internet (search "home full day cortisol DHEA saliva tests").

Saliva testing is accurate and easy. We have been thrilled with the information it has given us, allowing us to help people at a whole new level. You'll collect saliva in little tubes four or five times in one day: once in the early morning, once midmorning, once midafternoon, once late at night, and another in the middle of the night if you tend to wake up for more than a few minutes throughout the night. Then you'll mail your kit to the lab. If your test results show hormone levels that are overly high or overly low, you will know which kinds of repair strategies to implement. (This is important, because choosing the wrong strategy could make you worse.)*

We use labs that provide the test kits, and that actively educate health professionals on how to understand test results. Many health professionals, even holistic ones, are not yet acquainted with this invaluable tool and effective remedies for restoring the adrenals to their optimal function. See pages 362–363 for a list of saliva-test providers and consultants.

TEST RESULTS: FINDING YOURSELF ON THE STRESS MAP

When your adrenal-stress saliva test results come back, they will tell you some fascinating things about how stress is affecting you now.

Stage I of Adrenal Exhaustion. Here levels of your stress-coping king, cortisol, are abnormally high for part or all of the day and night. You may still have energy, perhaps too much of it, because your emergency stress response is over-amped. You may not be sleeping well or restfully if your cortisol levels are high at night (when they should be shutting down) or in the morning (when they should be just rising for the day, not left on all night). You may have lost your appetite and even be losing weight. High cortisol lowers your mood-elevating serotonin and sleep-inducing melatonin, and it cannibalizes your own muscle and bone for emergency fuel. You may be getting sick a lot as your defense team drops its heavy immune-protective responsibilities, because it literally can't cope anymore. You may be hypervigilant and/or unable to relax or rest. While cortisol will be too high in this stage, its backup, DHEA, will sometimes have become worn down to subnormal levels.

Stage II of Adrenal Exhaustion. Your stress-fighting cortisol supplies have finally run low, but they haven't run out yet. For a year or so, both

---

* There are a number of labs in the United States and abroad that do saliva testing and have done it for twenty years, As for being an accurate measure of body chemistry, the World Health Organization has published a paper indicating that saliva testing is now the gold standard for hormone testing.

cortisol and DHEA will hover in the low-normal range, leaving you tired and stressed, but functional.

Stage III of Adrenal Exhaustion. Now both your cortisol and DHEA levels are in the bottom of the low-normal range most or all of the day. Your energy is low. You can tolerate very little stress. This situation is far more common than you might suspect.

One of our clients, Monique, was a highly skilled nurse who worked in a hospital that required all of its nurses to work twelve-hour shifts. She became alcoholic under the stress (she came from an alcoholic family that could not handle stress well). When she came to us, she was irritable, weepy, hopeless, and exhausted. She had a lovely family and had been going to AA for a year and loving it, but she could not keep from drinking on her way home from her long work shifts. She felt better on the supplements right away and quit drinking for a month with no problem—until she went back to work. She took another medical leave while we waited for the results of her cortisol and DHEA levels to come back. When they did, all her scores were *very* low.

Now she is doing fine, even after she gets off work. She takes her breaks regularly and has protein-carb snacks. She gets to sleep by ten o'clock most nights, exercises moderately, goes to her supportive AA meetings, meditates, and has fun with her young daughter. Without the testing and the specially targeted supplements you're about to be introduced to, she would never have been able to stay sober, employed, or happy.

Note: Since more than 90 percent of alcoholics are hypoglycemic, blood sugar and adrenal-stress evaluation and treatment are essential for recovery.

RECOVERING FROM OVERSTRESS: USING SUPPLEMENTS TO RESTORE YOUR ADRENAL FUNCTION

The many hormones the adrenals generate are powerful. For the most successful treatment, work with a competent health care professional on this hormone-regulating mission.

THE SUPPLEMENTS THAT PROVIDE
GENERAL SUPPORT

Among your basic supplements (see chapter seventeen) and your blood sugar stabilizing supplements are several products that will help restore your adrenal function. Vitamin C and the B vitamins are top helpers. In fact, 90 percent of the vitamin C you take in is used by your adrenals, and the vitamin B complex is just as important.

Your basic multivitamin/multimineral, taken with meals, and your basic vitamins B and C, taken between meals, will supply your body with adrenal support all day. C and B complex vitamins are water soluble and do not store in the body, unlike proteins, fats, minerals, and fat-soluble vitamins. The kidneys quickly excrete any excess. Because of the rapid turnover of these vitamins, a lower dose and more frequent intake assure a steady supply of stress-reducing, adrenal-supporting nutrients.

A note on B Complex sublingual supplements: The highly recommended GABA Calm by Source Naturals that dissolves under your tongue contains the sweetener sorbitol and flavoring to cover the unpleasant B vitamin taste. If you are diabetic or sensitive to any of these sweeteners, use comparable products in capsules.

It is usually important to take extra amounts of vitamin B_5 (pantothenic acid) in the early repair process and over the next few months. B_5 allows the adrenals to make more of their antistress (and anti-inflammatory) cortisol. It also burns away excessive cholesterol and triglycerides in the blood. Take 100 to 500 milligrams with meals, depending on the extent of your stress. Take one bottle and stop to see if you still need more than you get in your basic B complex and multi. If you continue to be overstressed, take another bottle's worth.

Another top stress buster is the amino acid GABA, your brain's natural Valium. It can be very relaxing, even at only 100 milligrams, because it deactivates the stress hormones. Try the 500-milligram size if you need more, especially at bedtime. The aminos theanine and taurine have similar effects. A mildly relaxing homeopathic formula called Calms Forté can provide milder soothing effects.

If these supplements help but do not completely restore your stamina and allow you to face stressful situations without feeling strained, drained, or overwhelmed, it's time to move on to the ultimate destress protocol. Our most deeply stressed and exhausted clients take the basic supplements with the special blood sugar stabilizers and stress busters, and add the ultimate adrenal repair supplements, and are *very* glad they do. (You'll only need all this for a few months.)

THE ULTIMATE ANTISTRESS SUPPLEMENTS

Note: These supplements are potent. Please consult an expert while using them.

If your adrenals are in Stage I and your cortisol levels are too high, try:

✦ An amino acid supplement called phosphorylated serine (Seriphos).* It works by reducing the ACTH (pituitary) messages that order the adrenals to release emergency amounts of cortisol and DHEA. We have seen it help with many problems, like intractable insomnia, that do not respond to melatonin, tryptophan, or GABA.

✦ The cortisol-lowering champ, hydrolyzed casein, is also very effective. We often combine it with Seriphos. (Note: this product can give discomfort to people who don't tolerate milk well.)

✦ Vitamin B$_1$ in your multi and extra B complex have the remarkable ability to prevent cortisol excess or lower it in Stage I, as well as raise levels that are too low in stages II and III.

DHEA. For Stage I, II, or III of adrenal exhaustion, if DHEA is too low according to your saliva test:

The hormone DHEA serves as a backup to cortisol in responding to stress and immune system needs, and tests often show that it needs to be supplemented in stress-exhausted people. Your test results will clearly show whether or not you'll need supplements of DHEA. We have seen some chronically fatigued clients respond to DHEA within a week.

Note: DHEA caution: Do not take DHEA if you have hormonally linked illness, such as breast or uterine cancer, endometriosis, or prostate cancer. Monitor your testosterone and estrogen levels if you are taking DHEA, because it can build up the levels of these hormones.

---

* Phosphatidylserine is a similar supplement available in health food stores, but it's not nearly so effective as Seriphos.

Since DHEA is a root hormone that can convert to testosterone and to estrogen, women should watch for acne or the growth of facial hair as signs that it's time to cut down or stop (but retesting can let you know that it's time to stop before such symptoms appear).

Both men and women should watch for headaches, stomach discomfort, light-headedness, and excess throat mucus.[7]

Adrenal Glandulars

Please be cautious about taking whole glandular adrenal supplements, which include the adrenal medulla. The adrenaline made in the medulla can make your problem worse by overstimulating you, adding to your stress level and further exhausting your adrenals. On the other hand, if you're low in adrenaline, this additional adrenaline will provide much-needed energy.

If your adrenals are in Stage II or III, your levels of cortisol are dropping abnormally low. Here are some remarkably helpful supplements to try.

Cortisol. Our clinic's must successful remedy for low cortisol, that is, chronic stress exhaustion, is a product called IsoCort, made by Bezwecken. It contains low doses of cortisol, and its benefits can be felt right away without side effects. Take it at the time(s) of day that your cortisol levels are low, starting with low doses and going up as needed. IsoCort is easily found on the Web, at dietcure.com as well as other sites. Stronger bioidentical, prescription cortisol is also available as Cortef. William McK. Jeffries, M.D., in *Safe Uses of Cortisol*, explains how low doses of Cortef (2.5 to 5 milligrams) two to three times per day can be gently supportive. This dosage adds up to the same 10 to 20 milligrams a day of cortisol that your adrenal glands should normally produce themselves.[8] In periods of severe cortisol deficiency, more is needed.

Cortisol can convert to natural cortisone. Too much conversion can cause the "moon face" (classic symptom in which the face swells up to be round, like the moon) and other high-cortisone side effects, but only at very high doses (100 milligrams or more per day). We have had hundreds of clients use one or the other low-dose form of cortisol for a few months with no adverse side effects and dramatic benefit. Both forms of cortisol can temporarily fill in for your own depleted hormone and rest your adrenals so that they can regenerate, at which point cortisol supplementation will no longer be needed.

Your adrenals' cortisol levels naturally rise highest in the morning and drop gradually through the day and night. Supplementation should restore this normal rhythm as well as mimic cortisol surges when stress hits you.

Licorice. If you have normal to low blood pressure you can raise your cortisol levels in a hurry by using the surprisingly potent herb licorice, in the form of licorice root capsules or liquid extract (glycyrrhiza is the name of the chemical in licorice that has this pro-adrenal effect). Excessive amounts of licorice can be toxic, but your dose won't go near the toxic level, which is more than 100 milligrams of glycyrrhiza per day. Reduce or stop your dose as you no longer need it; for example, if your appetite decreases, if you feel jumpy, or, especially, if you get insomnia, heart palpitations, or increased blood pressure.

Try licorice root whole or as an extract. It should be taken right before the times your cortisol drops. If you take licorice after three P.M., your sleep may be affected. Do not get the licorice without glycyrrhiza, the only ingredient in it that builds up cortisol. Do not take for more than three months.

Caution: If you have high blood pressure or high estrogen levels, use cortisol itself instead of licorice, which can raise both.

Pregnenolone. This root hormone of your adrenals is used to produce all of your hormones. Supplementing with it can take another burden off your adrenals.

Caution: Do not use pregnenolone if you are taking progesterone in any form, particularly as a cream, without first testing your progesterone levels. Do not use it if you have high levels of progesterone or if you are hyperthyroid. Monitor your symptoms and hormone levels.

THE COMPLETE ADRENAL REPAIR PROTOCOL

SUPPLEMENT	AM	B	MM	L	MA	D	BT*
❏ Pantothenic acid, 100–500 mg	__	1	__	1	__	__	__
❏ GABA (or theanine), 100–500 mg as needed for relaxation	__	__	1	__	1	__	1

Ultimate Support Supplements:

(Consult a professional for exact doses; these potent supplements need monitoring.)

For Stage I adrenal exhaustion/elevated cortisol (after saliva testing for cortisol); do not use in acute anorexia:

❏ Seriphos (1–3 capsuls) 4–5 hours *before* any cortisol spikes. Max 3 per day. Stop one day per month.

❏ Hydrolyzed casein, 250 mg. Add 1-2 capsules at the time of any cortisol spike if Seriphos is not helpful enough.

For stages I, II, and III of adrenal exhaustion:

	AM	B	MM	L	MA	D	BT*
❏ Vitamin B_1 (thiamine), 100 mg†	__	1	__	1	__	1	__

For Stage I, II, or III, if DHEA levels are too low:

	AM	B	MM	L	MA	D	BT*
❏ Females: 5–10 mg DHEA capsules or sublingual drops	__	1 dose	__	__	__	1 dose	__
❏ Males: 10–15 mg DHEA capsules or sublingual drops‡	__	1 dose	__	__	__	1 dose	__

Take DHEA at the end of meals. Start with the lower dosage for 1 week to check your responses.

For Stage II or III; choose one, if cortisol levels are too low:

❏ IsoCort (by Bezwecken) 1–5 pellets, or as recommended, when cortisol is low.

❏ Licorice root capsules or liquid licorice root extract (10–40 mg), at or before your cortisol drops. Stop after three months, maximum.

❏ Cortisol (by prescription), e.g., Cortef. Take as recommended during the time of day when cortisol is low.

❏ 5–20 mg pregnenolone per day, as recommended, at the end of your meals, if testing indicates.

*AM = on arising; B = with breakfast; MM = midmorning; L = with lunch; MA = midafternoon; D = with dinner; BT = at bedtime.

† If you have more than one imbalance that calls for extra vitamin B_1, do not take more than 300 mg per day as an additional single nutrient supplement, in divided doses of 100 milligrams.

‡ The micronized capsule form of DHEA and pregnenolone is much more potent than the non-micronized form, but less potent than the drops.

All are available at dietcure.com or (800) 733-9293.

RETESTING AND ADJUSTING YOUR SUPPLEMENTS

While it can be helpful to supplement as needed with DHEA or pregnenolone in capsules or as tinctures (which contain either glycerin or alcohol), it should be done under a health practitioner's care and *only* after thorough testing. These are powerful hormonal supplements (licorice is powerful, too). If your levels of cortisol, DHEA, estrogen, progesterone, or testosterone get too high because of supplementing with cortisol, licorice, DHEA, or pregnenolone, you could develop serious new problems. If you already unknowingly have too much estrogen, progesterone, or testosterone, you could make a potentially hazardous hormonal imbalance worse.

My advice is to test all of your sex hormone levels before using licorice, DHEA, or pregnenolone. After treatment starts, retest cortisol, DHEA, and any excessively elevated or deficient sex hormones. Retest in sixty to ninety days and again in six months. (See chapters six and fourteen for more on sex hormone testing.)

Your retests will guide you in knowing when to decrease and eliminate your cortisol, licorice, DHEA, or pregnenolone, as well as any sex hormone supplements.

ADDRESSING STRESS LONG-TERM

Now look at your lifestyle and destress it. Anything that will rest and calm you can help restore your adrenals.

+ Cutting out meal skipping and refined carbohydrates, which tax your adrenals, is crucial.
+ Get counseling for emotional stress, if you need to.
+ Don't overexercise.
+ Learn to relax at least twice a day.
+ Breathe deeply.
+ Take baths.
+ Get massages.
+ Learn stretching to help you relax, such as yoga or tai chi.
+ Get at least eight hours of sleep every night. Have a light bedtime snack, if you tend to get hungry then or during the night.
+ Take long, quiet vacations every year.
+ Get away on weekends as much as possible.
+ Do not overwork or push yourself on a regular basis.

See the section on relaxation in chapter twenty-one for more destressing suggestions.

All of these helpful efforts aside, there will more than likely be many times when your stress levels will rise too high again. Life's challenges, including the stressful American diet, are a constant threat to maintaining our physical and emotional balance. But you can learn to keep ahead of it by using your blood sugar and adrenal-repair supplements, foods, and lifestyle changes.

ACTION STEPS

1. If you suspect diabetes or severe hypoglycemia, get your blood sugar and insulin levels tested and consult with a knowledgeable M.D., N.D., or D.O.
2. Take the blood sugar stabilizing and adrenal-repair supplements along with your basic supplements.
3. To keep your blood sugar level stable:
   - Don't skip meals.
   - Avoid sweets and white flour products.
   - Eat at least three solid meals per day. Don't let more than four hours go by without food.
   - Whole-food (low-carb) snacks may be needed in midmorning, midafternoon, and at bedtime.
   - Eat a substantial breakfast (at least 25 percent of the day's food intake).
   - Stay away from refined sweets, starches, alcohol, caffeine, and NutraSweet. (It should be easy because of your supplements.)
4. If you have symptoms of adrenal exhaustion, consult a health care professional and test your adrenal function. Use saliva testing for cortisol and DHEA levels. If you are having hormonal problems or taking any hormones, you should also test the levels of your sex hormones.
5. Reduce, then eliminate your blood sugar and adrenal-repair supplements as you no longer need them.

Readings

Richard K. Bernstein, M.D., *Dr. Bernstein's Diabetes Solution: The Complete Guide to Achieving Normal Blood Sugars*, 4th Edition (Boston: Little, Brown & Co., 2011).

Sarah Brewer, M.D., *Natural Approaches to Diabetes: The Complete Holistic Guide* (London: Piatkus Books, 2010).

Kathleen DesMaisons, Ph.D., *Potatoes Not Prozac: Simple Solutions for Sugar Sensitivity* (New York: Simon & Schuster, 2008).

William McK. Jeffries, M.D., *Safe Uses of Cortisol* (Springfield, IL: Charles C. Thomas Publisher, 2004).

Robert H. Lustig, M.D., editor, *Obesity Before Birth: Maternal and Prenatal Influences on the Offspring* (New York: Springer, 2010). Also search "Sugar: The Bitter Truth" on YouTube for a fascinating explanation of how high-fructose sweets create obesity.

Susan Mitchell, Ph.D., and Catherine Christie, *I'd Kill for a Cookie: A Simple Six-Week Plan to Conquer Stress Eating* (New York: Plume Books, 1998). This is a good guide to the causes and cures of stress eating.

Geraldine Saunders and Dr. Harvey M. Ross, *Hypoglycemia: The Classic Healthcare Handbook* (New York: Kensington, 2002).

William G. Timmins, N.D., *The Chronic Stress Crisis* (Bloomington, IN: Author House, 2011).

James L. Wilson, N.D., D.C., Ph.D., *Adrenal Fatigue: The 21st-Century Stress Syndrome* (Petaluma, CA: Smart Publications, 2001).

Resources

SUPPLEMENTS

All supplements included in this chapter are available through our clinic's order line, (800) 733-9293, and at dietcure.com.

Call Boiron for its homeopathic adrenal cortex of various strengths at (800) 264-7661 or visit boiron.com.

SALIVA TESTING LABS

See Resources at the end of chapter twenty-one, "Essential Support."

TWELVE

Thyroid Solutions

B y now you've read chapter four and have identified your own low thyroid symptoms and which of the two common types of thyroid dysfunction—hypothyroidism or thyroiditis—you might have. In this chapter you'll learn what to do once you've found a helpful physician and the test results confirming your diagnosis have come back. Then you'll be ready to try thyroid-targeted nutrients or the right prescription medication.

FINDING A PHYSICIAN

Find a physician through one of the holistic medical associations (see pages 360–361), and look for one who knows about the work of Broda Barnes. Barnes was an M.D. who spent his entire career studying and treating thyroid dysfunction. This brilliant holistic pioneer strongly promoted a thorough evaluation of both thyroid and adrenal function, and the use of Armour (natural animal, or glandular) thyroid medication.

Keep in mind that whomever you see, you will still have to master the information in this chapter to be sure you get the best care. Recovery Systems is the only clinic in the country that I know of that specializes in the holistic treatment of eating, mood, and addiction problems and the role of thyroid dysfunction in these problems. You can't expect a health care provider seeing a wide range of problems to have the specialized information that you will get from reading this book.

Most good holistic M.D.'s or D.O.'s will have valuable experience and ideas to add to the thyroid solutions I describe in this chapter. (N.D.'s are not typically as helpful in treating thyroid problems as they are in treating the other problems that I discuss in this book.) My advice is to ask your doctor to follow the suggestions here before, or at the same time as, exploring any other treatment options. For example, many physicians are eager to suggest iodine, but for those with Hashimoto's especially, this can be a big mistake, which I'll discuss later. It will also be important to find one who keeps an open mind on the animal versus synthetic medication question. For example, people with Hashimoto's thyroiditis do better on synthetic thyroid meds.

THE ADRENAL LINK

Many of my clients seem to have exhausted adrenals as well as malfunctioning thyroids. If you tend to be tired and overwhelmed in the afternoon, if you tend to be overly alert at night, have dark circles under your eyes, are easily stressed (among the other symptoms listed in chapter three on page 50), your adrenals may be the primary problem.

The adrenals are energizing partners of the thyroid. If the thyroid fails, the adrenals get overworked and run down. The result is the stressed "tired but wired" sensation that we often associate with having too much fight-or-flight adrenaline in our system. If excessive stress has caused the adrenals to go into permanent overdrive, the thyroid will automatically turn down in an effort to calm the system. Furthermore, at this point the adrenals cannot regulate the immune system properly, and immune system problems such as thyroiditis can result. See chapters three and eleven on diagnosing and treating adrenal exhaustion, and get your adrenals tested at the same time that you get your thyroid tests.

What to Request of Your Physician

1. A review of the symptoms and history that you have identified, including at least three underarm temperatures.
2. A manual examination of your thyroid gland.
3. An ankle reflex test.
4. Blood tests for thyroid function (described in detail in chapter four); TSH, free T_4, free T_3, reverse T_3, two thyroid antibody tests, plus basic blood work (a CBC, SMAC panel, and ferritin [sensitive iron] level). You'll need the last three tests to determine if you, like so many people with thyroid problems, have some form of anemia (low iron, or ferritin

under 100, low B_{12}, and/or low folic acid). Also included
are cholesterol levels, which are often elevated in people
with thyroid trouble.
5. For adrenal function, a saliva test and orthostatic blood
pressure readings.

Once you've had your blood drawn, you'll go home and focus
on getting the foods and supplements you'll need for the next two
weeks, until all the lab test results are back and you can return to
your doctor for test results and treatments.

NUTRITIONAL STRATEGIES

EAT PLENTY OF NUTRITIOUS FOOD

Make sure that you start consuming adequate amounts of high-quality
food and using the basic nutritional supplements. (See chapters seventeen and eighteen.) If you have a mild thyroid problem, this nutritional
boost alone may correct it.

To treat both low thyroid and thyroiditis, be sure you eat the following every day:

+ **Vegetables:** At least 4 cups. Do not rely on lettuce alone, because of
  its bulk, but eat a variety of colored veggies. (Cabbage, spinach, ruta-
  baga, broccoli, cauliflower, and turnips can inhibit the thyroid, so be
  sure to eat less of them if you have hypothyroidism.)
+ **Protein:** At least 20 grams (3 to 4 ounces of lean meat, fowl, or fish)
  or more *per meal* (see protein content table on page 270).
+ **Healthy fats:** At least 2 tablespoons per day of good oils in foods
  such as avocado, nuts and seeds, extra virgin olive or coconut oil,
  and butter.
+ **Carbohydrates:** Be moderate in the amounts of fruit, potatoes,
  squash, and beans that you take in each day. Two servings of fruit per
  day plus ½ to 1 cup, one or two times per day, of other carbohydrates
  is usually adequate.
+ **Avoid soy,** if indicated, **and gluten:** As little as 3 to 4 tablespoons of
  soy milk per day can powerfully suppress your thyroid function and
  lower your metabolic rate.[1] Wheat, rye, oats, and barley contain the
  gluten that is known to trigger thyroiditis.

Caution Regarding Pregnancy

If you boost your thyroid function, you are likely to become more fertile, because the thyroid can stimulate reproductive hormonal function quite dramatically. A 52-year-old nurse who had never conceived had a surprise pregnancy when her thyroid was treated. She was elated, but you should be very careful if you want to avoid pregnancy.

WEIGHT AND THYROID RECOVERY

Some of you are undereating because your thyroid is so sluggish that you gain weight on normal or even subnormal amounts of food. You'll find that on the kinds of foods I'm recommending you'll be able to eat more. Sometimes it takes a while to get your thyroid and metabolism going. But then you'll gradually increase your calories and still lose weight. Getting enough protein, the builder of muscle and mind, is particularly important, because low thyroid keeps you from benefiting fully from the protein food you eat, and many of you skimp on protein, anyway. You'll notice the difference right away: you'll feel more energetic and stronger overall.

DRINK PURIFIED WATER

Water is an invaluable nutrient, and you need about eight 8-ounce glasses of it a day. But you may run into problems when you drink tap water, because chlorine (or chloramine), fluoride, bromine, and hydrocarbons, which are found in most water supplies (including hot tubs and swimming pools), can suppress thyroid function. Research and consider purchasing filtration devices that can eliminate some or all of these contaminants. Filtration systems can be installed for your whole house or just under the kitchen sink. Pitchers and faucet attachments are also available. All filtration devices have limitations. Reverse osmosis may be the most effective.

The purity of bottled water is hard to judge. Plastic bottles emit biochemicals into the water (fake estrogens are of particular concern, as they can create hormonal imbalances that are linked to breast cancer). Although expensive, spring water in glass bottles may be best, its purity, too, must be verified. Well water should be carefully analyzed for high nitrate levels due to agriculture, hydrocarbons leaking from gas stations in the area, and high levels of such natural toxins as arsenic.

AVOID STIMULANT DRUGS

You may have been using drugs for energy, especially caffeine. Work with the Amino Acid Therapy Chart in chapter nine if you need to kill your cravings for these substances. If you are too tired without stimulants even after using L-tyrosine, you may have to wait until you get on some thyroid medication before your energy will rise enough to allow you to be comfortable off of them.

WHEN THE TEST RESULTS COME BACK

Once you've been eating well and taking your basic nutritional supplements for two weeks, you should get your test results back. Talk to your doctor about what to do next if you are unsatisfied with the results you've been getting from the dietary changes and basic supplements. Although more than 90 percent of our clients stop any overeating or food craving and begin to feel better by this point, many need to add medication to their programs once their test results are in.

SIMPLE LOW THYROID (HYPOTHYROIDISM)

Your symptoms, basal temperatures, ankle reflex, and a thorough panel of blood tests should tell you if you have simple low thyroid function (hypothyroidism). Three quarters of my clients who suffer from low thyroid function have classic hypothyroidism—their temperatures and their energy are low but their weight is usually high.

Elizabeth suffered from mild hypothyroidism. She was an athletic 32-year-old strawberry blonde in recovery from a past eating disorder that had taken its toll on her body, as had many years of overwork and a stressful marriage and divorce. Elizabeth came to Recovery Systems after her energy had dropped and she had begun to gain unneeded weight. She was blood-tested by our M.D., who found that her thyroid scores were below normal. He offered her a prescription for thyroid medication, but advised her to talk to one of our clinic's nutritionists first. At the nutritionist's suggestion, Elizabeth increased the amount of protein and vegetables she was eating and began taking the amino acid L-tyrosine and a thyroid-boosting supplement containing kelp, animal thyroid gland, and herbs; she also took the six basic supplements we recommend.

She immediately regained her energy and vitality. In fact, she had to cut down on her dose of L-tyrosine and the thyroid booster in just a few weeks, because they soon made her overly energized. We have since learned that over-the-counter thyroid boosters sometimes contain active hormones, although this is illegal.

THYROIDITIS: WHEN YOUR IMMUNE SYSTEM IS ATTACKING YOU

If you suffer from the second, more complex thyroid affliction, Hashimoto's autoimmune thyroiditis (HAIT, or Hashimoto's), in which your thyroid is attacked by your immune system, your thyroid antibody test results will usually show it. A needle biopsy can be done for a definitive answer if you and your doctor are unsure.

If you have HAIT, first you'll need to do everything you can to calm down your hyperactive immune system. It will help to eliminate from your diet any foods that you are allergic to (see chapters five and thirteen), because continual allergic reactions provoke your immune system into hyper attack mode. *Wheat and other gluten-containing grains are specifically known to cause thyroiditis.* You will also need special supplements or medicine.

A THYROIDITIS STORY

The story of Dina's thyroiditis is a typical one. When I first met Dina, she was 34 years old, thin, and pale, with huge black circles under her eyes. She was very knowledgeable about nutrition and had been able to recover on her own from both anorexia and bulimia, which were an integral part of her life as a ballet dancer. She was working part-time and going to graduate school, but her energy was poor, she slept very badly, and she was stressed and hypersensitive. "I'm just one raw nerve," she told me.

Dina's problems started at age 14, about the time her periods began. She had recently been given a TSH test and scored in the high-normal range, but she was declared to have no thyroid problem and told that no further investigation was needed. Twelve months later, Dina began having seizures and waking up in the night feeling suffocated, which terrified her. That was when she called us, and we sent her to an M.D. with a comprehensive list of thyroid tests to request. The results were astonishing. Her thyroid antibodies, which should have been under 10, were over

20,000! Her blood test scores for anemia were off the scale as well. She was diagnosed with severe autoimmune thyroiditis. In fact, she had had it for twenty years, ever since she had stopped being alert and calm and became tired and wired at age 14. Touching her neck, her doctor could feel a lump of scar tissue on her thyroid (no prior doctor had ever examined her).

Dina began her thyroiditis treatment with a strong dose of Synthroid, which made her symptoms worse. Next she was put on animal thyroid and, though she lost her appetite, she began to gain three pounds a week. Because of these adverse symptoms she was switched to very small amounts of Synthroid and Cytomel. She immediately dropped back to her original weight. Her dosages were gradually increased in tiny increments. In addition to these two medications, Dina took vitamin B_{12} shots and iron for her anemia, a rich multimineral and multivitamin for other thyroid-support needs, omega-3 fish oil as an anti-inflammatory, vitamin C with bioflavonoids, and vitamin E. She was assisted by a gifted Chinese acupuncturist, who gave her regular treatments with needles and herbs for her weak adrenals and insisted that she cut back on her heavy exercise for a while. All this brought her thyroid-antibody score from 20,000 to 1,700 in six months. In one year it was down to 298. More important, she began glowing with health and vitality and was able to return to regular exercise. She gained five pounds of muscle, but her dress size stayed the same.

Curing her thyroiditis had another unexpected effect. Dina had been an A student until her thyroiditis hit at age 14. On her thyroid-repair plan, she regained her concentration and proudly revealed to me that one of her graduate school professors had told her that her recent paper was the best he had ever read.

Thyroiditis is a very serious condition that can eventually destroy the thyroid gland and adversely affect every cell in the body. Dina had to continue working closely with her M.D. on her medication dose, but her office visits became much less frequent after the first year. Unfortunately, by the time her thyroiditis was diagnosed, her confused immune system had destroyed her thyroid gland entirely, so she will need to stay on medication for life.

SUPPLEMENTS FOR THYROID PROBLEMS

Because you've had an impaired thyroid, you haven't been able to absorb nutrients from your food very efficiently. Whether you suffer from hypothyroidism or thyroiditis, the extra nutrients found in the supplement plan (laid out in chapter seventeen) will help you now, and they will help you even more later as your improved thyroid function increases your absorption over the next few months.

Cautionary note: Wait until your test results are back before trying tyrosine or iodine. You may have thyroiditis, which calls for calming the thyroid, not boosting it. If taking these boosters makes you agitated, stop them.

To boost low thyroid function, try the following. (Note that some thyroid-boosting mixtures contain these boosters and may include herbs as well, or you can buy the boosters separately.)

✦ **L-tyrosine.** This amino is the primary food that the thyroid uses to make all of its hormones. L-tyrosine is probably the body's most energizing food, because it's the source of not only the thyroid hormones but the body's natural stimulants adrenaline, testosterone, norepinephrine, and dopamine—collectively known as the catecholamines. Low thyroid can drive many people to a dependence on stimulating drugs such as caffeine and cocaine as their own natural energizers run down. Many of you have come to need coffee all day long to keep going, or sweets to give you a lift, or in some cases drugs such as Dexatrim or ephedra, or even cocaine, to really get you moving. Tyrosine is the nutrient that relieves you of your need for these fake energizers. It can often jump-start the thyroid.

If your problem is just a mildly underactive thyroid, you'll feel the effects of tyrosine right away. Taking 500 to 2,000 milligrams before breakfast will usually eliminate your coffee cravings right away, too. Usually two to four 500-milligram capsules in early morning and midmorning (separate from meals) is enough to get you reenergized. You can take the same amount of tyrosine in midafternoon, if it doesn't keep you awake.

	AM	B	MM	L	MA	D	BT*
❏ L-tyrosine, 500–1,500 mg, 1–3 times/day	1–3	__	1–3	__	1–3	__	__
❏ glandulars or homeopathics	__	__	__	__	__	__	__

*AM = on arising; B = breakfast; MM = midmorning; L= lunch;
MA = midafternoon; D = dinner; BT = bedtime.

✦ **Thyroid glandulars.** These low-potency supplements are made from the thyroid glands of animals. Unfortunately, by law, their active hormones have been removed, though they still do help some people, if taken in the morning before breakfast and midmorning, and along with L-tyrosine (which is often included).

✦ **Homeopathic thyroid.** A microscopic yet potent glandular; ask health food stores or homeopathic practitioners about these remedies. They have benefited some of our clients.

✦ **Iodine.** You'll get some in your basic multivitamin, and you are already getting some iodine in salted foods (even salt without iodine added may contain some iodine). Don't add more unless you've tried and failed using the other methods I describe here. Iodine can trigger problems such as prolonged palpitations and insomnia, especially in those with Hashimoto's thyroiditis.

THYROID MEDICINE

At Recovery Systems, we have seen several thousand people successfully use many different kinds and doses of medication for both kinds of thyroid problems. For both hypothyroidism and thyroiditis, many physicians exclusively prescribe Synthroid, or another brand of bioidentical T_4, like Levoxyl or levothyroxine. This sometimes works well, but we have seen many cases in which they were not beneficial. In these cases, other forms or combinations of thyroid medication have been much more effective.

Most holistic doctors much prefer to start with the original and most natural thyroid medication: glandulars containing active animal thyroid hormones. Pigs are the animals with the most humanlike thyroid glands. One difference: the ratio of the key thyroid hormones, T_3 to T_4, in pigs (4:1) is not the same as it is in humans (10:1). That may be one reason that animal thyroid does not work well for everyone. This porcine thyroid comes in several forms: Armour, Westhroid, and Nature-Throid (fewer additives), and particularly pure compounded varieties. When you start on thyroid medication, be patient. Finding the right medicine and the right dose takes time and care. It can be difficult to determine how long each experimental course of medication should go on before the next higher dose or different medication should be tried. Some people feel benefits within days of their first dose. Others take weeks or even months to find the right dose or combination. This process is well worth the time. Be patient but persistent. Perhaps your doctor will be willing to give you a schedule to follow on your own for increasing your doses at certain intervals, if your initial lower doses aren't strong enough. Or he or she may want to retest first before increasing.

Do you have trouble swallowing pills, especially tablets or large capsules?

This is not unusual for people with a thyroid problem, because the throat can become congested and the thyroid gland can actually swell and hamper your swallowing capacity. Look for liquid, powder, or sublingual forms of the supplements you'll need. If necessary, you can blend them in a smoothie; you won't notice them. Or you can stir them into a little applesauce and/or mashed banana for between-meal doses. They'll be easier to swallow as soon as your throat congestion clears.

CHOOSING AND EXPERIMENTING WITH MEDICATION

Here are the thyroid medication choices:

✦ Glandular (porcine) sources of the primary thyroid hormones T_3 and T_4 are made from pigs' thyroid glands. Brands include Armour, Nature-Throid, and Westhroid. The latter two contain fewer additives. Compounding pharmacies' customized formulations can be even purer. (Compounders create medicines tailored to specific patient needs by doctors' orders.)

✦ Synthetic T_4; for example, Levothroid, Levoxyl, and Synthroid. There can be some surprising differences in the way you react to different types of T_4. Try them all if necessary.

✦ Synthetic T_3 (such as Cytomel), the most active, potent form of thyroid medication, is preferable when RT_3 is high..

✦ Synthetic combinations of T_3 and T_4, which provide the same 4:1 ratio of T_4:T_3 as the animal sources; for example, Thyrolar.

✦ Avoid any T_4 when RT_3 is high (even in glandulars).

The animal-derived thyroid medications contain not only T_3 and T_4 but also T_1 and T_2. T_2 may be needed to prevent dry skin and problems with fibrous breast and uterine cysts. Our female clients seem to divide evenly into those who do well with bioidentical synthetic hormones and those who do well on the more complex bioidentical glandular sources. I have observed that male clients seem to do better on the glandular medications.

Working with your physician, choose a type of medication and a starting dosage, then monitor your reactions closely. If there is no response, your doctor can raise the dose gradually. If there is still no improvement at the highest safe dosage (i.e., when you begin to experience adverse reations), your doctor will need to try another kind of medication and see how you fare on that.

The standard medical procedure is to start with synthetic T_4. If T_4 medications alone don't help much, more potent T_3 medications such as Cytomel may be added. You may not have to be on thyroid medication for life. Consult with your physician after the first year to see about going off it, but most of our clients have not been able to do without it.

TREATMENT FOR THYROIDITIS

Everyone I have worked with who has had elevated thyroid antibodies on their test results has needed medication in addition to improved nutrition and, often, acupuncture. The most successful pharmacological protocol for thyroiditis that we have seen includes a combination of synthetic T_4, typically with T_3 (usually Cytomel). These synthetics are simpler and less likely to cause an allergic reation than those dirived from animals. Doses start very low and fluctuate based on test results. You may need to work closely with your doctor on adjusting your doses over an extended period of time.

Nathan Becker, M.D., a well-known San Francisco endocrinologist, found, after many years of treating thyroiditis with carefully monitored doses of T_4 alone, that adding small doses of Cytomel, if needed, improved his results. We have worked with several of his patients and can verify the success of this approach. He also says that 30 percent of his patients can eventually go off of their medications because the treatment causes the immune system to stop attacking the thyroid gland, allowing the gland to function more normally, especially if gluten has triggered the problem and the patient is now strictly avoiding it. (See chapter five.)

We have seen a few women diagnosed with thyroiditis who were put on glandular thyroid medication gain weight until they switched to synthetic T_4 (with or without Cytomel or other bioidentical synthetic T_3). But our former consultant Richard Shames, M.D. (author of *Thyroid Power*), says that he has occasionally seen women with thyroiditis who do *better* on animal thyroid. It's an individual matter, so keep trying until you find the right solution for you.

Avoid iodine: serious adverse reations to supplemental iodine (even to kelp tablets) are very common among Hashimoto's sufferers. One of our clients took iodine for one week and had insomnia and palpitations for two years.

Low Thyroid Function and Anemia

Low body temperature can mean low hemoglobin. If your test results show you have anemia, you'll need B_{12}, B_1, iron, and/or folic acid. Weekly B_{12} shots taken over the course of several months can quickly help improve your energy and mood if you also have pernicious B_{12} anemia, which occurs when you don't have adequate B_{12} and is common among people with thyroiditis. Thyroiditis blocks our digestion of B_{12}. B_1 anemia also responds to extra B_1. Minerals are also crucial for thyroid function in general, and especially crucial for thyroiditis, so be sure you're taking a good multivitamin/multimineral. Finding extra-absorbable iron can be difficult. Try Slow Fe (available over the counter in drug stores) or Niferex (available only by prescription). Eat liver!

ADVERSE EFFECTS OF THYROID MEDICINE AND IODINE AND OTHER CONCERNS

You will probably be told in advance by your physician to reduce or stop your thyroid medication if any adverse symptoms show up and to come in for an appointment right away to change your dosage or type. We rarely see any serious adverse symptoms, only the mild, though marked, changes listed below.

Common Adverse Symptoms of Thyroid Medication

✦ A wired, agitated, hyper feeling
✦ Heart palpitations (If you have this symptom, check your adrenals, too.)
✦ Sleep disturbances
✦ Feeling overheated
✦ Diarrhea

LONG-TERM EFFECTS OF THYROID MEDICATION

Are you afraid that thyroid medication will cause your gland to atrophy and never function on its own again? I have been reassured by many thyroid specialists that this does not happen, and I have personally watched many people go off of thyroid medication after a year or longer on it. Most of them return to the level of function that they had prior to going on the medication. Some have had better function on their own after a period on thyroid medication. None of them had worse function, but they *have* often been very tired for a week or two after getting off their medications.

If your gland has been destroyed by thyroiditis or radiation, or for other reasons just cannot function on its own, you will need to take medication for life. Dr. Broda Barnes discovered this from patients who had been forced, by cancer or overactive thyroids, to have their thyroid glands removed surgically. He reports in *Hyporthyroidism* that they all died young of heart disease unless they were put on thyroid medication. Dr. Barnes learned that the right amount of thyroid medication was extraordinarily heart protective, but that (particularly in older people) a heart weakened by years of hypothyroidism must have the medication slowly introduced, as palpitations can result if too large a dose is used at the start.

Without adequate minerals as supplements, too much thyroid medication over a long period of time might demineralize your bones. (Discuss monitoring your bone density with your doctor.) Yet taking the minerals calcium and iron within an hour or two of taking thyroid meds can interfere with their absorption. Try nighttime mineral dosing, since you won't need to wait to eat or take mineral supplements, and some research shows them to be more effective taken at night, especially if you already have some bone loss.

WHAT IF I HAVE ALREADY BEEN TREATED FOR A THYROID PROBLEM, BUT I DIDN'T GET BETTER?

Many women come to our clinic saying, "Oh, yes, I thought it was my thyroid, but I'm on medication [usually Synthroid], and I'm still tired. I guess my weight problem must be caused by something else."

Usually the real problem is the medication. Of course, it helps a lot to eat plenty of high-quality thyroid-activating vegetables and protein, and take supplements such as L-tyrosine. An evaluation of adrenal function sometimes reveals a crucial deficiency that, when treated, improves some of the symptoms too. But what may really be needed is a better dosage, type, or combination of medication.

Many doctors who don't look carefully at symptoms use a standard dose of Synthroid. Then they test to see that the score on a single test indicator (usually TSH) has gone down, and if so, quit attending to their patients' complaints. Then they resort to the same old "just get on a diet" advice.

More attentive, holistic physicians retest more indicators (free T_3 and T_4, and antibodies if thyroiditis has been diagnosed). They also test in the morning, before thyroid meds have been taken. If the test scores improve, they want to know by how much. Being on thyroid medication should cause test results to show strongly normal results (not low or even midrange results). They are also likely to be convinced by patients' continuing symptoms that, test scores aside, the thyroid may still not be functioning properly. This often prompts them to suggest a trial of a different dose or type of medicine, or a trial of iodine (if Hashimoto's is *not* the problem).

THYROID MEDICINES AND ALLERGIES

Are you allergic to corn or milk? Armour (animal) thyroid contains corn, and Synthroid contains milk sugar and acacia (from a tree that many people are allergic to). Check with your doctor, because thyroid medicines for food-sensitive people can be specially prepared through compounding pharmacies, which prepare medicines to the specific order of an M.D. or D.O. Compounders can also eliminate chemical coloring, binders, and additives. All major metropolitan areas have compounding pharmacies. (For more on these pharmacies, see Resources at the end of chapter twenty-one.)

Be sure to address any other imbalances right away, especially *candida* and gluten allergies. Both of these imbalances can block your recovery from low thyroid and thyroiditis, as can mercury overload (if you have been eating fish such as tuna or swordfish regularly, or have many metal fillings).

ACTION STEPS

I. Thoroughly review your symptoms, your own history, and your family members' history, as per chapter four. Check your morning underarm temperature at least three times to see if it is under 97.8 degrees.

2. Choose a health care professional to work with. A holistic M.D. or D.O. who specializes in thyroid and other endocrine problems would be ideal. See chapter twenty-one for more suggestions on finding a physician. Request a review of your symptoms and history and complete testing as described in this chapter and in chapter four.

3. Avoid thyroid-suppressing drugs and chemicals. If weight gain started with an SSRI, use *The Mood Cure* to find alternatives.

4. Basic nutritional support:
   - Water: Daily, drink eight or more 8-ounce glasses of filtered water.
   - Food: Follow the guidelines in this chapter and in chapter twenty for increasing your intake of vegetables, protein, whole carbs, and healthy fats. Remove gluten and soy with Hashimoto's.
   - Supplements: Take the basic supplements outlined in chapter seventeen and the extra supplements as per the charts in this chapter.

5. When your test results come back and you know whether you have hypothyroidism or thyroiditis, follow the directions in this chapter for using nutrients, medicine, and diet.

6. If you are going to take medication, work with your physician until you have the right medication at the right dose. Continue paying attention to your symptoms and taking your basal temperature.

7. Try tapering off your medication in a year or two in consultation with your physician.

8. Keep a food-medication-mood log to monitor your progress (see chapter twenty-two).

Readings

Barry Durrant-Peatfield, M.B., B.S., LRCP, MRCS, *Your Thyroid and How to Keep It Healthy* (London: Hammersmith Press, 2006).

Richard Shames, M.D., and Karilee Halo Shames, Ph.D., R.N., *Thyroid Power: Ten Steps to Total Health* (New York: William Morrow, 2002).

Richard Shames, M.D., and Karilee Halo Shames, Ph.D., R.N., with Georjana Grace Shames, L.Ac., *Thyroid Mind Power: The Proven Cure for Hormone-Related Depression, Anxiety, and Memory Loss* (New York: Rodale Books, 2011).

Mark Starr, M.D., *Hypothyrodism, Type 2: The Epidemic* (Irvine, CA: New Voice Publications, 2011).

Lawrence C. Wood, M.D., David S. Cooper, M.D., and E. Chester Ridgway, M.D., *Your Thyroid: A Home Reference*, 4th edition (New York: Ballantine Books, 2005). Good but basic.

Resources

See chapter twenty-one for information on physician referrals.

Homeopathic thyroid: Boiron and Hylands have thyroid formulations found in health food stores, or contact a homeopathic pharmacy; for example, call (888) 427-6422 or visit homeopathy2health.com.

THIRTEEN

Overcoming Addictions to Allergy Foods

By now you realize that while you love your favorite foods, they may be creating unacceptable problems such as asthma, migraines, low energy, or constipation—not to mention unneeded weight gain. In this chapter you'll learn how you can test for these allergies—at home, in the lab, or in the doctor's office. More important, you'll eliminate your interest in them using anti-craving supplements to make the transition to your new eating habits deprivation-free.

When you learn what allergies you have, don't despair about never being able to eat normally again. Along with lists of foods to avoid, I'll provide lists of foods you can eat that you probably never thought of, foods you might end up enjoying a lot.

TESTING FOR ALLERGIES

HOME TESTING

The easiest, fastest, and cheapest way to test for allergies to wheat, rye, oats, barley, and/or cow's milk products is to do a home test. Dr. John E. Postley, a Columbia University professor, made it clear in *The Allergy Discovery Diet* that the home test is also the most accurate way of all to identify food allergies. Here are important cautions for home testing:

◆ Keep a detailed food-mood log to monitor the testing process (see chapter twenty-two).

◆ Reintroduce only one food or food group at a time.

◆ Wait two full days between tests of different foods. For example, if it turns out you are allergic to wheat, wait two days before you try rye. The reason for this is that sometimes you can get delayed allergic symptoms hours or days after your test. If that delayed reaction hits on the day that you try the next food, you won't know which food is the problem. Some people have problems only with wheat, not with all gluten-containing grains. If wheat is not a problem, the other three gluten-containing grains—rye, oats, and barley—are not likely to be troublemakers either, and you probably don't need to test them.

◆ Do not dismiss any adverse reactions, as you may be tempted to do.

◆ Women should test after their period and before PMS.

Here's how to do the test:

Days 1 to 7: Making the Break. Do not consume any of the foods that you have decided to test (either cow's milk products or the gluten-containing grains). Review the material in chapter five to remind yourself of hidden sources of these allergens so that you don't accidentally consume them. The supplements recommended at the end of this chapter will make sure your detox is short and mild, so don't dread this testing period. It won't be like any of the diets that you've endured. You won't miss the foods you eliminate, and by Day 5 (if not before) you should be feeling better than you have in a long time. You may notice quick weight loss in this first week.

Day 8: The Challenge. On the eighth day, notice whether any of your bothersome symptoms have gone away. Then eat a regular serving of one test food for breakfast and again at lunch. For example, if you're testing for a milk allergy, have some milk at breakfast and a glass of milk with lunch. Make a note of how you feel. Also note your oral temperature, any food cravings, your mood, energy, digestion, respiratory symptoms, bowel function, appetite, skin changes, headaches, sleep patterns, and any and all information that your body imparts. You may have a very strong reaction, such as a migraine if you're prone to them. If you get only a little tired, bloated, or headachy after your challenge meals, don't ignore it. If you gain weight or start craving foods again, don't be surprised. It's not a coincidence.

When testing the gluten-containing grains, test first with wheat (bread, pasta, or another very plain form of wheat), because it is the grain highest in gluten and will therefore give you the clearest results. Do not eat any more of the food or food group for the next two days (after waiting two days, you can test another gluten-containing grain). Allergic reactions to milk products and gluten-containing foods can be very similar, so you'll get a clearer response to your testing if you eliminate both, then reintroduce them one at a time to see which one is the problem, or whether they are both problems. If it feels too overwhelming to let go of milk products and the gluten-containing grains all at once, start with testing and removing the grains first.

Do not eat any more of your confirmed allergy foods as you go on to test others. It can help to test your foods while you are with someone who can help you notice your reactions. I've noticed many wives turn out to be the best observers of their husbands' changing symptoms.

If you have no leftover adverse symptoms from your first challenge, you can test another food. If you determine, after reintroducing grain and milk, that you need to avoid one or both of them permanently, you can expect to feel better for as long as you stay away from them. If you suddenly feel bloated or tired or achy again, you'll know that you've inadvertently consumed your allergen. Or perhaps you'll eat a little of one because of convenience or pressure when there's nothing else available on the menu or everyone's indulging in a traditional holiday treat—and you'll experience some of your old symptoms for a while. But they'll fade, and you can use two tablets of Alka-Seltzer Gold to get rid of them quickly.

Trust your body's messages. They will tell you what works and what doesn't.

OTHER WAYS OF TESTING FOR FOOD INTOLERANCES

At Recovery Systems, we do other types of testing when allergy symptoms persist even after the big-three allergens have been eliminated and challenged. What follows are the methods we've found to have value, though none is perfect.

Although allergy testing methods have improved over the years, it is typical to get some inaccurate information along with the accurate. Allergy to gluten-containing grains seems to be the hardest to identify, partly because some of the defending antibodies (SIgA) measured are so often destroyed by the adverse impact of gluten and casein on the tissues that create the antibodies.

TESTING OPTIONS

Antibody Testing. Blood tests for IgG (delayed-reaction antibodies) vary in effectiveness. The anti-gliadin (i.e., gluten) test is inconsistent, even at labs which identify other food allergens well. Adding a test for transglutaminase sometimes helps. A stool test (e.g., from EnteroLab) for gluten (and milk) may be more sensitive, is easier for children, and may be ordered online.

Immunolabs. This blood test measures IgG antibodies unusually well and has been used successfully by our, and many other, clinics for years.

Simple Pulse Test. Monitor your pulse to see if it increases or decreases by 12 to 20 beats right after eating a particular food.

Applied Kineseology (NAET or BioSET). This procedure determines if your muscle strength declines when you are exposed to certain foods. (Treatments based on this testing can help eliminate some allergic reactions while retaining the actual foods in your diet. It can be a long process, but we've seen some miraculous results.)

Small Intestine Biopsy. We used to think that this was the most accurate way to diagnose celiac disease (the most extreme version of gluten intolerance). It involves sedation and swallowing a tiny tube, which extracts a small sample of the intestinal wall. The sample is removed for viewing under a microscope. Unfortunately, the sample may be taken from a nearby, undamaged area and result in misdiagnosis.

AVOIDING ALLERGY-ADDICTORS

IF YOU NEED TO AVOID GLUTEN OR WHEAT

Becoming wheat- or gluten-free can alleviate your low energy, depression, agitation, digestive disturbances, cravings, and more very quickly. You will not continue to feel deprived, even though you need to avoid many (mostly nutritionally negligible) foods, because there are so many delicious foods you *can* eat. Also, there are easy substitute foods that you'll love. I enjoy eating very much and always have, yet I haven't had gluten-containing food for more than ten years.

Common Gluten-Containing Foods to Avoid

Additives	MSG (monosodium glutamate), HVP (hydrolyzed vegetable protein), TVP (textured vegetable protein)
Bread	yeast, quick bread, muffins, scones, corn bread, buns, white or wheat bread, pancakes, bagels, biscuits, pizza, croissants, crackers, pretzels
Grains	wheat, rye, barley, oats, spelt, kamut, teff
Meat, poultry, fish	breading or batter on fried fish, fried chicken, corn dogs; anything floured before frying (to brown); dishes prepared "en croute" or "stuffed"
Pasta and others	macaroni, noodles, spaghetti, orzo, couscous, bulgur wheat, seitan (used as a protein source; it is 100 percent gluten)
Pastries	cookies, biscotti, cake, pie, crumb toppings, cobbler, doughnuts, brownies
Possible problem foods	quinoa and amaranth (There is some debate on whether or not these are gluten-containing grains. Our clients have not had problems with them.)
Sauces	Mornay, cheese sauce, béchamel, white sauce, gravy, some soy sauces
Soups	barley and wheat varieties of miso soup, cream soups, bouillon, soups with bread in them (such as French onion), soups with pasta (minestrone, chicken noodle, and others)

Hidden Sources of Gluten

You probably wouldn't think to avoid these foods, but all *can* contain gluten.

+ French fries (often dusted with flour before freezing)
+ Croutons on salad

+ Chinese crispy noodles (except rice noodles)
+ Processed cheese (like Velveeta)
+ Dumplings
+ Most soy sauce
+ Mayonnaise
+ Ketchup
+ Some salad dressings
+ Distilled vinegar (If the label just reads "vinegar," it is probably grain vinegar. Stick to wine vinegar, apple cider vinegar, or balsamic vinegar.)
+ Caramel color
+ Modified food starch
+ Malt or malt flavoring
+ Sulfites
+ Foods made in the same fryer as breaded foods
+ White and whole wheat flour tortillas

Read labels! The label for bakery products or mixes must read "gluten-free," not just "wheat-free," unless wheat is the only grain that causes problems for you. Don't get overwhelmed; just eat simply. Make sure that you do not consume allergens hidden in a recipe or disguised as something else. Ask whether there is wheat or white flour in any restaurant food. "Wheat" is often used to designate "whole wheat" as opposed to "white" flour, but white flour is made from wheat that has had its brown parts removed; therefore, it contains gluten.

What to Eat Instead of Food Containing Gluten If you're gluten intolerant, you must avoid gluten permanently. Benefits will begin almost immediately, but it will take months for your intestinal lining to completely heal. Any exposure can restart the damage. Stick to the safe grains, such as corn, rice, buckwheat, millet, quinoa, and amaranth.

Many ethnic cooking styles are corn- and rice-based. Suppose you lived in South America, where corn and beans are staples in wonderfully tasty dishes. Or you lived in Asia, with the rice, vegetables, fish, coconut milk, and other foods used in all those richly varied cooking styles. It's easy to avoid gluten in those parts of the world, and it can be easier here than you might think. There is a cornucopia of hearty, luscious eating possibilities. For carbohydrates, instead of the gluten-containing grains formerly in your diet, use potatoes, yams, squash, taro, and all kinds of root vegetables. There are even creative recipes and ready-made mixes for pancakes, muffins, and yeast bread that are delicious. A bread machine can be used to make tasty gluten-free breads, like the one you'll find in chapter twenty, "Menus, Meal Ideas, and Recipes."

Safe Gluten-Free Foods

Additions	nuts, seeds, beans, or dried vegetables sprinkled on salads, soups, and other dishes
Bread	made from rice, bean, and potato flours; corn tortillas; all-rice crackers
Grains	corn, cornmeal mush, grits, brown rice, basmati rice, wild rice, creamy rice hot cereal
Grains tolerated by many gluten intolerants	millet, quinoa, amaranth, buckwheat
Meat, poultry, fish	sautéed, roasted, stewed, or braised (if not floured first); broiled, steamed
Pasta and others	made from rice, corn, and quinoa flours; polenta
Sauces	béarnaise, hollandaise, and others, *if* they are thickened with cornstarch, arrowroot, or gluten-free flour, like rice, potato, or garbanzo
Soups	split pea and potato, if no other thickeners are added; clear-broth soups: chicken rice, vegetable beef, and others
Sweets	fruit
Vinegar	apple cider, balsamic, and wine vinegars

See chapters eighteen, nineteen, and twenty for even more suggestions of fresh, delicious, nutritious foods you can enjoy.

Gluten Intolerance and Anorexia or Bulimia

Please do not remove gluten (or any other possible allergen) from your diet, even for a week, unless you can keep a commitment to replace the nutrients and the calories you'll be losing with gluten-free foods. The bloat and constipation so often caused by these grains may have played a role in your starting to "feel too fat" and to diet despite probably being at normal weight. Removing gluten may help in your recovery, but *only* if you are able to continue eating and keeping down at least as much as you are now. *Please don't use allergen elimination as a new opportunity to undereat.*

AVOIDING SUGAR

Sugar can be extracted from many foods—corn, barley, sugar beets, sugarcane—and is called by many names. Here's a list of words from the Diabetes Friends Action Network (DFAN) that will let you know that a food contains sugar.

Common Sugar Forms

WORDS ENDING IN -OSE:

 ✦ Dextrose
 ✦ Fructose
 ✦ Galactose
 ✦ Glucose
 ✦ Lactose
 ✦ Levulose
 ✦ Maltose
 ✦ Sucrose

WORDS ENDING IN -OL:

 ✦ Mannitol
 ✦ Sorbitol
 ✦ Xylitol

OTHER SUGARS

 ✦ Beet sugar
 ✦ Brown sugar
 ✦ Cane sugar
 ✦ Confectioners' sugar
 ✦ Corn sugar
 ✦ Corn sweetener
 ✦ Granulated sugar
 ✦ High fructose corn syrup
 ✦ Honey
 ✦ Invert sugar
 ✦ Isomalt
 ✦ Maltodextrin
 ✦ Maple sugar
 ✦ Maple syrup
 ✦ Molasses
 ✦ Raw sugar

+ Sorghum
+ Turbinado sugar

FOODS TO AVOID IF YOU ARE INTOLERANT TO COW'S MILK

What to avoid here depends on whether you react badly to lactose or to other contents of these foods, like the protein casein.

+ Butter and artificial butter flavor
+ Buttermilk
+ Casein and caseinates (sodium, potassium, magnesium, calcium, or ammonium)
+ Cheese
+ Cottage cheese
+ Curds
+ Galactose (a lactose by-product); this one's a problem for relatively few people, but be aware of the potential
+ Hydrolysates (casein, milk protein, whey, whey protein)
+ Lactose (often sodium stearoyl lactylate), lactalbumin, lactoglobulin, and other ingredients that begin with *lact-*
+ Milk
+ Milk solids (curds)
+ "Natural ingredients" (Sometimes this refers to dairy products or by-products. Call the manufacturer—an 800 number is usually listed on the packaging—for further information.)
+ Sour cream, sour cream solids, sour milk solids, whey yogurt

Common Foods That May Contain Milk Products

+ Bread
+ Canned tuna (Watch for "hydrolyzed caseinate." You'll have better luck with tuna packed in water.)
+ HVP (hydrolyzed vegetable protein; may use casein in processing)
+ Kosher pareve desserts (may contain casein from nonanimal sources)
+ Margarine
+ Medicines and vitamins (It's common to put lactose in coatings and binders; this is especially true of homeopathic medicines.

Be sure to alert your physician and pharmacist about your allergy.)

✦ "Nondairy" products of all kinds ("Nondairy" is not the same as "milk-free." It can contain as much casein as whole milk and still meet the dairy industry's definition.)

What to Eat Instead of Cow's Milk Products For some, but not all, goat's and sheep's milk products are good substitutes. (Use the elimination-and-challenge test to find out.) They are delicious and more easily digested than cow's milk products. Goat's or sheep's milk feta, a pungent, crumbly white cheese, is available almost everywhere. (Feta can also be made from cow's milk. Read the label carefully.) Goat's milk is available in supermarkets as well as health food stores, and it comes fresh, canned, and powdered. Goat's and sheep's milk yogurt (both fresh and powdered) are available at most health food stores, as are many kinds of cheese—feta, chèvre, Parmesan, ricotta, cheddar, and Monterey Jack. Cheese made from goat's or sheep's milk is made and prized in many parts of the world.

Butter, which is low in lactose, can be tolerated by some people. Ghee (clarified butter) contains no lactose or milk protein at all. Coconut oil can be used in most recipes in which you would use butter. (Look for organic versions, which do not contain antibiotics or pesticides.)

For a milk substitute, use coconut milk rather than soy milk, which is hard to digest, usually sweetened, and, like most soy products, now suspected of causing health problems. Or make your own delicious milks out of nuts or seeds that have soaked in water overnight. The next day, rinse them and blend them with a little water until you make a cream. Dilute it with more water if you like—yummy, and very nutritious. (See the recipe for Seed or Nut Milk on page 327.)

You can substitute any liquid, including water, in recipes that call for milk. These substitutions can be delicious. For example, in sauce recipes, meat or poultry broth or vegetable juice can substitute for milk, giving the dish a distinctive flavor.

Instead of	Use
1 cup milk	1 cup water
1 cup milk (for baking)	1 cup water + 2 tablespoons coconut milk
Light cream	Thick seed or nut milk (see page 327)
Heavy cream	Meringue (egg whites beaten until stiff) or coconut milk, refrigerated to thicken
Sour cream	Goat yogurt (if you can tolerate it)

Instead of	Use
Cream cheese	Creamy goat cheese (if you can tolerate it)
Condensed milk	Powdered goat milk plus water (Add a little water at a time until the mixture is the same thickness as condensed milk.)

SUPPLEMENTING FOR RECOVERY FROM ALLERGY-ADDICTION

TO STOP CRAVINGS FOR SUGAR, DOUGH, AND CHEESE

The most important amino for eliminating cravings for gluten, milk products, and sweets (including chocolate) is DLPA (or DPA, if DLPA is too energizing). It builds up your endorphin levels, which gives you the comfort you've been getting from the allergy-addictors. For sweet and starch cravings, you'll also benefit from chromium (the blood sugar normalizing mineral included in your Master Supplement Plan) and may need the blood sugar stabilizing amino acid L-glutamine, which also helps heal any digestive damage from gluten or milk (it even helps with AIDS diarrhea and gastrointestinal burns after radiation treatments for cancer). Check the Amino Acid Therapy Chart on pages 122–123 to choose any other amino you might need to totally eliminate cravings (e.g., 5-HTP or tryptophan can help with afternoon and evening carb cravings as well as constipation).

	AM	B	MM	L	MA	D	BT*
❑ DLPA (or DPA), 500 mg for cravings. See pages 122–123 if cravings persist.	1–2	__	1–2	__	1–2	__	__
❑ Aloe vera liquid, 4–8 oz, George's or Professional's Care brand, for healing from digestive or bowel discomfort.	1	__	__	__	__	__	1
❑ Vitamin C powder, 1,000 mg; or Alka Seltzer Gold, as needed for allergic reactions on reexposure.	__	__	__	__	__	__	__

*AM = on arising; B = with breakfast; MM = midmorning; L = with lunch; MA = midafternoon; D = with dinner; BT = at bedtime

MILK INTOLERANCE

Lactase (e.g., Lactaid) is an enzyme product available from your drugstore that helps the body digest milk sugar. It comes in three strengths and is to be taken with the first bite of milk-based food. Of course, lactose-free milk is available everywhere, and cheese, yogurt, and kefir are available, too.

Note: If your problem is the casein or whey (i.e., the protein in milk), lactase will not relieve your symptoms. In that case, you are only safe with ghee. Many people fall into this category.

FOR ALLERGIC REACTIONS THAT CAUSE DIGESTIVE DISTRESS

The aloe vera plant heals the damage to the "skin" of your digestive tract in the same way it can heal your external skin. Aloe juice can get sluggish bowels moving normally, too. Look for George's or Professional's Care brands. They are the only ones that concentrate the white, tasteless core of the plant, which is the most healing and least irritating of its parts.

FOR QUICK ELIMINATION OF ALLERGIC REACTIONS TO FOOD OR INHALANTS

Use two Alka-Seltzer Gold as needed during detox week for headaches or digestive discomfort. Use it anytime you have an adverse reaction to a food. Or use 1,000 milligrams of vitamin C powder in the ascorbate form, as needed initially or for accidental reexposure after detox and elimination.

ALLERGIES ARE STRESSFUL: REPAIRING DEEPER DAMAGE

If you are allergic to common foods such as the big three, your body might have been engaged in a struggle every day for most of your life. This chronic stress has strained you in ways beyond the obvious postnasal drip, stomach bloating, or food cravings. You have been dealing with constant assault, and the troops are probably very tired. Thankfully, taking the supplements and changing your diet will relieve the pressure that your immune system and stress emergency system have been under. But if you continue to feel a lack of vitality and to have a tendency to feel too easily overwhelmed, please consider a simple test for adrenal-stress function. If your adrenals (your stress and immunity guardians) are worn too low, you won't be able to revive them without a special supplement protocol that can be determined only after you get your saliva test results. (See chapters three and eleven.)

ACTION STEPS

1. Review your symptoms, as discussed in chapter five, and decide which foods you are probably allergy-addicted to.
2. Do your home elimination and reintroduction tests. Keep a food-mood log to record the process.
3. Start on your DLPA and other anti-craving supplements as well as your basic supplements and any digestive-repair supplements needed.
4. Learn how to avoid any of the big-three foods you have adverse reactions to, and how to enjoy all the other foods that you can eat without injury. See chapters nineteen and twenty for suggestions on shopping and preparing food without sugar, gluten, or milk products.
5. Consider getting some of the testing I describe on page 194, especially if you think you might have intolerances to foods other than the big three.
6. Check your adrenal-stress symptoms if you benefit by removing any of the big-three allergy foods but continue to feel worn out and overwhelmed (see chapters three and eleven).

You may not believe it now, but you will soon find that avoiding these foods, though inconvenient, will become second nature. Feeling so much better will keep you motivated. What's more, you'll still enjoy eating!

Reading

Nancy Appleton, Ph.D., *Lick the Sugar Habit* (New York: Avery, 1988).

Kenneth Bock, M.D., and Cameron Stauth, *Healing the New Childhood Epidemics: Autism, ADHD, Asthma, and Allergies* (New York: Ballantine Books, 2008).

Ellen W. Cutler, D.C., *Live Free from Asthma and Allergies: Use the BioSET System to Detoxify and Desensitize Your Body*, Revised Edition (Berkeley, CA: Celestial Arts, 2007).

William Davis M.D., *Wheat Belly* (New York: Rodale, 2011).

Nicolette M. Dumke, *The Ultimate Food Allergy Cookbook and Survival Guide: How to Cook with Ease for a Food Allergy Diet and Recover Good Health* (Louisville, CO: Adapt Books, 2006).

——, *Food Allergy and Gluten-Free Weight Loss: Control Your Body Chemistry, Reduce Inflammation and Improve Your Health* (Louisville, CO: Adapt Books, 2011).

Ann Louise Gittleman, Ph.D., CNS, *Get the Sugar Out: 501 Simple Ways to Cut the Sugar Out of Any Diet*, 2nd Edition (New York: Three Rivers Press, 2008).

Peter H. R. Green, M.D., and Rory Jones, *Celiac Disease: A Hidden Epidemic*, Revised Edition (New York: William Morrow, 2010).

Bette Hagman, *More from the Gluten-Free Gourmet: Delicious Dining Without Wheat*, 2nd Edition (New York: Henry Holt, 2000).

Danna Korn, *Gluten-Free Kids: Raising Happy, Healthy Children with Celiac Disease, Autism, and Other Conditions*, 2nd Edition (Bethesda, MD: Woodbine House, 2010).

Shari Lieberman, Ph.D., CNS, FACN, with Linda Segall, *The Gluten Connection: How Gluten Sensitivity May Be Sabotaging Your Health—And What You Can Do to Take Control Now* (New York: Rodale Books, 2007).

Devi S. Nambudripad, M.D., D.C., L.Ac., Ph.D. (Acu.), *NAET: Say Good-Bye to Your Allergies* (New York: Delta Publishing, 2003).

Vikki Petersen, D.C., C.C.N., and Richard Petersen, D.C., C.C.N., *The Gluten Effect: How "Innocent" Wheat Is Ruining Your Health* (Sunnyvale, CA: True Health Publishing, 2009).

William H. Philpott, M.D., and Dwight K. Kalita, Ph.D., *Brain Allergies: The Psychonutrient and Magnetic Connections*, 2nd Edition (New York: McGraw-Hill: 2000).

John E. Postley, M.D., with Janet Barton, *The Allergy Discovery Diet: A Rotation Diet for Discovering Your Allergies to Food* (New York: Doubleday, 1990).

Doris Rapp, M.D., *Is This Your Child?: Discovering and Treating Unrecognized Allergies in Children and Adults* (New York: William Morrow, 1992). By a holistic allergist.

Rudy Rivera, M.D., and Roger Davis Deutsch, *Your Hidden Food Allergies Are Making You Fat* (Roseville, CA: Prima Lifestyles, 2002).

MAGAZINES

Gluten-Free Living
glutenfreeliving.com; (800) 324-8781

Living Without: The magazine for people living with allergies and food sensitivities
livingwithout.com; (800) 424-7887

Other Resources

ORGANIZATIONS

Celiac.com
www.celiac.com

Feingold Association of the United States
feingold.org
For important allergy perspectives, especially on ADHD.

Dairy Free Zone
nondairy.org
Whether you're allergic to milk or are lactose intolerant, you'll find lots of recipes and useful tips here.

Simply . . . Gluten-Free
simplygluten-free.com

REFERRALS TO PRACTITIONERS

The American Academy of Environmental Medicine
aaemonline.org; (215) 862-4544
For holistic allergy testing and treatment resources and holistic medical referrals.

The International Society for Orthomolecular Medicine
http://orthomed.org/isom/isom.html
For referrals to holistic allergy specialists.

TESTING

ALCAT Worldwide
alcat.com; (800) 872-5228
Blood testing for food and other sensitivities.

EnteroLab
enterolab.com; (972) 686-6869
Stool testing for gluten, milk, and other allergies.

Immuno Lab
http://www.immunolabs.com/patients/contact-us; (800) 231-9197
Blood testing for food allergies.

FOURTEEN

Hormone Help

As debilitating as your PMS or menopausal reactions might be, if you follow the advice in this chapter you may be completely free of any adverse symptoms in a few months. By your *very next* period, if you have a few weeks' running start with the right nutrients and foods, your PMS problems—from food cravings to cramps, bloating, and mood swings—could be entirely gone. Menopausal mood swings, food cravings, and weight gain can desist quickly, too. But other menopausal symptoms (like low energy and hot flashes) can take somewhat longer to eliminate.

If you are suffering from PMS, you'll learn how foods, supplements, and herbs can balance your hormone levels and eliminate your symptoms. If you are perimenopausal or menopausal, or have PCOS (polycystic ovary syndrome, page 93), you will learn how to test your hormone levels and find herbal options and natural low-dose hormone replacements to alleviate your symptoms. I'll also describe how acupuncture and stress management can help rebalance your hormones and how to find hormone-balancing helpers.

HORMONAL FOOD CRAVINGS

Do you experience powerful cravings for sugar and fat before your period or as you approach menopause? Most of these hormonally inspired food cravings will disappear when you stop eating "drug" foods. Chocolate, sugar, refined flour products, caffeine, and NutraSweet all contribute to hormonal mismanagement. They have to go if you are going to escape PMS or menopausal cravings and weight problems. I know that it is not enough to tell you to just quit eating these foods, but if you start taking the supplements I recommend, you will lose interest even in chocolate.

Once your cravings are gone (and it won't take long), you will feel satisfied, not deprived, by highly nutritious food. Green, purple, yellow, and red vegetables will delight you. Seafood, chicken, eggs, and meat will satisfy and please you. You will enjoy, but not overeat, wholesome carbs such as beans, potatoes, rice, and polenta.

The trouble is that addictive, druglike foods are everywhere; we call them convenience foods. It can be inconvenient to eat well, but it is more inconvenient to have PMS and hot flashes! It takes time to prepare fresh food or to find healthy places to eat. You will need to make it a priority, because the time you have now is being spoiled by the hormonal imbalances that are probably being magnified by your current diet in a real vicious cycle: unbalanced hormones make you overeat, and overeating further unbalances them.

AMINO ACIDS TO STOP FOOD CRAVINGS AND MOODINESS

These nutrients are just what you need to break the cycle. Whether you are pre- or postmenopausal, amino acids will reduce your sugar cravings and mood swings. These nutrient heroes are described in more detail in chapters one and nine, but I'll summarize here. Hormonal changes, particularly drops in estrogen and progesterone and rises in stress hormones, can radically reduce the supply of all of your four mood-enhancing brain chemicals: serotonin, endorphins, catecholamines, and GABA. The following aminos will build them right back up:

✦ **Glutamine** stops hypoglycemic (low blood sugar) cravings for sweets, starches, and alcohol and is mildly calming.

✦ **5-HTP (or tryptophan)** is particularly needed for afternoon and evening cravings during PMS. Many studies have made it clear that low serotonin, common during the week (or two) before menstruation, is a primary cause of irritability, negativity, depression, and insomnia. Chocolate and other drug-carbs can indirectly trigger a brief serotonin surge (at a high price, as we mentioned earlier). Using 5-HTP or L-tryptophan, the brain's natural serotonin fuels, is a much more effective way of raising levels. Because the low estrogen that inhibits serotonin in PMS can also be a factor in menopause, these aminos can help menopausal women, too.

✦ **GABA supplements** can relax your muscles, like a natural Valium, to help with cramps and stress.

✦ **D-phenylalanine (in DLPA or DPA)** will increase your endorphins, which have also been shown to drop during PMS. This helps explain why some of us experience so much painful cramping and emotional teariness around menstruation. If the DLPA is too stimulating, order DPA by itself.

✦ **Tyrosine,** a stimulating amino acid, can help a lot with caffeine and chocolate cravings.

See the Amino Acid Therapy Chart (pages 122–123) and decide which aminos you will need, based on your particular mood symptoms.[1]

FOR CRAVINGS AND MOOD SWINGS; USE AS NEEDED							
	AM	B	MM	L	MA	D	BT*
❑ L-glutamine, 500 mg	1–2	__	1–2	__	1–2	__	__
❑ 5-HTP, 50 mg	__	__	1–2	__	1–2	__	2
(or tryptophan, 500 mg)							
❑ GABA, 100–500 mg	__	__	1	__	1	__	1
❑ DLPA, 300–500 mg *or*	1–2	__	1–2	__	1–2	__	__
DPA, 200–500 mg	1–2	__	1–2	__	1–2	__	__
❑ L-tyrosine, 500 mg	1–2	__	1–2	__	1–2	__	__

*AM = upon rising; B = with breakfast; MM = midmorning; L = with lunch; MA = midafternoon; D = with dinner; BT = at bedtime.

TAKE YOUR BASIC SUPPLEMENTS

Many research studies have confirmed that even the moderate doses of nutrients in multivitamins/-minerals can provide dramatic improvements in PMS and help in menopause. Along with an improved diet, the Diet Cure's Basic Supplement Plan, in chapter seventeen, will provide all the extra nutrients you'll need to decrease or eliminate PMS symptoms: the B vitamins (especially B_6) and the minerals calcium, magnesium, and zinc all play a role. Most of us are deficient in these nutrients because we have not been eating enough fresh, whole foods and our produce comes from mineral-depleted soils. Another of your basic supplements, fish oil, can also help stop PMS symptoms. If it doesn't, evening primrose oil will. PMS, among other things, is a nutrient-deficiency problem, but such deficiencies can be easily rectified.

EAT WELL AND STOP DIETING

You will need to eat at least three times a day from now on. By eating more vegetables, protein (such as meat, fish, and eggs), and good fats (e.g., butter and olive oil); eliminating caffeine, sweets, and white flour starches such as white bread, cereal, and noodles; and taking your supplements, you'll find yourself free of carb cravings and weight gain, even premenstrually, within two months. Keep in mind that too many high-carb/junk foods and any dieting will keep you hormonally unbalanced. One example: The insulin that is triggered by too many carbohydrates lowers testosterone in men, who gain fat and lose muscle and sex drive as a result. Insulin does the reverse in women, raising testosterone levels, thus contributing to male-pattern (abdominal-only) weight gain and polycystic ovary syndrome, among other things (see adverse effects of high and low testosterone on page 93).[2]

The combination of supplements and improved eating does the trick for 75 percent of Recovery Systems' clients under 40 who suffer from PMS. Many of our clients with clockwork PMS seven to fourteen days a month suddenly find themselves menstruating without any of the usual warning signals: no cravings, no weeping, no rages, no sore breasts or bloating, and no cramping. If you still have premenstrual cravings or mood swings after two months, the following information may help with any remaining, stubborn problems. If it doesn't, hormone testing and more potent balancing strategies are in order.

Watch for your body's reaction to the proteins you feed it. Some of us seem to be genetically programmed to do best with animal protein, despite our vegetarian or health ideals. Remember that red meat is the only source of easily absorbed iron and zinc, two minerals that are very important if you are menstruating. Many of our vegetarian clients dream of hamburgers before their periods each month—their bodies are sending them a message to get more iron and zinc. Be sure to supplement with these two minerals if you are vegetarian *and* menstruating.

The Soy Story

Does the soy story have a happy ending?

Once upon a time researchers found that women of the Far East had low breast cancer rates. Why? Was it that they ate soy products? Was it that they ate 20 percent more calories than we do? Was it because they ate few refined, processed foods and more vegetables? Less fat? Less animal protein?[3]

Somehow soy became the focus of the excitement. Soy is a *very* complex bean that contains many nutrients. Some of these nutrients, the phytoestrogens, act like estrogen, fooling our cells. One cup of tofu provides the estrogen equivalent of one dose of Premarin,[4] the potent estrogen brew made from horse urine. Initially it was suggested that soy might be protective against breast cancer, osteoporosis, and Alzheimer's in menopause. But this is all in question now.

Many U.S. children are now becoming vegetarian and using soy all their lives. Yet low estrogen is not a problem in youth, especially for boys. We don't need more estrogen then. What does soy do to females who are not close to menopause or low in estrogen? These are some of the questions about soy. Some disturbing answers:

1. Despite their relatively high soy intake, Japanese women have *much* higher rates of osteoporosis than we do (one in three versus one in eleven). Moreover, bone-mass deterioration begins in Japanese women at age 20, not at age 35, as in the United States.[5]
2. Soy increases the growth rate of cancerous breast cells in women (in vivo) and in test tubes (in vitro).[6]
3. Soy increases progesterone activity and breast cell growth in menstruating women.[7]
4. Soy decreases thyroid (T_3) and DHEA levels in menstruating women and others (both of which are central to energy, health, and weight maintenance) as well as lowering levels of estrone, LS, and FSH (female reproductive hormones).[8]
5. One study found soy to be a factor in disturbances in menstruation in a group of premenopausal women.[9]
6. Infants of both sexes who are fed soy milk later develop hormonal abnormalities such as obesity, diabetes, early

menstruation, or delayed male genital development, having been exposed to 13,000 to 22,000 times the amounts of estrogen complex that breast-fed babies have been exposed to.[10]

The upshot is that factors other than soy likely contribute to good health in the Far East (where it is used primarily as a condiment, not an entrée). Remember that all people on simpler diets (and with simpler lives) have much better health than we do in the United States, and most of them do not use soy (especially now that most of it is genetically engineered).

If you are eating soy, be aware that, in addition to slowing down the thyroid, it is very difficult to digest. Soy sauce, miso, and tempeh are fermented products easier for the stomach to break down than tofu, soybeans, soy milk, and soy protein powders, which are not fermented and often cause stomachaches. We don't recommend that people force down soy products that they can't digest, that they don't really need, and that may actually prove to be harmful to them.

OTHER SUPPORTIVE SUPPLEMENTS

HERBAL HELP FOR PMS

The six basic supplements and the aminos usually stop junk-food cravings so that you can start eating well. This stops PMS in 75 percent of sufferers under 40. If you continue suffering from PMS, try adding an herbal formula that includes the herbs vitex or chasteberry, which have been used and extensively researched in Europe and the United States with good results. You can find them at your health food store.

THE ENDOMETRIOSIS SOLUTION

Try miraculous proteolytic enzymes, like Vitalzym, for the excruciating menstrual cramping of endometriosis. These potent (but not hormone-altering) enzymes quickly gobble up the problematic endometrial tissue! One of our staff members with PCOS that included terrible endometriosis had tried two surgeries and several medications before she discovered Vitalzym. After twenty years of suffering, with a very healthy diet and these enzymes she was cured in two months.

HERBS IN MENOPAUSE

Our clients have tried many herbal formulations that feature dong quai and black cohosh. They are easy to find in health food stores and they often make women feel so much better, typically eliminating hot flashes and night sweats. Research confirms this and even finds that black cohosh protects against osteoporosis. Black cohosh, sold under the name Remifemen, is now the highest-selling alternative for menopausal hormone depletion in Germany, Australia, and the United States. It is the main ingredient in many popular products like Change-O-Life, from Nature's Way. Dong quai is China's chief female tonic. But these herbs may not fully normalize your hormonal functions; you may still be low in estrogen, progesterone, testosterone, or DHEA or otherwise out of balance. Please get your hormone levels and bone integrity tested to find out.

SPECIAL HORMONE-REBALANCING SUPPLEMENTS							
SUPPLEMENTS (as recommended)	AM	B	MM	L	MA	D	BT*
Herbs For PMS:							
❏ Vitex	—	—	—	—	—	—	—
Herbs for Menopause:							
❏ Dong quai	—	—	—	—	—	—	—
❏ Black cohosh	—	—	—	—	—	—	—
Most potent bioidentical hormone protocols:							
❏ Progesterone	—	—	—	—	—	—	—
❏ Estradiol	—	—	—	—	—	—	—
❏ Estriol	—	—	—	—	—	—	—
❏ Testosterone	—	—	—	—	—	—	—
❏ DHEA	—	—	—	—	—	—	—
❏ Pregnenolone	—	—	—	—	—	—	—

*AM = on arising; B = with breakfast; MM = midmorning; L = with lunch; MA = midafternoon; D = with dinner; BT = at bedtime.

MORE ALTERNATIVES: ACUPUNCTURE, STRESS REDUCTION, HOMEOPATHY

Acupuncture. Acupuncturists can help tremendously by prescribing hormone-balancing herbs and ordering hormone tests. They even have well-documented success with infertility. (By the way, the needles don't usually hurt.)

Julie learned firsthand the curative effects of acupuncture. She had been in menopause for two years. She ate well and had been using hormone creams for two years. Most of her hot flashes and insomnia had disappeared as a result, but a large and uncomfortable fibroid tumor had not subsided. Because we had seen acupuncture help with hormone-related problems, including infertility and the side effects of chemotherapy after breast cancer surgery, we suggested she try it for her fibroid. She went to an acupuncturist who specialized in women's health problems. After two sessions in which the acupuncturist used fifteen painless needles in her pubic area, the fibroid and its symptoms subsided and did not return. The acupuncturist told Julie that similar treatments for fibroids are successful about 50 percent of the time.

Exercise, Relaxation, and Sunlight. Descending estrogen levels during PMS and menopause bring important feel-good brain chemicals down with them: serotonin and endorphins. Exercise can help, but you have to almost kill yourself to get a short-lived endorphin high. Fortunately, the supplement DLPA raises endorphin levels easily to keep mood up and food cravings down. Serotonin levels will rise nicely, though only temporarily, after moderate exercise. The supplements 5-HTP and tryptophan will keep your levels up much longer than exercise will, so you won't have to suffer from depression if you can't exercise. Sunlight (or therapeutic lamps, 3,000 lux or brighter) will raise serotonin levels, too. So exercise outdoors in winter without sunglasses whenever you can. Raising serotonin helps with food cravings and mood swings, as well as insomnia in PMS and menopause (see pages 14 and 124).

Menopausal exercisers can lose some of their new abdominal fat by building muscle. Muscle burns fat for a living; it uses fat as fuel for its activity. But we do put on abdominal fat in menopause for an excellent reason: we need it to create the special fat-generated estrogen, called estrone, to replace the estrogen that used to come from our ovaries. Don't get too buff; we were meant to soften with age. And don't try to solve this abdominal "problem" with a tummy tuck unless you're prepared to start using the Vivelle patch or other supplemental estrogen. We've seen two women who got very depressed after literally cutting off their abdominal estrogen factory.

The Adrenal Connection

Stress can disrupt your hormonal life in newly understood ways. It is important to get saliva testing of your adrenal stress hormones, especially if you are in perimenopause or menopause. During these times your ovaries are making less estrogen and progesterone, and your adrenals are having to take over much or all of the job, on top of making twenty-four other hormones. The adrenals are mighty, but if they have to attend to too much stress, they can't do these additional jobs very well. The stress of junk-food eating, low-calorie dieting, and other health and life problems can exhaust your adrenals, reducing their ability to help your body cope with the demands of perimenopause, menopause, and other problems such as PCOS and infertility. Adrenal exhaustion is often the cause of hormonal deficiencies. Don't overlook it! See chapters three and eleven for more on stress and the adrenals and how to test these stress-hormone levels.

Stress will cause muscle to be lost (and bone, too). If you are tired after a workout, stress has probably worn out your adrenal glands, and you'll need to slow down your exercise program, at least for a while. Moderate exercise is actually a proven stress fighter. Don't forget that stress can destroy the hormones that should be coming from the adrenals (when your ovaries can no longer make them) to stop your menopausal symptoms. They can easily get rerouted to stress-coping functions instead. Anything that destresses you protects your estrogen, progesterone, testosterone, and DHEA levels. See chapter twenty-one for more on exercise, relaxation, and stress busting.

Homeopathy: If you have tested your hormones and found imbalances, but you decide that you do not want to use even bioidentical hormones, you might consider homeopathic remedies. They are well laid out in *Menopause and Homeopathy*, by Ifeoma Ikenze, M.D., a Harvard-trained holistic women's health expert. Find a homeopath with sex hormone balancing experience.

TEST YOUR HORMONES WHEN PMS
OR MENOPAUSAL SYMPTOMS
JUST WON'T GO AWAY

If you've experienced little or no relief from your PMS or other symptoms after two months on the preceding program, I suggest you have your hormone levels tested. Since serious hormonal imbalances can begin ten years before menopause (and sometimes earlier), I encourage hormone testing at any sign of adverse hormonal change, so common now in women over 40 that it has been given a name: perimenopause. For example, if you've never had PMS before and you suddenly start experiencing it, or it worsens, or your periods start getting heavier, crampier, or more irregular, you should test your hormones levels. I think many women are shocked at how early their periods can now become sporadic or absent.

You could experiment, trying first an estrogen supplement and then, if that doesn't work, a progesterone supplement. Both are available in natural (i.e., bioidentical), easily absorbed, plant-based products. But I don't recommend this. I would much prefer that you test your hormone levels before you do anything else. You know from chapter six what symptoms to watch for, so you'll have an idea of what your hormone tests should reveal. Sex hormone testing is an imperfect technology, especially for menstruating women, who are harder to evaluate than menopausal women, and men, as their hormone levels change so much. Be sure to start a detailed food/mood/sleep/energy/cramping log on test days and for at least a month in addition if your symptoms vary a lot. (See chapter twenty-two.)

Always retest six months later if you start taking any hormones, or anytime you experience symptoms of hormonal imbalance. Continue to retest.

Blood and Saliva or Urine Testing. Blood tests for estradiol, progesterone, testosterone, pregnenolone (available only as a blood test), DHEA, and others give you a rough idea of these basic hormone levels. They measure inactive (bound) as well as active (free) hormones. Unfortunately, the inactive ones are ten times more prolific but have no effect on you. There are blood tests for free hormones, but they are hard to find and more expensive. On the other hand, while saliva testing measures only the free hormones, the technology varies from lab to lab and so results are not always reliable. Twenty-four-hour urine testing identifies the most hormones, but it is very hard to interpret. (See Hertoghe's book, listed on page 224.)

Whatever testing you do, your results will be compared with the levels that are considered normal for the time of the month that you tested in. For stubborn PMS, we suggest a test while you are having symptoms. Your results will be measured against "normal" premenstrual (i.e., luteal) levels. If you are menopausal, you could continue having hormonal fluctuations each month for up to seven years after you stop having periods! How do you know? Do hot flashes vary? Do you still get days with swollen breasts or other PMS symptoms? Or are you like too many of our clients who say, "No variation. I have PMS now twenty-four-seven!" If you are beyond any signs of cycling, you could collect a single blood or saliva sample anytime.

Testing salivary hormone levels throughout an entire menstrual cycle.
Whether you are having regular menstrual periods or irregular peri-menopausal cycling, you can chart your course by collecting saliva samples on alternate days over an entire 28- to 36-day period. This provides a treasure trove of information. Some women have two ovulations per month, for example. Some have none. Some have plenty of estrogen or progesterone, except during PMS. This is information you should have. Your map will change as you get closer to menopause and experience new symptoms. Testing will help you understand and address these changes. Our clinic relies on it! Several labs do this, or an abbreviated form of it. (See chapter twenty-one, pages 362–363.)

Most saliva-testing labs will discuss your results with you by phone or refer you to practitioners in your area who will help you order, interpret, and treat your imbalances. They will also consult with health professionals by phone on your behalf. Be sure to retest within ninety days, and then every six months after you start your hormone supplements, until your levels and symptoms are optimal. Then retest annually or as needed.

Blood tests can be ordered through a cooperative physician or directly through online labs. Many kinds of practitioners can order and interpret hormone testing, but they can't all provide estrogen and testosterone, which are available only by prescription. So you'll definitely need a licensed M.D., N.P., D.O., or N.D. at some point if your hormone levels turn out to be abnormal. You may need to be assertive about getting tested (and using bioidentical HRT) if your physician is not holistic. Insist on a thorough testing-based and symptom-based assessment.

For test ordering information, see chapter twenty-one.

Sex Hormone Dysfunction and Your Thyroid

The interrelationship between the thyroid and sex hormone functions is decisive in several ways. The thyroid often falters during major sex hormone shifts: the start of menstruation, during pregnancy, or in menopause. Low thyroid can lead to sudden weight gain at any of these junctures. It can often result in miscarriage, infertility, heavy clotting, menstrual bleeding, lower sex drive, and other reproductive malfunctions. See chapters four and twelve for much more on how to recognize if low thyroid is a factor in your sex hormone imbalances and what lab tests to order.

Sex Hormone Tests: Blood and/or Saliva

Basics: For All:
   Estradiol
   Progesterone
   Testosterone (free and total)
   DHEA-S
   LH and FSH
   Sex hormone binding globulin (SHBG)
   Salivary adrenal cortisol testing as per chapters three and
      eleven
   Thyroid panel for infertility and unusual weight gain as per
chapters four and twelve
Menopausal Extras:
   Estriol
   Pregnenolone (blood only)
PCOS Extras:
   Estrone
   LH, FSH, and ratio
   Androstenedione
   Glucose/insulin (blood only)
   Ovarian ultrasound for cysts

Why Testing Is Important. Most of the hormone-troubled women who come to our clinic have never had their hormone levels tested, even the ones who are seeing gynecologists and on potent hormonal drugs! Premarin was, for years, prescribed for menopausal women at a whopping 625-milligram dosage regardless of symptoms or body size. Too often it raised estrogen levels too high. Why? It was not closely monitored, and low estrogen was not always a problem to begin with. Since the 2002 exposé on heart disease, breast cancer, and other serious health problems resulting from high doses of Prempro (Premarin and Provera), many doctors have gone to the other extreme—not giving *any* hormonal help.

Because your own body's hormones can become unbalanced in hazardous ways, you really must test them before you consider using any additional hormones, however natural. As several studies have shown, unnaturally high estrone, estradiol, and testosterone are implicated in breast cancer. Other studies show that low estriol is associated with breast cancer (as is low melatonin). Other tests may be recommended as well; for example, sex hormone binding.

Globulin, when elevated (e.g., by birth control pills), binds up, or inactivates, sex hormones. Advice on further testing should come from your experienced practitioner.

Testing Your Bones. Your bones hold secrets to navigating perimenopause and menopause osteoporosis-free. They will start shrinking slowly at age 35, then quickly for the first ten years of perimenopause, then slowly again. A non-radiation method is available using ultrasound technology to measure your current bone density, and a simple urine test, the Dpd test, will tell you if, and at what rate, your bones are now breaking down. This test can be repeated to make sure that your hormone-rebalancing program is working, and whether you'll need to increase your hormone supplements along with other bone-promoting strategies, like increasing minerals, protein, and weight-bearing exercise. High cortisol and low estrogen, progesterone, testosterone, or DHEA can all contribute to bone loss—another reason to be sure your stress and sex hormones are all in balance.

BIOIDENTICAL HORMONES:
THE MOST POTENT HORMONAL THERAPIES

If the dietary and supplement strategies just described fail, and you know from your symptoms and test results where the hormonal trouble lies, you'll need to get good experienced professional help in moving into a hormone-balancing experiment. Good help is getting easier to find, but be prepared for trial and error. Ask around for recommendations from patients who have had good results without months of frustration. You'll need to be very careful not to subscribe to rigid ideas about hormones. For example, there are whole camps of clinicians who are either anti-estrogen and pro-progesterone, or the reverse. There are those who advocate raising both hormones to *pre*menopausal levels and restarting menstrual cycles. Many would, like Suzanne Somers, seem to love it, but I don't know of any research confirming the advisability of it long-term.

Plant-based hormones used to be impossible to absorb by mouth, but the micronized (microscopic in size) forms, now routinely used everywhere, are fully absorbable. Some of these formulations are found in health food stores. All can be found in pharmacies as pills, troches, patches, and creams. Many compounders and pharmacies specifically cater to women's health needs. (Some are listed in the Resources for chapter twenty-one.)

Studies have found bioidentical progesterone to have none of the dangers of the nonbioidentical progestins, which are still found in birth control pills and drugs like Provera (of course, excessive, unmonitored doses, even of bioidentical hormones, could cause problems). Mare's urine is closer to human estrogen than progestin is to human progesterone (but what the mares suffer in the extracting!). Studies show that all types of estradiol, when taken with bioidentical progesterone, have proven safe if taken at appropriate doses and monitored.

In the past, Premarin and Provera were handed out in high doses without benefit of testing to help identify which, and in what amounts, they might be needed and safely used. A trend toward lower dosing has been under way since the publication of the shocking results of the studies I mention in chapter six, but testing and retesting is still not common practice, and progestins are still being prescribed, so be assertive.

There are three types of naturally occurring estrogen: estradiol, estriol, and estrone. Compounders can make a blend to your doctor's specifications. They can also tailor dosing and combine estrogens with other hormones if indicated. The hormone supplement 17beta-estradiol is readily available in pills and patches and has a good track record used alone, but combining it, as the body does, with comparable levels of estriol may be ideal. Adding estrone can be problematic. Do find an experienced clinician who does not rely totally on a pharmacist who has never met you.

Bearded Ladies and Balding Gentlemen: The Power of Hormones (Even the Most Natural)

You know personally how powerful hormones can be: just think of sexual arousal and PMS. Even plant-based bioidenticals are very potent, and they can be overused, creating imbalances that can be dangerous.

There is one other thing to be aware of. The pathways between hormones are not entirely predictable. For example, the very popular hormone supplement DHEA can easily convert to unneeded estrogen or testosterone. That is why women using DHEA (as well as testosterone and progesterone) can grow facial hair. (This can also happen in polycystic ovary syndrome or menopause as estrogen levels drop.) Yet if you are truly deficient and carefully monitored through symptoms and testing, DHEA supplementation can be a boon. A well-known L.A. radio host reported using DHEA and losing most of his luxuriant head of hair. It had raised his testosterone level too high and male-pattern baldness had set in with a vengeance. (It grew back when he ran out of the DHEA.)

Stop using and retest immediately any hormone if you begin to get adverse effects. It may be especially easy to absorb too much hormone through the skin. One of our clients used progesterone cream as body lotion, instead of the ⅛ to ¼ teaspoon recommended, and grew soft, downy sideburns. It took her several months off of progesterone to get rid of them and longer for salivary levels to drop to normal.

HRT for Perimenopause and Menopause. You will need to get the results of a full-cycle saliva test in order to figure out the perimenopausal mystery zone. Only a few saliva samples or a single blood test are typically needed for menopausal testing. If you turn out to have osteopenia or osteoporosis, help is available through weight-bearing exercise and supplementation with minerals, estrogen, testosterone, and DHEA, as well as vitamins D and K. Do research the drug Fosamax, though, before trying it. It can cause serious problems.

If your tests show that you are too low in one of the estrogens or testosterone, you'll need to work with a physician to bring up your levels. Watch for quick improvement of any adverse symptoms you're experiencing. For example, increased estrogen should soon stop hot flashes and mental fog, estriol suppositories stop vaginal dryness at once, and testosterone can quickly relieve certain kinds of depression and low libido. Retest regularly and at any sign of discomfort, to avoid both excess and deficiency.

If your cortisol and DHEA levels are low, this could be the real key to your hormonal problems, because it's a sign that your adrenals are too exhausted by stress to make adequate amounts of estrogen, progesterone, or testosterone. (Remember, in perimenopause and menopause, your adrenals take over as your ovaries produce less of these hormones.) Use the suggestions in chapter eleven to restore your adrenals to working order as soon as possible. Retest everything over the next few months to see if raising your cortisol and DHEA has brought your other hormones up to a point where you might be able to cut back on your HRT.

If your progesterone levels are too low, your doctor will suggest that you take progesterone, which can eliminate PMS or make you more able to sustain a pregnancy.

Where to Find Bioidentical Hormones. You can buy progesterone in creams, drops, and pills over the Internet, over-the-counter, and by prescription (e.g., Prometrium); the same is true for DHEA, pregnenolone, and estriol. Estradiol (e.g., the Vivelle patch) and testosterone are available only by prescription.

The strengths and combinations of hormones available, especially in compounding pharmacists' repertoires, are extensive, and they can be tailored to your needs. Compounding pharmacists will consult with you and your physician by phone about what and how much of any hormone to use, depending on your symptoms and test results. Be ready to call the compounding pharmacist yourself first, since many physicians don't seem to be aware that these compounders and their customized hormonal products and advice exist.

Compounders usually send out prescriptions through overnight mail. Beware of those who do not advise hormone testing before and after prescribing. (See chapter twenty-one for a list of resources for compounding pharmacies.)

Ideally, you'll work with a physician who is experienced and effective (and does not rely totally on pharmacists who are not clinicians and have never met you). But good hormone balancers are hard to find. Many women complain of long hormone replacement ordeals before their symptoms are relieved. But clinicians are getting better training all the time. (If naturopathic doctors [N.D.'s] are licensed in your state, they may be the best trained.)

If Your Levels of Any Hormones Are Too High. The following are suggestions that our clients' physicians often make:

✦ Stop taking any foods, herbs, or supplemental hormones that might be encouraging excess. For example, hormonal creams are especially suspect, and alcohol and soy raise estrogen levels.

✦ Increase the amount of vitamin C you are taking to 5 grams per day.

✦ Use a gentle fiber, like pectin, daily. Be sure to eat plenty of fiber-containing foods—fruit, beans, nuts, seeds, and crunchy vegetables. Fiber binds with and removes hormones (and heavy metals, like mercury).

✦ If testosterone is raising your spirits and energy but tests show it is converting to too much estrogen, cut the dose and try supplements such as DIM or citrin, which can block that conversion. Retest.

✦ To reduce excessive testosterone, as in PCOS, try the herb saw palmetto.

ACTION STEPS

1. Use the symptoms lists in chapter six to get a sense of which hormones may be out of balance.
2. Use supplements and herbs, acupuncture, or homeopathy for PMS, perimenopausal, and menopausal cravings, mood swings, and other adverse symptoms.
3. Follow the basic food recommendations—pay close attention to what to avoid as well as what to consume.
4. If the above recommendations don't eliminate your symptoms, work with an effective health care professional and get testing as per the suggestions in this chapter.

5. When results are in, decide which hormone supplements or prescriptions to try.

6. Keep track of your symptoms and retest to monitor your levels and adjust hormone replacement therapy as needed.

7. Get hormone testing, thyroid testing, adrenal testing, or bone-density testing as needed. Remember: Labs can err. Your symptoms rule.

Now that you have access to a hormone-balancing diet, supplements, herbs, acupuncture, comprehensive testing, and bioidentical hormones, you don't need to go on blindly suffering hormonal havoc. Your hormonally linked moods, cravings, infertility, hot flashes, acne, and cramps can be understood and relieved.

Readings

Thierry Hertoghe, M.D., with Jules-Jacques Nabet, M.D., *The Hormone Solution: Stay Younger Longer with Natural Hormone and Nutrition Therapies* (New York: Three Rivers Press, 2002). Re: urine testing.

Ifeoma Ikenze, M.D., *Menopause and Homeopathy: A Guide for Women in Midlife* (Berkeley, CA: North Atlantic Books, 1998).

Christiane Northrup, M.D., *Women's Bodies, Women's Wisdom: Creating Physical and Emotional Health and Healing,* Revised Edition (New York: Bantam Books, 2010).

Suzanne Somers, *Breakthrough: Eight Steps to Wellness* (New York: Three Rivers Press, 2009).

Elizabeth Lee Vliet, M.D., *It's My Ovaries, Stupid!* Revised Edition (Savvy Woman's Guide Publishing, 2011).

Resources

See chapter twenty-one for information on testing and compounding pharmacies and chapter seventeen for supplement-ordering information.

FIFTEEN

Yeast Elimination

If you've been on the aminos as per chapters one and nine and your diet has improved and you still have cravings for sugar, starch, or alcohol, accompanied by bloating and some of the other conditions described in chapter seven, read on. If you've already tested positive for the yeast *Candida albicans*, this is your chapter. Some of the other imbalances covered so far in this book have had relatively quick and straightforward solutions that can be implemented easily, often without professional advice or help. But yeast-overgrowth detection and elimination can be difficult. At Recovery Systems we've spent years developing techniques to get rid of yeast. At first there were really no effective natural remedies available in health food stores (we tried them all), so we had to go further afield in ordering supplements. In fact, our head nutritionist, Timothy Kuss, ended up creating two of his own products, because he could not find what he needed anywhere.

But now effective natural remedies are more readily available. What I have done in this chapter, with Tim's help, is point you to these supplements and describe the methods for killing yeast that we use at Recovery Systems. They may not all be available in stores, but they can be ordered through the Internet at dietcure.com and from other reputable websites.

I recommend that you work with a knowledgeable health professional on this problem if you can. All health professionals have their own ideas about what works best against yeast overgrowth. The information here will let them know what our nutritional staff has found most effective. Our methods kill the yeasts so gently that you won't feel uncomfortable in the process—and you won't have to restrict your diet as much as earlier protocols required. We used to think that starving the yeasts out by withholding all carbs was the way to go, but starving never works! In this case, the yeasts just overgrow again when essential healthy carbs eventually have to be reintroduced (for instance, instant bloat after the first apple).

To control yeast overgrowth, you must do five things:

1. Gradually but significantly reduce the yeast population of the body with supplements and/or pharmaceuticals.
2. Starve the yeasts by eating fewer carbohydrates (and raising protein and fat).
3. Strengthen the immune system.
4. Rebuild the health of the intestinal tract, which may have been damaged by an extensive yeast (or parasite) infection.
5. Eliminate parasites if you have both a yeast and a parasite infection (take a stool test to find out).

THE ANTI-YEAST EATING PLAN

Your diet holds the key to becoming yeast-free quickly. It is difficult, if not impossible, to overcome yeasts without avoiding or reducing certain high-carb foods that promote yeast overgrowth and emphasizing foods with potent anti-yeast qualities. The good news is that (1) anti-yeast supplements or meds are quite effective and allow you to eat a diet with fewer carb restrictions; and (2) this diet does not go on forever. As you kill off the yeast you can gradually start eating more healthy carbs again.

IMMUNE SYSTEM BOOSTERS

To control and conquer yeast, the best bet is to make the immune system as strong as possible. Try the following immune system boosters:

✦ A warm, dry home and plenty of sunlight help. Yeast thrives in wet, cold conditions in the home; it is less of a problem in hot, dry climates. Homes with little natural sunlight or that have mold or mildew promote yeast overgrowth. Get out and enjoy the sun every day to boost your natural immunity.

✦ Avoid exposure to toxins. Those that can lower immunity include chemical sprays and solvents as well as highly processed foods (you know, the ones that have ingredients on the label that you can't pronounce). Be sure to read chapter eighteen to bone up on the best foods for keeping your immune system strong.

✦ Exercise. Lymph, the fluid that removes bacteria from the body (our immunity fluid), doesn't move much unless we move our leg muscles and arm muscles.

✦ Relax. Any form of relaxing activity, whether it's meditation, yoga, massage, or doing something you love, such as gardening or walking in nature, actually boosts immunity. Test your adrenal function to see if stress has lowered it so much that it cannot support your immune system. See chapters three and eleven for testing and adrenal-repair information.

✦ Consume more garlic. Garlic, in food or as a supplement, boosts immunity overall as well as fights yeasts and parasites.

✦ Drink plenty of fluids. Purified water and teas such as ginger, pau d'arco, hyssop, spearmint, and raspberry all boost immunity. A ginger and pau d'arco blend is particularly therapeutic, and the ginger flavor makes the pau d'arco more appealing. If you don't like ginger, substitute spearmint instead.

RESTORE YOUR DIGESTIVE FIRE

According to traditional Chinese medicine, the digestive process is supposed to be a "hot" one. To break down food, the stomach requires ample hydrochloric acid and other digestive enzymes. When you have too much yeast, this digestive fire is squelched or reduced. An effective way to rekindle that flame is to use warming foods, such as ginger, oregano, cinnamon, cloves, and black pepper, all of which increase gastric secretions and assimilation of nutrients. Taking super enzymes with hydrochloric acid (HCl) helps too.

Cautionary note: Do not use these warming foods or HCl if you have an ulcer or tend to have stomach sensitivity, or if you find them too stimulating.[1]

Foods to Avoid

Alcohol	alcohol, alcohol-containing foods
Dairy	milk and cheese from cows, cottage cheese, sweetened yogurt (remember: the lactose in these foods is a form of sugar, which the yeasts feed on, and cheese is a fungal product, which encourages yeast growth); however, butter, ghee, and unsweetened yogurt are usually okay
Condiments	ketchup, mayonnaise, and barbecue sauce, among others
Fermented food products	apple cider vinegar, other vinegars (except rice vinegar), hops, malt, soy sauce, pickles, pickled vegetables
Fruits	Just in the first four weeks, you won't be able to eat any fresh fruit at all, let alone dried fruit or fruit juice (which I hope you will mostly avoid, even off the anti-yeast program).
Mushrooms	Forgo all these fungi except shiitake, reishi, and maitake, as they seem to fight yeast.
Processed meat	marbled meat, all processed and smoked meat, bacon, sausage, corned beef, ham, meat with MSG (because it causes meat cravings), and others
Starches	grains in general, bread, cookies, gravy, muffins, pancakes, pasta, sauces, tapioca, waffles, french fries, baker's yeast
Sweets	(things you won't eat anyway for your Diet Cure) candy of all kinds, soda pop, sugar (white, brown, raw), honey, molasses, turbinado sugar, maple syrup, rice syrup, sweeteners (malt, corn sweetener, date sugar, sucrose, fructose, high fructose corn syrup, mannitol, NutraSweet or aspartame, saccharine)

After the first four weeks, you can try introducing fruit and then increasing higher-carbohydrate foods such as beans and whole grains.

THE FIRST FOUR WEEKS

For the first four weeks, emphasize the nutrient-rich but yeast-discouraging foods listed here. It will help a lot to incorporate the foods at the bottom of the page, which are known to have anti-yeast and antifungal properties.

Safe Foods

Eggs	cooked at a low temperature
Legumes	beans, lentils, peas (one serving per day max)
Protein	antibiotic-free poultry, beef, lamb, fish
Vegetables	particularly steamed, lightly sautéed, and in salads
Freshly prepared soups	without cream or milk
Fresh nuts and seeds	preferably soaked in water overnight
Goat cheese, unsweetened yogurt made from cow's milk, and buttermilk	For those not dairy intolerant, they supply good bacteria and are not sweet.
Whole grains	basmati rice, millet, amaranth, quinoa, corn (only one moderate serving per day max)

Anti-Yeast, Antifungal Foods

- Avocado
- Broccoli
- Brussels sprouts
- Cabbage
- Coconut oil (non-hydrogenated) or full-fat coconut milk
- Collards
- Fresh lemon as a flavoring (to help the body detoxify)
- Garlic
- Kale
- Olive oil, flax oil
- Onions
- Spices such as cinnamon, cloves, oregano, rosemary, sage, thyme, turmeric

OTHER STEPS

+ Use flavorings such as onion, curry, and pepper (in moderation).
+ Use extra virgin olive oil and coconut oil or butter.
+ Be sure to drink eight 8-ounce glasses of water a day. Squeeze a little lemon juice into water and drink it before meals to support the liver in its yeast-expulsion effort. Other liquids to enjoy are vegetable juice and tea (pau d'arco, ginger, and/or spearmint).
+ Chlorophyll products, such as chlorella, spirulina, alfalfa, or barley greens, can be used as supplements or added into smoothies.

What Is the Recovery Process Like?

If you slip on the eating plan, don't despair; *just stay with the program*. You haven't blown it. The supplements will still be working.

As the anti-yeast supplements and your special diet kill off and neutralize the organisms, you should quickly lose your cravings, bloating, and other symptoms. However, occasionally the process of eliminating yeasts can cause adverse reactions such as diarrhea and flulike symptoms, which are caused when yeast organisms are killed quickly. If necessary, cut back or even stop the supplements for several days. These uncomfortable reactions usually don't last long. And on the supplement plan that we use now, these "die-off" reactions are very rare. But one of the reasons that I recommend you work with an experienced yeast-elimination expert is so that you'll have someone to talk to about the process. How long you need to stay on the anti-yeast program depends on how long yeast overgrowth has been present; the state and competency of your immune, digestive, and endocrine systems; and how closely you stick to the anti-yeast diet. It can take up to six months to overcome yeast overgrowth, but normally it takes from two to three months. How do you know it's gone? Retake the questionnaire after three months of your yeast-killing program. If you stop too soon, your yeast will just grow back and quickly cause carb/sweets cravings and make you feel bloated and miserable again. This had happened to many of our clients before they came to us.

AFTER THE FIRST FOUR WEEKS

Now add a piece of fruit and observe the response. If you bloat up and crave more sweet things after the experimental apple (or other fruit), wait another week or two before trying fruit again. The same goes for starchy grains and beans. Experiment and see for yourself. You'll usually be ready by week four to expand the amount of carbohydrates you can eat, at least a little.

Alcohol, sugar, and some other substances cannot be reintroduced. The only reason fruit can be added back in so quickly is the effectiveness of the anti-yeast supplements used in our program. Without them, fruit would have to be withheld for an additional four to six weeks or longer.

SUPPLEMENTS FOR PRUNING YEAST OVERGROWTH

Please note: This program is only for yeast and fungal infections that have gotten out of hand, not for the rare vaginal infection.

One of our yeast-recovery success stories is Risa, a blue-eyed brunette who played the violin professionally and who had suffered with chronic yeast infections. For three years they flared up every month before her period. She sometimes bloated so much that people thought she might be pregnant. She ate almost nothing but carbs and was spacey and miserable. Her score on the yeast questionnaire—the same one that you have on page 98—was 300. It's supposed to be under 100. On our anti-yeast program, she lost her cravings and most of her bloat in the first week. She used a special douche in addition to the oral supplements, so that by her next period she was free of her vaginal symptoms, too. When she retook the questionnaire, her score was 59!

Risa, like other Recovery Systems clients, took a combination of herbal remedies to fight her infection. A number of herbs exhibit potent and proven anti-yeast properties, but most herbalists agree that combination herbal remedies are much more effective than taking any one herb alone. Try to find a practitioner who has experience combining these herbs. The following herbs are generally available through health professionals, health food stores, and online, including at dietcure.com. Our clinic always includes these basics in anti-yeast protocols, adding additional products if needed.

INGREDIENTS FOR YOUR ANTI-YEAST SUPPLEMENT PROGRAM

✦ *Probiotics* (i.e., friendly bacteria). There should be trillions in the gut, particularly *lactobacillus* and *bifidus*, to prevent yeasts from taking over after good bacteria have been destroyed by antibiotics (along with the bad). Ask for the most potent available, ideally at least 50 billion per capsule with multiple strains; for example, NOW's Probiotic-10, or Flora Probiotic Plus, by Golden Health Products. The refrigerated variety is preferable, but probiotics that do not need refrigeration are invaluable for trips (they can help save your life in India!).

✦ *Pau d'arco.* This South American herb contains three anti-yeast compounds that are active against *Candida albicans* and fungi. Effective in tea, liquid extract, and capsules.

✦ *Grapefruit seed extract (GSE).* GSE kills yeasts and is nontoxic to humans. GSE, which comes in liquid concentrate form or in capsules, may also be used as a skin cleanser, gargle, douche, and as a traveler's aid to minimize gastrointestinal problems (it discourages parasites, too).

✦ *Garlic* inhibits microbes of all kinds, including yeasts and parasites. It is most active in raw form, fresh, on food, but it also may be taken in capsule form: one to three times daily, with meals. Most people use a combination of the two (three capsules is equal to a medium clove of fresh garlic). To help counter the powerful smell, chew one or more of the following herbal breath fresheners: parsley, fenugreek, or fennel.

✦ *Oregano oil* packs a wallop against a wide range of fungi and yeasts and has antiparasitic properties as well. *Caution:* Twenty-five percent of humans may tolerate only a small amount. That's why we now include it only in a mixed anti-yeast product such as NOW Foods' Candida Clear. (The same holds true for caprylic acid, another potent yeast killer.)

✦ *Biotin* is a B vitamin that helps stop sugar cravings and prevents yeasts from converting to the more damaging fungal form.

✦ *Ginger* gently inhibits both fungus and yeast while promoting friendly bacteria. Use fresh ginger to make tea or sauté in stir-frys.

ANTI-YEAST PROTOCOL

✦ *Upon arising:* Take 2 capsules of a combination of probiotics (50–100 billion) on an empty stomach.

✦ *With meals:* Take 1 to 2 capsules of grapefruit seed extract, 1 capsule of biotin (1,000 micrograms), 2 capsules or a small clove of garlic, and a product such as NOW Foods' Candida Clear, which combines oregano oil, pau d'arco, and caprylic acid.

✦ *Anytime:* Drink pau d'arco and ginger tea.

✦ *Bedtime:* Take 2 more capsules of probiotics.

Combine these yeast fighters with the foods described earlier. At Recovery Systems we use these nutrients and others that are not available in stores in a three-month protocol that you can order from us. (See dietcure.com.)

DRUGS THAT ERADICATE YEAST

When people do not respond to the herbal-based anti-yeast program, we refer them to a physician for a course of antifungal medication; for example, Diflucan (fluconazole), Nizoral (ketoconazole), or Sporanox (itraconazole). Yeast/fungal eliminating medications are usually taken daily for one to three months. Most people seem to do quite well on them, but some experience a die-off reaction in the third week. Be prepared for this; otherwise, you may conclude you're getting worse. To minimize die-off reactions, drink extra fluids, get plenty of vitamin C, and/or soak in a bath of Epsom salts (3 cups of Epsom salts to a bathtub of water). The liver-protecting herb milk thistle can help, too, if these drugs raise liver enzymes (we've never seen it). But for those with lots of bloating, nystatin or (oral) amphotericin B are sometimes added, as they exclusively work in the gut, while the others kill yeast throughout the body, including the vagina and sinuses. AIDS patients are often kept alive by these medicines that kill the opportunistic organisms we call yeast.

Yeasts That Won't Go Away

If you have been treated for a yeast overgrowth for three months or longer and you are not well on the road to recovery, one or more of the following conditions may be a factor that you'll need to discuss with a health professional:

✦ Parasites, or microbial organisms (giardia, amebas, and many others)

✦ Epstein-Barr virus (EBV), cytomegalovirus (CMV), or chronic fatigue syndrome associated with herpes or Lyme disease

✦ Hepatitis C

✦ Chronic gallbladder problems

✦ Allergies to foods listed on page 228, or adverse reactions to one or more of the anti-yeast supplements

It will take a few months and some hard work to get rid of your yeast overgrowth once and for all, but you should lose your cravings and start feeling better right away, which will encourage you to finish the kill-off meticulously. There is life after yeast!

ACTION STEPS

1. Get a blood and a stool test.
2. Find and organize your special anti-yeast foods and supplements along with the basic supplements listed in chapter seventeen.
3. Use an alternative pharmaceutical approach, if needed.
4. Follow the anti-yeast diet for four weeks.
5. After four weeks, gradually liberalize the diet.
6. If you don't respond, get parasite testing to rule out the possibility of a dual problem.

Reading

Ann Boroch, C.NC., *The Candida Cure: Yeast, Fungus, and Your Health—the 90-Day Program to Beat Candida and Restore Vibrant Health* (Quintessential Healing, 2009).

Resources

For help finding a health professional to test for and treat yeasts (or parasites), see the Resources for chapter twenty-one.

For an anti-yeast protocol that the Recovery Systems Clinic uses, call (800) 733-9293.

TESTING

Blood antibody testing for yeasts is done at most labs, but is not terribly accurate.

For stool testing for yeasts (and toxic bacteria) our clinic uses:
Genova Diagnostics for practitioners, (800) 522-4762.
Order two tests to be done at home three days apart.

For stool testing that also tests for parasites our medical consultant uses:
Metametrix Clinical Laboratory (DNA testing), (800) 221-4640, metametrix .com; or Doctor's Data labs, (800) 323-2784, doctorsdata.com.

SIXTEEN

The Fatty Acid Fix

Before we get to the cures, let's review the possible causes of your fat cravings: You could be after the pleasure that fats elicit because your endorphin levels are too low; you might be deficient in omega-3 or GLA from too much low-fat dieting or high omega-6 fat intake, or because your genetic needs for those fats are so high; or you may lack fat-digesting enzymes, have liver-gallbladder problems, or have intestinal parasites.

In this chapter you will learn about the supplements that can end the allure of greasy foods, improve liver or gallbladder function, and purge parasites, if necessary.

TESTING

Good blood testing (see page 362) can provide all the data that you'll need: Are your fatty acid and vitamin D levels optimal? Is your total cholesterol over 260 or under 170? Ill health appears above or below those levels. What is your ratio of LDL to HDL? It won't look good if your bad fat intake and, more important, your carb intake have been too high for a long time. But cutting the excess carbs will change that. We see cholesterol levels drop quickly at our clinic, just as studies on Dr. Atkins's diet have proven.

If you suspect a liver or gallbladder problem, get a physical exam, as well as a blood test for liver enzymes and for hepatitis A, B, and C. If you suspect a parasite, see page 105 for a symptom list and specific suggestions for testing (and treating).

WHO NEEDS THOSE CREAMY, CRUNCHY COMFORT FOODS?

That's what you'll probably say about ten minutes (I'm not kidding) after you try DL-phenylalanine (DLPA), the naturally comforting supplement that I rave about in chapters one and nine. DLPA helps raise the levels of your own powerful pleasure chemicals, the endorphins. It will help you to enjoy moderate portions of healthy fats instead of overdoing fried foods, cheese, and peanut butter. If, like me, you still can't be moderate about one or more of these fatty foods, the only solution is total abstinence—but with DLPA you won't care! Our clients don't call DLPA "the break-up pill" for nothing. Scan chapters one and nine to determine if DLPA is for you and at what dose.

FROM FISH TO NUTS: FOODS THAT RESTORE OMEGA FAT BALANCE

To be sure you are getting enough healthy fat and to get rid of fat cravings, optimize your intake of the essential fats. First, to restore omega-3 levels, eat the fish listed on pages 271–272 at least twice a week. These fish include wild salmon (especially the meat near the skin), sardines (especially those packed in their own oil), mackerel, and herring. *Not* tuna (a lean fish loaded with mercury). Avoid farmed fish, whose nutrient makeup is doubtful. Please also take the fish oil included in your basic supplements in chapter seventeen, if you have the "fishy" genetics I mentioned earlier. Flaxseed oil is high in ALA, the crude form of omega-3. It is very fragile, so keep it in the freezer (it won't solidify). You can also just throw some seeds from the freezer into your smoothies (great for keeping you regular, too).

Getting enough omega-6 fats is easy. Have a small handful of raw seeds or nuts (preferably soaked overnight and then rinsed to remove digestion inhibitors), put them in a breakfast smoothie with fruit and protein powder, or sprinkle them on a salad a few times a week. The most prized omega-6 oil is GLA—similar to omega-3 in its anti-inflammatory powers (it's great for PMS). GLA oil can be found as a supplement derived from the evening primrose plant or black currant seeds.

OILS

Almost all vegetable oils contain some of the two essential fats and many others in some ratio, but oils with a good balance of omega-3 to omega-6 are rare, and they're usually rancid by the time they're bottled, because they are so easily damaged by heat, light, and oxygen.

For your salads, use extra virgin olive oil (domestic is best). Although olive oil is low in omega-3's, it's even lower in omega-6 oils (which is good). It lowers cholesterol and does not block omega-3 function, as other vegetable oils do. Use it for cooking, but not frying. Hotter cooking, like frying, should be done with butter or coconut oil.

DARK GREEN LEAFY VEGETABLES

Dark green leafy vegetables are another source of omega-3. To eat more of these, try chard, kale, spinach, arugula, collards, mustard greens, and mesclun salad mix. If you haven't baked kale till it crisps, with sprinkles of olive oil and salt, you've missed a treat!

WALNUTS

Walnuts are the only nut besides the Brazil nut with enough omega-3 to balance omega-6 effectively. Most nuts and seeds are much higher in omega-6 than omega-3 oils. Eat walnuts only when they are fresh, in the fall and winter, unless they are left in the shell and cracked just before eating. You can try freezing them as well. The packaged, shelled variety get rancid faster than any other nuts.

FATTY FOODS TO FLUSH

Fats that we used to think were safer than butter are the fragile vegetable oils, like soy, canola, corn, and safflower, that become rancid quickly when exposed to heat and light in processing, even before bottling. They contain little omega-3 and lots of the omega-6 fatty acids—and we are all getting too much of them—contributing to the cardiovascular problems that are so common now. Unrefined, early press flax oil, available at health food stores in the refrigerator case, contain protective elements, like vitamin E, that keep it more stable. But otherwise avoid using these damaged oils at home, and ask for olive oil in restaurants.

Other problem fats are the chemically fried fats: the partially hydrogenated vegetable oils (that is, shortening) found in most packaged foods like cookies and crackers. Hydrogenated and even partially hydrogenated oils have been fried with hydrogen and metal for six to eight hours. This converts them from their natural liquid state into solid, indigestible trans fats, which are unquestionably linked to heart disease. (Why are these fats still served in our hospitals?) A trans fat is a mystery fat. Your body doesn't know what to do with it, so it gets slapped onto your artery walls, creating a crust of plaque.

Oils that are used repeatedly for deep-fat frying become health hazards, even if they are basically stable, like coconut or palm oils. Fried fats block or destroy the essential omega fats and the fat-soluble vitamins D, E, A, and K.[1]

So run from any fully or partially hydrogenated trans fats.[2] Read your labels! Avoid fried foods and most vegetable oils. Enjoy butter, ghee, coconut oil (and coconut milk), and extra virgin olive oil.

ALCOHOLISM, DEPRESSION, AND OIL

As I explained in chapter eight, if you are from a family that is Scandinavian, Irish, Scottish, Welsh, or coastal Native American, you are more likely to suffer from alcoholism and depression because of a lack of fish oils in your diet. Depression and cravings for alcohol, as well as fat, can respond to the use of fish oil.[3] If you belong to one of these groups but do not want to use fish oil, use flax and algae oils together as described. *Note:* Alcoholics often also benefit from evening primrose oil high in GLA.

MORE SUPPLEMENTS THAT CAN STOP YOUR FAT CRAVINGS

✦ Try 100 mg EPA/DHA twice daily in **fish oil** for a few months while you slash your high O-6 vegetable oil intake. If your fatty acid test then shows you to be deficient in DHA or EPA and you don't eat fish, I suggest you continue to take fish or cod liver oil (like Carlson's cod liver oil with reduced vitamin A) and retest in six months. Flax caps are a good option for some, but others cannot break down this high Omega-3 vegetable oil into DHA and EPA, and must get them directly from fish or low-potency algae oil. Red and brown seaweed are the only other direct sources.

  If you are a vegetarian or can't digest the fish oil caps, flaxseed oil is the next closest thing to fish oil (only without the already-converted EPA and DHA that some genetic types need). But you can supplement your flax oil by ordering supplements made from DHA-rich algae oil. A dose of 100 milligrams twice per day (at breakfast and dinner) gives the same DHA as that in two fish oil capsules.

✦ **Lipase** is the specific digestive enzyme that helps you break down the fats you eat. You can find it as part of a complete digestive enzyme supplement that also includes enzymes that help digest proteins and carbohydrates. But you can get it by itself, too. Look for a product containing lipase with at least 8,000 USP units.

✦ The nutrients that are most crucial for helping you to utilize all of your essential and other fats are included in the Basic Supplement Plan. Vitamins A and E (both fat-soluble vitamins) work together with vitamin C and the mineral selenium to protect all the fats in your body from oxidation (that is, rancidity). Vitamin A is especially instrumental in keeping your skin moist and oiled. Most of the oils that you use have had their protective vitamin E removed so that they'll look pretty in their clear bottles. You'll have to put vitamin E back in. Selenium may have earned its reputation as a cancer fighter from its ability to guard the layer of fat around every one of our bodies' cells. All the B vitamins enhance the effectiveness of the omega oils that you take in.

Note: There is some controversy about the purity and safety of fish oil supplements as this oil is very fragile and full of sea-borne toxins that must be removed. (This is why I prefer your eating smaller, wild, cold water fish instead, whenever possible.) Avoid high doses long term, unless you have specific health problems that require them. Taste-test for freshness: bite open a caplet and make sure it is not very fishy tasting.

LIVER, GALLBLADDER, AND PARASITE SOLUTIONS

Consult a holistic health professional about any liver or gallbladder problems. Acupuncturists, in particular, can often be very effective in diagnosing and treating them. They are actually the only health professionals I know of who can successfully treat the liver for hepatitis C and help with liver cirrhosis, too (though milk thistle and SAM-e also have a good track record there). When we see symptoms of liver problems, the first thing we do is suggest an herb that has convinced even the medical community that natural methods can be remarkable: milk thistle. This herb can be very helpful to the liver in its vital job of filtering toxic or useless substances out of our bodies. If it is clogged with toxins, the liver can't process fats properly. Try 300 milligrams of milk thistle twice a day to see if that heavy feeling after eating fatty foods fades. For pale stools (low bile output) use artichoke extract. Lecithin caps or granules and ox bile help emulsify fats for those of you who have lost your gallbladders.

If you think you may have parasites, see page 105 for a symptom questionnaire and directions for stool testing and treatment.

SUPPLEMENTS

	AM	B	MM	L	MA	D	BT*
☐ DLPA	1-2	—	1-2	—	1-2	—	—
☐ Omega-3 (fish oil caps with DHA and EPA), 1,000 mg	—	1	—	—	—	1	—
OR:							
☐ Flax oil caps, 1,000 mg *or*	—	1	—	1	—	1	—
Algae oil, 100 mg	—	1	—	1	—	1	—
For Liver and Gallbladder Problems:							
☐ Milk thistle, 300 mg	—	2	—	—	—	2	—
☐ Artichoke extract	2		—		—		—
☐ Lecithin granules, 1 tsp	—	1	—	1	—	1	—
As a Fat-Digestion Aid:							
☐ Lipase, at least 8,000 USP units	—	1	—	1	—	1	—

*AM = on arising; B = breakfast; MM = midmorning; L = with lunch; MA = midafternoon; D = with dinner; BT = at bedtime.

ACTION STEPS

1. Try DLPA to stop comfort-fat cravings.
2. Eat fish at least twice a week and/or take omega-3 fish oil (and/or flax oil).
3. Avoid hydrogenated fats, vegetable oils (except extra virgin olive, coconut, and palm oil), and fried foods.
4. Try milk thistle, artichoke, lecithin, or ox bile for symptoms of liver or gallbladder trouble.
5. Test for and treat any liver or parasite problems.
6. Get acupuncture for liver or gallbladder problems.

Readings

Dr. Mary Enig and Sally Fallon, *Eat Fat, Lose Fat: The Healthy Alternative to Trans Fats* (New York: Plume Books, 2006).

Ann Louise Gittleman, M.S., with J. Maxwell Desgrey, *Beyond Pritikin: A Total Nutrition Program for Weight Loss, Longevity, and Good Health* (New York: Bantam Books, 1996).

Michael Murray, N.D., and Joseph Pizzorno, N.D., *Encyclopedia of Natural Medicine*, Revised 2nd Edition (New York: Three Rivers Press, 1997).

Uffe Ravnskov, M.D., Ph.D., *Fat and Cholesterol Are Good for You* (Sweden: GB Publishing, 2009).

Donald Rudin, M.D., and Clara Felix, *Omega-3 Oils: A Practical Guide* (New York: Avery, 1996).

Artemis P. Simopoulos, M.D., and Jo Robinson, *The Omega Diet: The Lifesaving Nutritional Program Based on the Best of the Mediterranean Diets* (New York: HarperPerennial, 1999).

Gary Taubes, *Good Calories, Bad Calories: Fats, Carbs, and the Controversial Science of Diet and Health* (New York: Anchor Books, 2008).

Resources

For directions on how to contact holistic health practitioners, see Resources in chapter twenty-one.

SUPPLEMENTS

Fish oil capsules are widely available, as are flax. Vegetarians can supplement their flax oil by ordering supplements made from DHA-rich algae oil. Call Martek Biosciences Corporation at (800) 662-6339 (Dietary Supplements). Martek sells to both retail and practitioners.

Part III

Your Master Plan
for the Diet Cure

SEVENTEEN

Your Master Nutritional Supplement Plan

Up until now, you've been identifying your body's imbalances and learning how to use supplements to correct each of them nutritionally. Now it's time to put it all together in a Master Supplement Plan. Your Master Supplement Plan will be laid out in two parts: (1) the basic supplements that you'll be taking regardless of which imbalances you have and that you'll need to take long-term; and (2) the special repair supplements targeted at specific imbalances, which you'll be taking short-term.

Every one of the supplements recommended in this book will be listed here in this chapter. The basic supplements list will include suggested amounts. The special repair supplements list will be left blank so that you can fill it with the amounts you decide to take, based on the recommendations in Part II, chapters nine through sixteen.

I have tried to list supplements that you'll be able to find in health food stores, through mail order sources, and in some drugstores. Starred (*) supplements need to be special-ordered (by you or through your health consultant) because they cannot usually be found in stores or catalogs. I have listed these less accessible supplements only when I knew of no other supplement that works well for the particular purpose. This doesn't mean that good options don't exist, but that at our clinic we have not discovered or used them. These less accessible supplements or any of the exact supplements we use for our clients can be ordered from dietcure.com or the order line that our clinic uses: (800) 733-9293.

YOUR MASTER SUPPLEMENT PLAN

You'll need to take quite a few supplements at first. Then over the next three to twelve months, as you establish consistently more nutritious eating habits, you'll cut down to the six most basic supplements. These you should probably continue to take permanently. You should always reintroduce your special repair supplements if you need them temporarily to get you over any rough times.

THE BASIC SUPPLEMENTS

I have been alluding to the basic supplements throughout the book because they really are the basis for your Diet Cure, the support for your Master Food Plan. The broad collection of supplements included in these basics are intended to restore any nutrient depletions you have (we all have them) and to keep your nutrient levels strong permanently.

One of our nutritional consultants has been doing very detailed diet analyses for years. She has never found any diet, including the rich and healthy diets of superathletes, that meets 100 percent of the essential nutrients at even the minimal Recommended Daily Allowance (RDA) levels. (The RDA was the original U.S. governmental standard for preventing severe nutrient deficiencies, like scurvy. The standard for actually establishing health is called the Dietary Reference Intake, DRI, and is much higher.) There are just too many obstacles—among them heat, light, age, processing, and inadequate soil—between you and the amount of nutrients it takes to keep you happy and healthy.

YOUR BASIC MULTIPLE VITAMIN AND
MINERAL SUPPLEMENTATION

This basic collection of vital nutrients is intended to be safe enough to take permanently yet potent enough (in combination with your new foods) that they can actually correct some of your imbalances without any additional, more targeted repair supplements. Good multivitamins and minerals are the crown jewel of your Basic Supplement Plan. Look at the results of just two of many studies on the use of multis like the one you'll be taking (for the rest of your life, I hope):

1. A study of four hundred women found that taking a multi resulted in a 50 percent lower risk of having babies with any congenital abnormality.[1]
2. A ten-year study of nine hundred people found that taking a multi lowered the risk of colon cancer by half.[2]

Our clinic used and discarded dozens of multis over the years as better formulations appeared, until we finally found one that satisfied us. This supplement, True Balance, is wonderful for most people who need a Diet Cure. The high amounts of chromium, biotin, and the herb gymnema are the unique ingredients that make True Balance so effective for eliminating carb cravings and blood sugar imbalances. Many health food stores and supplement mail order houses carry it. In case you need an alternative to True Balance, I will also list two other multis our nutritionists have determined to be of high quality. So that you'll know exactly what a good multi is, I'm going to lay out the contents of all three multis. Get your knowledgeable supplement specialist to help you make sure that you get a multi that is equivalent in quality to these three. Unfortunately, it is impossible to get enough of the nutrients you need in good multis without taking four to six of them per day. If you just can't manage to take a lunchtime dose, you could take half the daily dose at breakfast and half at dinner.

You'll see in the following chart just how many valuable nutrients are packed into a good multi. But even the best multis plus the best foods can't provide enough of certain nutrients. The chart also includes the amounts of four basic nutrients you'll need to take in addition to your multi. When selecting a multi, keep in mind that men and menopausal women who regularly eat red meat should avoid more than 18 milligrams of added iron. (Menstruating women can handle more iron safely because they are always losing excess in menstrual fluid.) For details on why you need each of the vitamins and minerals in your multi, read *Dr. Atkins' Vita-Nutrient Solution*, by Robert C. Atkins, M.D.

WHAT IS A GOOD MULTI?

NUTRIENT CONTENTS FOR SUGGESTED DOSE PER DAY			
Brand	TRUE BALANCE	MY FAVORITE MULTIPLE	ALLERGY MULTI
Number suggested per day	4 capsules:	6 capsules or 4 tablets:	6 capsules:
❑ Vitamin A		5,000 IU	10,000 IU
❑ Beta carotene	5,000 IU	5,000 IU	15,000 IU
❑ B_1 (thiamine)	60 mg	50 mg	25 mg
❑ B_2 (riboflavin)	30 mg	50 mg	25 mg
❑ B_6 (pyridoxine)	33 mg	50 mg	50 mg
❑ B_{12}	80 mcg	50 mcg	100 mcg
❑ Niacin	70 mg	50 mg	
❑ Niacinamide	70 mg		100 mg
❑ Pantothenic acid	120 mg	50 mg	50 mg
❑ Biotin	3,200 mcg	300 mcg	150 mcg
❑ Folic acid	800 mcg	400 mcg	400 mcg
❑ PABA		50 mg	25 mg
❑ Choline	30 mg	50 mg	25 mg
❑ Inositol	30 mg	50 mg	25 mg
❑ Vitamin C	240 mg	250 mg	1,000 mg
❑ Vitamin D_3	250 IU	400 IU	400 IU
❑ Vitamin E	400 IU	400 IU	400 IU
❑ Chromium	800 mcg	200 mcg	200 mcg
❑ (Chromium needed in addition to multi)	(None)	(600 mcg)	(600 mcg)
❑ Calcium	200 mg	1,000 mg	1,000 mg
❑ (Calcium needed in addition to multi)	(300–500 mg)	(None)	(None)
❑ Magnesium	240 mg	400 mg	500 mg
❑ Potassium	100 mg	99 mg	99 mg
❑ Zinc	30 mg	25 mg	30 mg
❑ Manganese	5 mg	2 mg	10 mg
❑ Copper	1.8 mg	2 mg	2 mg
❑ Vanadium	18 mcg		
❑ Selenium	125 mcg	50 mcg	200 mcg

Brand	TRUE BALANCE	MY FAVORITE MULTIPLE	ALLERGY MULTI
☐ Iodine		150 mcg	
☐ Boron		200 mcg	
☐ Molybdenum		50 mcg	500 mcg
☐ Iron		Optional 18 mg	10 mg
☐ L-carnitine	30 mg		
☐ Bioflavonoids		150 mg	
☐ Gymnema silvestre	100 mg		

NAME OF MANUFACTURER	NAME OF MULTIVITAMIN MINERAL PRODUCT
1) NOW Foods	True Balance* (no iron)
2) Natrol	My Favorite Multiple capsules/tablets; My Favorite Multiple capsules/tablets without iron
3) Twinlab	Allergy Multi Caps (little iron)

All three of these are available from most health food stores (or they can be ordered for you). Internet sources are legion, and some have very good prices. You can also order these multis and any other supplements I mention in this book from dietcure.com, or call (800) 733-9293.

Trouble Swallowing Pills?

Those of you who hate swallowing pills can find sublingual, chewable, powdered, and liquid supplements through knowledgeable health practitioners and employees of good health food stores. Your trouble swallowing may be due to an enlarged thyroid (the thyroid gland sits in your throat). That's been the case with a number of our clients. Check chapter four to see if you have other low-thyroid symptoms.

Basic Magnesium and Calcium. Even very good multis, such as the three I've presented here, rarely contain enough of the minerals calcium and magnesium. These two minerals are too bulky to fit into a multi capsule or tablet along with all the other nutrients, since you need quite a bit of both. True Balance lacks sufficient levels of both calcium and magnesium. Twinlab's and Natrol's contain enough calcium but not enough magnesium.

Calcium's importance for building and protecting bone is now well established, but you may not know that calcium also helps with sleep and protects against colon cancer. Calcium has an inseparable mate, the mineral magnesium, which is deficient in 80 percent of us yet is even more vital than calcium. It protects us from heart attacks, Alzheimer's, constipation, low blood sugar, diabetes, eating disorders, chronic fatigue, low thyroid, PMS, and osteoporosis (to name only a few of its 325 benefits). Also, like all minerals, calcium and magnesium need to come from easily absorbed sources. (This is particularly important for magnesium, which can otherwise cause diarrhea.) Reliably absorbed minerals are chelated; that is, they are bound to tiny amino acids that transport them into your bloodstream. Solgar, Carlson, and other brands provide superior Albion-chelated calcium and magnesium.

Calcium and magnesium are listed right underneath your multi on your Basic Supplement Plan, which follows. Calcium is to be taken with breakfast *or* lunch, while magnesium should be taken at dinner.

Special Note for Vegans

If you eat *no* animal products, including fish, chicken, milk products, and eggs, your Basic Supplement Plan may not give you all the extra nutrients you'll need. Check your multi's contents against the following suggested amounts of key nutrients, and get any extra supplements you'll need to get up to these levels. Vegans (and vegetarians) should both test iron and ferriten levels and get a CBC test.

Vitamin B_{12}	500–1,000 mcg daily
Vitamin D	1,000–2,000 IU daily
	(more if testing indicates)
L-carnitine	1,000–2,000 mg daily
Zinc	25–50 mg daily
Selenium	100–200 mcg daily

Basic Vitamin B Complex. All eight imbalances require the B complex vitamins for repair and permanent balance maintenance. The B content of your multi won't be high enough to do the job without extra B complex for the first few months.

Coenzymated vitamins are already bound to the necessary amino acid and mineral cofactors. Many companies now make B complex using the most bioavailable, or coenzymate, forms of the vitamins. Or you can use an ordinary, low-potency B complex. Note: Premenopausal women need 4 milligrams of folic acid (i.e., vitamin B_9) per day to prevent birth defects. There is a form that is absorbed even when a genetic defect in folic acid metabolism makes the common form ineffective. It's called the L-5-MTHF (metafolin) form. It can be found alone or in the B-complex products mentioned above.

After the first three months, drop the extra B complex. The B's included in your basic multivitamin will suffice, since you'll be eating lots of fresh vegetables and other whole foods that contain B vitamins.

SUPPLEMENT PLANS BY CHAPTER

THE MASTER SUPPLEMENT PLAN

Basic Supplement Plan

Supplement	AM	B	MM	L	MA	D	BT*
❑ Multivitamin/mineral	—	2	—	(2)†	—	2	—
❑ Calcium, 250–350 mg	—	1	—	1	—	—	—
❑ Magnesium, 200 mg	—	1	—	—	—	1	—
❑ B complex, 10–25 mg	1	—	—	1	—	—	—
❑ Vitamin C with bioflavonoids, 1,000 mg C and 200–500 mg bioflavonoids	—	1	—	—	—	1	—
❑ Chromium, 200 mcg (not needed with True Balance)	—	2	—	—	—	2	—

Special Repair Supplements

Supplement	AM	B	MM	L	MA	D	BT*
Chapter Nine: Refueling Your Brain with Amino Acids							
❑ L-Glutamine, 500 mg	—	—	—	—	—	—	—
❑ GABA, 100–500 mg‡	—	—	—	—	—	—	—
❑ L-tyrosine, 500 mg	—	—	—	—	—	—	—

Supplement	AM	B	MM	L	MA	D	BT*
❏ L-phenylalanine, 500 mg	—	—	—	—	—	—	—
❏ DLPA, 500 mg *or* DPA, 500 mg	—	—	—	—	—	—	—
❏ 5-HTP (5-hydroxytryptophan), 50 mg *or* L-tryptophan, 500 mg	—	—	—	—	—	—	—
❏ St. John's wort, 300 mg	—	—	—	—	—	—	—
❏ Complete essential amino acids, 750 mg,	—	—	—	—	—	—	—
e.g., Total Amino Solution by Genesa	—	—	—	—	—	—	—

Chapter Ten: Nutritional Rehab for the Chronic Dieter

Anorexics and bulimics add the following supplements:

	AM	B	MM	L	MA	D	BT*
❏ Liquid zinc (only Ethical Nutrients' Zinc, Metagenics' Zinc Tally, *or* Biotics' Aqueous Zinc), 40 mg	—	—	—	—	—	—	—
❏ George's Aloe Juice, 4–8 oz	—	—	—	—	—	—	—
❏ Emergen-C Lite packets, 1,000 mg C with electrolytes (*instead* of the basic C)	—	—	—	—	—	—	—
❏ Stronger electrolytes, if needed							
❏ Vitamin B_1 100–200 mg$	—	—	—	—	—	—	—
❏ Vitamin B_6 100 mg	—	—	—	—	—	—	—

Chapter Eleven: Balancing Your Blood Sugar and Reviving Your Adrenals

	AM	B	MM	L	MA	D	BT*
❏ L-glutamine, 500 mg	—	—	—	—	—	—	—
❏ Biotin, 1,000 mcg (if not taking True Balance multi)	—	—	—	—	—	—	—
❏ Chromium, 200 mcg (if not taking True Balance Multi)	—	—	—	—	—	—	—

Adrenal Support Supplements

	AM	B	MM	L	MA	D	BT*
❏ Pantothenic acid, 100–500 mg**							
❏ Vitamin B_1, 100 mg$	—	—	—	—	—	—	—

Add as per your health professional's recommendation:

	AM	B	MM	L	MA	D	BT*
❏ IsoCort *or*	—	—	—	—	—	—	—
❏ Licorice							
❏ Cortisol (by prescription as Cortef) 2.5–7.5 mg	—	—	—	—	—	—	—
❏ DHEA	—	—	—	—	—	—	—

Supplement	AM	B	MM	L	MA	D	BT*
❏ Pregnenolone	—	—	—	—	—	—	—
❏ Seriphos	—	—	—	—	—	—	—
❏ Hydrolyzed casein	—	—	—	—	—	—	—

Chapter Twelve: Thyroid Solutions

Thyroid Boosters (if you have hypothyroidism but not thyroiditis)

❏ L-tyrosine, 500 mg	—	—	—	—	—	—	—
❏ Thyroid glandulars or homeopathics	—	—	—	—	—	—	—

Chapter Thirteen: Overcoming Addictions to Allergy Foods

❏ DLPA or DPA	—	—	—	—	—	—	—
❏ Professional's Care aloe vera juice	—	—	—	—	—	—	—
❏ Alka-Seltzer Gold or vitamin C powder	—	—	—	—	—	—	—

Chapter Fourteen: Hormone Help

For PMS

❏ Evening primrose oil	—	—	—	—	—	—	—
❏ Vitex	—	—	—	—	—	—	—
❏ Vitalzym	—	—	—	—	—	—	—

Herbs for Menopause

❏ Dong quai	—	—	—	—	—	—	—
❏ Black cohosh	—	—	—	—	—	—	—

Ultimate Hormonal Protocols

Add as per professional recommendation:

❏ Progesterone	—	—	—	—	—	—	—
❏ Estradiol	—	—	—	—	—	—	—
❏ Estriol	—	—	—	—	—	—	—
❏ Testosterone	—	—	—	—	—	—	—
❏ DHEA	—	—	—	—	—	—	—
❏ Pregnenolone	—	—	—	—	—	—	—

Chapter Fifteen: Yeast Elimination

(See separate lengthy protocol for yeasts at the end of chapter fifteen.)

Chapter Sixteen: The Fatty Acid Fix

❏ Fish oil (omega-3) or flax oil (ALA)	—	—	—	—	—	—	—

Supplement	AM	B	MM	L	MA	D	BT*
❏ Evening primrose oil	—	—	—	—	—	—	—
❏ Lipase, at least 8,000 USP	—	—	—	—	—	—	—
❏ Milk thistle (silymarin) *and/or*							
❏ Artichoke	—	—	—	—	—	—	—
❏ Lecithin granules, 1 tsp	—	—	—	—	—	—	—
❏ Parasite protocol (as per page 104)							
Other Supplements							
❏ _____	—	—	—	—	—	—	—
❏ _____	—	—	—	—	—	—	—
❏ _____	—	—	—	—	—	—	—

*AM = on arising; B = with breakfast; MM = midmorning; L = with lunch; MA = midafternoon; D = with dinner; BT = at bedtime.
†If you are taking True Balance or My Favorite Multiple tablets, it won't be necessary to take any at lunch, as there are only four a day to take.
‡GABA Calm, by Source Naturals, and True Calm, by NOW, combine GABA with the calming amino taurine.
§If you have more than one imbalance that calls for extra vitamin B, do not take more than 300 milligrams per day as an additional single-nutrient supplement, in doses of 100 milligrams.
**e.g., Source Naturals' GABA Calm or Country Life.

Basic Vitamin C with Bioflavonoids. In nature, vitamin C and bioflavonoids are always combined; they work best together that way as antioxidants that help prevent cancer, heart disease, asthma, and stress burnout, among other things. Our nutritionists generally recommend 2,000 to 3,000 milligrams per day—no more than what you'd get if you added two 1,000-milligram doses to the vitamin C in your multi.

Chromium. Chromium is a mineral that eliminates sugar cravings by improving your blood sugar balance, relieving stress, and helping to build muscle. Take extra doses to bring yourself up to 800–1,000 micrograms a day total (there's some chromium in the multi) for at least three months until your cravings are gone for good. (If you use True Balance or GlucoBalance as your multi, you won't need this extra chromium.)

Please make several copies of the Master Supplement Plan I've provided here and write in pencil, so that you can revise your plan over time as you change doses and start dropping supplements that you no longer need or start trying new ones. Review chapters nine through sixteen and fill in each special supplement section that pertains to you, based on the suggestions in the relevant chapters.

Supplements are foods and inherently safe. But like foods, not all nutritional supplements are needed by everyone, nor do they all agree with everyone. We are each unique, biochemically and genetically. Our reactions to supplements vary accordingly. In addition, supplements have gone through an elaborate pharmaceutical preparation process that leaves some tiny impurities that bother a few people. If you tend to be sensitive to medications or have many food sensitivities, you may already know whether you can or can't tolerate nutritional supplements. About one in one hundred clients at our clinic has some adverse reaction to a supplement even though he or she obviously needs it. More have adverse reactions, such as mild headaches, to supplements they don't need. Unpleasant reactions to supplements can indicate a liver problem that needs attention. Milk thistle (300 milligrams with breakfast and dinner) often sets it right.

So although supplements are rarely dangerous, they often let you know quickly if they are not appropriate for you. If, for example, at first you love magnesium for its relaxing and laxative effect but then begin to experience loose bowels, it's time to cut the dose.

Nutritional supplements are known for their safety, but there are some exceptions. If you have any concerns or questions, consult with a knowledgeable health professional before starting your supplement program. Your Master Supplement Plan will not provide overdoses of any nutrients, but I'd like you to know which nutrients could conceivably cause adverse symptoms at excessive doses:

Are Your Supplements Safe?

The U.S. death rate due to prescription and over-the-counter medications: 106,000 per year (290 deaths per day), according to the *Journal of the American Medical Association* in April 1998.[3] Since then it has increased 65 percent.

The U.S. death rate due to supplements: no deaths in 2008, according to the 2009 report by the American Association of Poison Control Centers.

IMPORTANT SUPPLEMENT PRECAUTIONS

VITAMINS AND MINERALS

Iron. This may be the only truly hazardous supplement. Just a few adult-dosage pills can kill a child. We used to think that men and menopausal women shouldn't take iron without careful supervision of their heart function, but recent studies have questioned iron's involvement in heart problems. With more than 18 milligrams per day, constipation and stomach upset can occur. At more than 100 milligrams per day, fatigue and weight loss can occur. A blood test for ferritin (sensitive iron) levels will rule out any problems.

Vitamin A. Doses above 50,000 IU can cause dizziness, blurred vision, headache, and nausea. If you're pregnant, too much or too little can cause birth defects.

Vitamin B$_3$ (niacin). Doses as low as 300 milligrams in one sitting can cause headache, nausea, low blood pressure, and a brief hot flush. Doses over 2 grams may cause liver damage.

Vitamin D. Vitamin D is actually a powerful hormone. Daily doses above 1,000–2,000 IU may cause nausea, headache, fatigue, diarrhea, skeletal pain, dry mouth, loss of appetite, and possibly irreversible kidney and heart problems. The sun is a better way to get vitamin D in the summer, before putting on sunscreen. For those with fair skin, ten to twelve minutes of exposure to the sun (on each side) is about all you can do safely. For those with darker skin, up to 120 minutes total may be okay before applying sunscreen.

Zinc. High doses (over 50 milligrams) cause nausea, anemia, dizziness, and lower immunity and HDL (good cholesterol), and they block copper absorption.

Vitamin B$_6$. More than 250 milligrams per day for prolonged periods can cause temporary nerve damage.

Selenium. More than 800 micrograms per day causes brittle hair and nails, dizziness, fatigue, nausea, diarrhea, and liver disease.

Copper. More than 2 milligrams (the RDA[†]) can cause nausea, head-ache, and jaundice.

Magnesium. More than 1,000 milligrams per day can cause diarrhea, low blood pressure, and nausea.[4]

AMINO ACIDS

You should consult a physician before taking *any* amino acids if:

- ✦ You have lupus.
- ✦ You have a serious physical illness.
- ✦ You have severe liver or kidney damage.
- ✦ You have an inborn error of amino acid metabolism (e.g., PKU).
- ✦ You have an overactive thyroid or Hashimoto's thyroiditis.
- ✦ You have an ulcer (aminos may be too acidic).
- ✦ You are pregnant.
- ✦ You are taking many medications.
- ✦ You have schizophrenia or other mental illness.

---

†   Recommended Daily Allowance.

If you:	You should consult a physician before taking:
have high blood pressure	tyrosine, DL-phenylalanine, L-phenylalanine
take MAO inhibitors	tyrosine, DL-phenylalanine, L-phenylalanine,
	L-tryptophan, 5-hydroxytryptophan (5-HTP)*
are hyperthyroid (or for some who have Hashimoto's thyroiditis)	tyrosine, DL-phenylalanine, L-phenylalanine
get migraine headaches or have melanoma	tyrosine, DL-phenylalanine, L-phenylalanine
take SSRIs (selective serotonin reuptake inhibitors), SNRIs (serotonin/norepinephrine reuptake inhibitors) or other drugs, like phentermine, that can activate serotonin	L-tryptophan, 5-hydroxytryptophan (5-HTP)*
have bipolar disorder (e.g., manic depression) or lymphatic cancers	L-glutamine (and fish or flax oil), tyrosine, DLPA, and phenylalanine (or SAM-e) can lift depression but can also trigger mania.
have very low blood pressure	GABA, taurine, niacin
have asthma	tryptophan, 5-HTP, *melatonin

If you are being treated for any serious illness or are on any medications, consult with your doctor about taking amino acids. Should you get permission from your doctor to try amino acids but experience discomfort of any kind taking them, discontinue them.

TAKING YOUR SUPPLEMENTS

Once you are clear on which supplements to take and have used the suggestions here and in chapter nineteen to purchase them, you'll be ready to start taking them.

✦ Whether you have one or more than one imbalance, you can start taking all of your rebalancing supplements at once, unless you are very sensitive and reactive to supplements (then introduce slowly).

✦ Watch your reactions to the supplements carefully.

✦ If there is a range of doses given, please start with the *lowest* dose of all of your supplements. Do this just to make sure you have no adverse reaction.

✦ If you've tried your supplements at the lowest dose and tolerated them well but got little benefit from them, go up to the next highest dose and watch your reactions again. But don't take more than the maximum doses recommended here without expert consultation.

✦ Record your body's responses in your food-mood log (see page 369) to help tune in and track progress or problems. If you've had a positive reaction to an amino acid at the lowest dose, for example, you may find that a higher dose is too much. (Most of our clients do better on the higher doses.)

✦ If you have any adverse symptoms (e.g., headache that starts only after certain supplements), check the troubleshooting tips that follow and stop taking, or lower the dosage of, the supplement that is the most likely culprit. If the symptoms don't stop quickly (within twenty-four hours), stop all supplements, and when the symptoms have disappeared, reintroduce your supplements one by one until you find the culprit. (Our clients have had to do this only very rarely.)

✦ To keep track of what you're taking, it can be very helpful to lay out your supplements in either small labeled plastic bags or plastic pill organizers with dividers designed to hold them all for several days.

✦ For help in adjusting your doses of supplements for best effect, read chapter twenty-two carefully, where I walk you through your first few weeks on your supplements. If you mistakenly take your breakfast, lunch, or dinner supplements without food, your multi may nauseate you.

✦ If you forget your between-meal supplements, just take them with your next meal. Don't skip them. They'll still work, just not quite as well.

✦ It can be hard to remember to take the supplements between meals. Use an alarm or a computer reminder.

Supplement Troubleshooting Table

Troubling Symptom	Supplements That May Be Implicated
Stomachache	hydrochloric acid (HCl), B complex, amino acids, fatty acids

Troubling Symptom	Supplements That May Be Implicated
Headaches	L-tyrosine, DLPA, L-phenylalanine, L-tryptophan, DHEA
Diarrhea	magnesium, vitamin C
Nausea	B complex, 5-HTP
Light sensitivity	St. John's wort
High blood pressure	licorice, L-trosine, L-phenylatamine, Isocort
Jitteriness	L-tyrosine, L-phenylalanine, DLPA, licorice, IsoCort, thyroid supplements
Acne, oily skin	DHEA
Insomnia	L-tyrosine, L-phenylalanine, DLPA, and sometimes 5-HTP, licorice, IsoCort, thyroid supplements, and fish oil

ELIMINATING YOUR SUPPLEMENTS

Once you have corrected your imbalances and your symptoms are gone, you can begin to experiment with going off your special repair supplements, one at a time. If your symptoms come back, you'll know that you still need that particular supplement for a while longer. Eliminate it again in a month and see what happens. Continue to do this until you no longer need any of your special repair supplements, but be ready to take them again short-term during stressful times, should you need to, in the future. Continue with your basic supplements. Experiment with varying your multi once or twice a year by trying a new one when your old multi runs out, to get a different ratio of nutrients. Notice any differences in how you feel after you buy your new multi.

In the next chapter you'll get some help in buying your Diet Cure supplies and getting ready to go into action.

Readings

Robert C. Atkins, M.D., *Dr. Atkins' Vita-Nutrient Solution: Nature's Answer to Drugs* (New York: Simon & Schuster, 1998). An interesting and readable tour of basic supplements.

Eric R. Braverman, M.D., et al., *The Healing Nutrients Within* (Laguna Beach, CA: Basic Health Publications, 2003). A complete guide to amino acid therapy.

Robert Crayhon, M.S., *The Carnitine Miracle: The Supernutrient Program That Promotes High Energy, Fat Burning, Heart Health, Brain Wellness, and Lon-*

gevity (New York: M. Evans and Co., 1998). This is good for vegetarians in particular.

Shari Lieberman, Ph.D., CNS, FACN, and Nancy Bruning, MPH, *The Real Vitamin and Mineral Book: The Definitive Guide to Designing Your Personal Supplement Program*, 4th Edition (New York: Avery, 2007).

Michael T. Murray, N.D., *Encyclopedia of Nutritional Supplements: The Essential Guide for Improving Your Health Naturally* (New York: Three Rivers Press, 1996).

Julia Ross, M.A., *The Mood Cure* (New York: Penguin Books, 2003).

Krispin Sullivan, C.N., *Naked at Noon: Understanding Sunlight and Vitamin D* (2011). Available at sunlightd.org.

Resources

See chapter nineteen (pages 317–318) for complete information on sources for all the supplements that I recommend in this book and list in this chapter. The simplest way to start may be to order anything you can't find locally at dietcure.com under "Order Books, Nutrients, and CDs" or call (800) 733-9293. Otherwise you'll be ordering supplements from several different sources. I suggest you do that later, when you know for sure which supplements you'll be reordering and feel up to comparison shopping.

EIGHTEEN

Your Master Eating Plan

A Nutritional Survival Guide

B efore I go into detail about how you can best feed yourself, I want to try to free you from the question "How *much* nourishing food should I eat?" I don't believe that there is one answer for everyone. We are each unique, especially in the United States, where our activity levels and genetic ancestries are too varied to be calorically predictable. What we do know is that twenty-first-century-style commercial American food has created unprecedented weight and health problems for much of the entire world. *Any* of the refined sugars, starches, and fats that comprise it could be hazardous to you, depending on your unique tolerance level. We also know that eating too little healthy food is hazardous. The World Health Organization has determined that below 2,100 calories, women begin to experience starvation. For men it's below 2,300 calories.

Proportion is the other important consideration. On the next page you'll see an illustration of what the proportions of your nutritious fare will look like. Your plate will be crowded with delicious foods. But what, exactly, should be included?

WHAT IS THE IDEAL MEAL?

DIET CURE PLATE

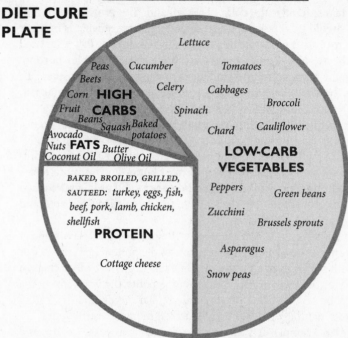

Lettuce

Peas
Beets
Corn **HIGH CARBS**
Fruit
Beans
Avocado Squash Baked potatoes
Nuts **FATS** Butter
Coconut Oil Olive Oil

Cucumber
Celery
Spinach

Tomatoes
Cabbages
Chard

Broccoli
Cauliflower

LOW-CARB VEGETABLES

Peppers
Zucchini

Green beans

Brussels sprouts

Asparagus

Snow peas

BAKED, BROILED, GRILLED,
SAUTÉED: turkey, eggs, fish,
beef, pork, lamb, chicken,
shellfish
PROTEIN

Cottage cheese

TYPICAL DINNER PLATE

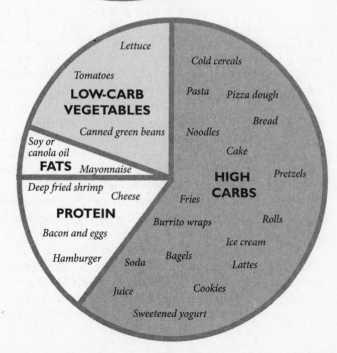

Lettuce

Tomatoes

LOW-CARB VEGETABLES

Canned green beans

Soy or canola oil
FATS Mayonnaise

Deep fried shrimp
Cheese
PROTEIN

Bacon and eggs

Hamburger

Cold cereals
Pasta Pizza dough
Bread
Noodles
Cake

HIGH CARBS

Pretzels

Fries
Burrito wraps
Rolls
Ice cream
Soda Bagels
Lattes
Juice Cookies

Sweetened yogurt

To start, take a look at the palm of your hand. The protein portion of the meal should be about palm-size: about a quarter of what is on your plate. High-protein foods include meat, chicken, turkey, fish, eggs, and cottage cheese. Next comes the low-carbohydrate vegetables portion, which ideally takes up more than half of your plate: lettuce, asparagus, tomatoes, broccoli, cabbage, celery, cucumbers, kale, and spinach to mention a few.

Reserve a corner of the plate for the high-carb vegetables, grains, legumes, or fruits, including potatoes, yams, polenta, beans, and rice. Finally, allot a small percent of your plate to the compact oils used to prepare or flavor foods, whether in the form of butter on your potato or a few tablespoons of extra virgin olive oil on your salad or in your cooked veggies (this is in addition to the fat in your fish, chicken skin, nuts, and avocados).

What about priority? Where to start? Begin your meal with some of the low-carb veggies (e.g., salad) and some of the protein (e.g., poultry or lamb). Both will contain some wholesome fats (e.g., olive oil or chicken skin). When you've taken the edge off your appetite, dig into some of the starchier food on your plate. Then eat as you like. You'll find that eating in this order naturally reduces undue interest in higher-carb foods.

Here's an example: If your favorite dinner is a steak, potato, and salad, I encourage you to enjoy this American favorite. Your steak should be about the size of your palm (takes up almost a fourth of your plate). Don't just have a little side salad—have a salad loaded with a variety of vegetables, at least three to four times the size of your meat (if you have cooked vegetables, they should be about twice the size of your meat, but salad is bulkier). Have a moderate-size potato. For fat, enjoy butter on your potato and olive oil dressing on your salad. Start with some salad and steak. Then move on to some potato.

But don't go hungry! If you feel you want more food, have it. Just have it roughly in the proportions I've just described. If you want extra-high-carb foods on a regular basis, without balancing protein, ask yourself, "Is this a more ideal proportion for me or am I out of balance?" You'll find the answer in how you feel after your meals: strong and content or heavy and dissatisfied. If the latter, make sure you're taking your chapter one aminos to stop carb cravings.

The ideal proportion of protein to healthy carbohydrate varies somewhat from one person (or meal) to another, but our most successful clients are the ones who eat three meals, each with 20–30 grams or more of protein, and at least four cups of low-carbohydrate vegetables and two fruits a day, plus several tablespoons of healthy fat. To this nutrient-rich base, they add whatever extra healthy carbs, fats, and proteins they need. Once your cravings are gone, you can decide how much potato, avocado, butter, or apricots feels satisfying. I want you to find out for yourself what your ideal foods and amounts are. The Diet Cure is designed to give you the freedom and confidence to do just that.

Now that you're clear on what to eat and in what order, the last critical factor in your Master Eating Plan is *when* to eat:

1. Never skip meals. Skipping breakfast in particular automatically slows metabolism and induces afternoon and evening food cravings and overeating.
2. Eat three substantial, balanced meals per day—morning, midday, and evening.
3. Eat breakfast within one hour of arising. Eat at least 25 percent of your day's calories at breakfast, the only meal that speeds up calorie burning. You may be like many of our clients, who stop all compulsive eating simply by adding a solid and early breakfast. If you can't stand to eat in the morning, at least drink a healthy smoothie. (See smoothie recipes in chapter twenty, "Menus, Meal Ideas, and Recipes.")
4. Eat lunch no more than four to five hours after breakfast and dinner no more than four to five hours after lunch.
5. If you sag (i.e., get tired, weak, or grouchy, or crave carbs) between meals, have well-balanced snacks. Prepare fruit or vegetables with proteins (for example, apple and nuts or cheese), as per chapter twenty. Add a bedtime snack if you eat dinner early and get hungry or cravey later.
6. Plan to get to sleep close to 10 P.M. (with the help of tryptophan, 5-HTP, and/or melatonin, if necessary). Getting to sleep early often takes care of late-night munching and helps you wake in time to make a nice breakfast. (If getting to sleep is a more serious problem, see the sleep chapter in my book *The Mood Cure*.)

NUTRITIONAL SURVIVAL TRAINING

There are only six nutrient groups essential to life. In order of importance, they are water, protein, fat, carbohydrate, mineral, and vitamin. Many billions of advertising dollars are spent each year to entice you to buy processed food devoid of anything but cheap, damaged carbs and fats that provide you with *none* of the nutrients you require to survive and thrive. Food marketing preys on your emotional needs, with Coca-

Cola promoted as "the real thing," and products that are loaded with refined flour and sugar promoted as healthy because they are "low-fat."
More important is the fact that this industry has knowingly increased
the addictiveness of its products, just as the tobacco industry did—and
even more lethally!

Yet at no other time in history have so many truly nutritious foods
been available, and we know more about foods and their effects on the
body than ever before. We're starting to realize that the most important
element in the prevention and treatment of disease is diet and lifestyle.
But we've also been getting conflicting information for years about what
foods are good and what foods are bad. Though most of us know that we
need vegetables and fruits, we don't know for sure what else to eat, and
we've become so addicted to commercial carbs that we've largely lost our
taste for these or any other healthier foods.

The first sixteen chapters of *The Diet Cure* teach you how to free
yourself from the tyranny of addictive foods. In this final section you'll
learn about what to eat instead. These next three chapters will teach you
about why you'll need which foods and why to avoid others, and they'll
give you specifics about what you can cook, order at a restaurant, or
snack on between meals.

This chapter is a basic survival course in nutrition. Let's start by
looking at a summary of the foods that will maximize your health. Then
we'll learn more about each of these nutrient-dense foods. Finally, we'll
go to the rogue's gallery of foods to avoid and examine the downside of
being vegetarian.

Your Daily Food Guide

This rough guide will help you to keep track of whether you
are consuming enough of the right kinds of foods in your meals
and snacks.

Protein
20–30 concentrated grams per meal from poultry, meat, fish,
eggs, or cheese (or less concentrated beans, nuts, or seeds)

Low-Carbohydrate Vegetables
At least 4 cups per day of zucchini, cauliflower, green beans,
carrots, spaghetti squash, turnips, beets, kohlrabi, eggplant, mushrooms, chard, turnip greens, kale, or other low-carb choice:

+ 6 spears asparagus = ½ cup
+ 1 head broccoli = 1½ cups
+ 1 salad tomato = ⅔ cup
+ 3 stalks raw celery = 1 cup
+ 1 cup raw salad greens (leaf lettuce, romaine, cabbage, spinach, arugula, etc.) counts as ½ cup when calculating the 4 cups per day

High-Carbohydrate Foods*
Legumes
Up to 1 cup per day (more for vegetarians and fast metabolizers, or in winter):
+ 1 cup = ½ can of garbanzo, black, kidney, refried, or navy beans
+ 1 cup = 8 oz. split pea soup or lentil dahl
+ 1 cup = ⅓ cup dry beans measured before cooking

High-Carb Vegetables
1 to 2 cups (cooked or raw equivalent) per day:
+ 1 cup = 8 oz. cooked butternut or acorn squash, yams, Jerusalem artichoke, pumpkin
+ 1 cup = 1 potato (approx. 4" x 2")
+ 1 cup = 1 sweet potato (approx. 5" x 2")

Fruits
2–4 servings per day (best eaten between meals):
+ 1 serving = one medium apple, nectarine, or peach
+ 1 serving = ½ grapefruit or ⅛ cantaloupe
+ 1 serving = 1 cup berries, cherries

Whole Grains
Up to 1 cup (cooked or equivalent) per day of rice, polenta, corn, quinoa, millet, buckwheat, etc. (More for vegetarians and fast metabolizers, or in winter):
+ 1 slice bread or 1 6" corn tortilla = ½ cup

Fresh Nuts and Seeds
Up to ⅓ cup 3 times a week (vegetarians and fast metabolizers will need more of this rich source of fat, protein, and vitamins):
+ ¼ cup = 1¼ oz. almonds, pine nuts, or sunflower seeds
+ ¼ cup = 2 oz. pumpkin seeds
+ ¼ cup = 4 tbs. tahini (sesame butter)

Additional Fats
At least 3 tablespoons per day of extra virgin olive oil, coconut oil, or butter/ghee

Liquid
Eight or more 8-ounce (1-cup) portions of filtered water, herb tea, or mixed vegetable juice (not pure carrot, which is overly sweet)

---

*For weight loss, a maximum of 2 fruits, 2 cups total of high-carbohydrate vegetables, legumes, or grains, and up to ¼ cup nuts/seeds works best.

PROTEIN, FAT, AND CARBOHYDRATE— THE ONLY FOODS THERE ARE

PROTEIN: NUMBER ONE

In Greek, the word *protein* means "of primary importance." Protein supplies your body's building blocks, the amino acids, which are so critical to constructing and maintaining the healthy structure of the body, from its muscle to its hormones and even its genes. Foods containing protein have different kinds and amounts of amino acids. Our bodies require twenty-two different amino acids for proper function. A complete protein contains nine essential amino acids: tryptophan, lysine, methionine, valine, leucine, isoleucine, phenylalanine, threonine, and histidine.* These nine amino acids are essential because they *must* be derived directly from our diets. Our bodies cannot manufacture them from other aminos. High-carb-consuming, protein-deficient mothers produce children with built-in weight and health problems.

Certain foods supply all the essential amino acids in sufficient amounts. These foods are called complete proteins—meat, fish, poultry, eggs, milk, and cheese. Plant-based proteins are missing one or more amino acids and are called incomplete proteins. But two or more plant-based proteins can be combined to create a complete protein; for example, beans combined with whole grains, nuts, or seeds. But these vegetable sources provide only a fraction of the total volume of protein found in animal sources.

---

*   In addition, arginine is considered essential in infancy.

In reaction to previous generations' overconsumption of red meat, protein, like fat, has gained a bad reputation. But most people no longer eat three-inch-thick steaks as we did in the 1960s! We've gone to the other extreme. We tend to be protein malnourished now. Adults normally require between 60 and 100 grams of protein on a daily basis. Bodybuilders, heavy exercisers, and those under great stress require more.

Red Meat: What's the Beef?

It's time to rethink our contempt for meat and potatoes and our fear of red meat. Although much maligned, red meat is highly nutritious: It's a great source of protein, and its fat content includes vitamin D and the essential omega-3 and -6 fats along with safe, blood-sugar-stabilizing saturated fats. (See page 272 in the "Fat: More Friend Than Foe" section of this chapter for more on the benefits of saturated fat.) Perhaps the most uniquely beneficial content of red meat is its extraordinarily assimilable forms of zinc and heme iron. The non-heme form found in vegetables is much harder to absorb. One hundred percent of iron in veggies is non-heme. Pale meats (e.g., chicken or turkey breast) contain a third to half the heme iron of beef. Many female vegetarians dream about burgers monthly, and all vegetarian athletes find it harder to heal injuries without the zinc from red meat.

Buffalo, venison, beef, lamb, and goat have been staples of the human diet for thousands of years. Particularly when these red meats were wild and range fed, their consumption was associated with excellent health and weight. The current care and feeding meted out to these mammals is certainly no worse than that accorded chickens. But somehow poultry has escaped the stigma. It's probably because it contains half the fat. But, as you'll see, that's not necessarily a good thing.

True, conventionally raised American meat contains antibiotics, pesticides, and hormones used as growth stimulators. But so do chickens and milk! Less fatty parts contain fewer of these toxins, which are stored in fatty tissues, but neither organic nor range-fed meats pose such problems at all. A 2007 study dispelled the myth of red meat causing colon cancer.[1] A 2010 study confirmed that it is processed meats that are the real problem, with a 42 percent increased risk of heart disease and 19 percent increased risk of diabetes when consumed daily.[2]

Both meat and poultry cooked rare can harbor dangerous *E. coli* bacteria, and if exposed to high heat, they contain ten times the amount of the cancer-causing chemical heterocyclic amine than when cooked at medium heat. Use a meat thermometer to be sure the inside reaches 180 degrees; this way, you'll avoid both extremes. Or use a Crock-Pot (see page 323 ["Slow Cookers" in chapter twenty]).

With blood type A—low in hydrochloric acid—there is a tendency to have trouble digesting beef. Taking enzymes that contain HCl can eliminate the problem.

For more on the benefits of red meat, see the meaty Weston A. Price Foundation site, westonaprice.org

PROTEIN IN COMMON FOODS

Food	Quantity	Protein in Grams
Beans	1 cup	15
Bread	1 slice	2–3
Buttermilk	1 cup	8
Cheese, firm	1 ounce	6–10
Cheese, soft	1 ounce	2–4
Corn	1 cup	4
Cottage cheese	1 cup	25–30
Eggs	1	6–7
Fruit	1 (apple, banana, orange, etc.)	1
Meat, poultry, fish	3–3½ ounces	17–27
Milk	1 cup	8–9
Nutritional yeast	1 tablespoon	8
Nuts	¼ cup	2–7
Oatmeal, cooked	1 cup	6
Rice, cooked	1 cup	6
Seeds	1 ounce	6
Yogurt	1 cup	8–9

EGGS

Disparaged for decades, eggs have now made a comeback. They are one of the most nutrient-rich foods of all, and they are an excellent source of protein, minerals, B vitamins, and excellent, highly digestible fats. Research suggests only those people with both high cholesterol and high triglycerides need to limit their eggs to four per week. Those with high cholesterol only (not high triglycerides) are not adversely affected by eating even two eggs per day. So about 80 percent of the population can enjoy eggs with no limitations. When they are poached or soft- or hard-boiled, eggs are particularly healthful because the yolk stays intact, which prevents oxidation. Choose eggs from free-range chickens, those that do not live in a tiny space in their own filth and don't have to be fed antibiotics to prevent disease. The yolks are bright orange, not pale yellow!

MILK PRODUCTS

These foods are nicely balanced, containing carbohydrate (milk sugar) and good fat as well as protein, especially organic and full-fat varieties. Only cottage cheese is equal in protein content to meat and fish, but Greek yogurt is close. (Other cheeses, e.g., cheddar, would provide equal protein, if we could tolerate enough of their 70 percent fat content.)

SEAFOOD

All fish offer an easily prepared and digested protein that is also rich in minerals, such as iodine, and essential fatty acids—particularly the highly beneficial but rare omega-3 oils. In general, the fattier the fish, the greater the omega-3 content. Fish oils have general anti-inflammatory qualities, reduce clotting, maintain the nervous system, and help lower cholesterol and triglyceride levels. High omega-3 sources include:

+ Salmon
+ Mackerel
+ Herring
+ Sardines
+ Anchovies
+ Lake whitefish
+ Lake trout
+ Sable

+ Conch
+ Halibut
+ Oysters
+ Bluefish
+ Calamari (squid)

Deep-ocean fish have not been subjected to the hormonal and anti-biotic onslaught that land animals raised as food are, but they now have more residues of pollutants such as mercury than freshwater fish or shallow-water seafood such as scallops, shrimp, clams, oysters, and lobster. Mercury is concentrated in large fish like tuna and swordfish, so choose smaller fish. Farmed fish are being subjected to antibiotics and other toxins. Keep those fish to a minimum, as farming practices worldwide vary so much.

PROTEIN POWDER: TRY PEA, RICE, OR WHEY

Better alternatives to soy or egg protein powder (I'd rather see you eat real eggs), these protein powders contain 12–15 grams of protein per tablespoon, almost no carbs, and no sugars. They have a higher protein value than soy, are easier to digest, and mix very well in a variety of foods, blender drinks, and smoothies. Whey is best for those who tolerate this milk protein well. Ask your health food store owner about them, but don't have protein powder more than once a day, as it's harder on the kidneys than real food protein.

FAT: MORE FRIEND THAN FOE

Over a third of your total calories will come from foods such as avocados, olive oil, butter, meat, and fish. Eating this way won't make you feel heavy or gain weight. (It's carbs that do that.) Fat will actually help you lose (if needed), by making you feel satisfied rather than continuing to eat indefinitely because you don't ever feel really complete. And good fat will help you to burn fat more effectively. Every cell in your body needs its coat of fat to protect what's inside. Every cell needs a *good* coat, not a moth-eaten, leaky one, so enjoy your healthy fats. And don't worry about weight gain. Dr. Atkins and numerous studies proved long ago that fat is not the top villain in weight gain—refined sweet and starchy carbohydrates have that dubious honor. History attests to this as well. When we ate more fats (traditional, safe fats such as butter) and less sugar, our weight and health were ideal. In fact, going low fat has had no beneficial effect on women's rates of heart disease, stroke, or cancer.[3]

Believe it or not, fat truly *is* beneficial to your health. It is the most abundant substance in the body, next to water, and an engineering masterpiece. Fat provides twice as much energy as carbohydrates, so it gives us a long, smooth energy source to keep us strong and steady all day. This reduces carb craving, because when blood sugar levels drop, fat can be burned instead of carbs for energy. Fat is vitally important for the energy, health, and structure of every cell in the body. Your brain is 60 percent fat!

OMEGA-6, -3, AND -9 OILS

One of the two essential fats, omega-3, is so rarely found in what we eat that most of us are dangerously deficient in it. The most concentrated omega-3 sources are fish, fish oils, flaxseed, and the increasingly popular chia seed, which protect us against many dangers, including cardiovascular disease. That's why you'll be eating oceanic (low in mercury and wild) fish and/or flaxseeds two times a week, plus using 2,000 milligrams of fish oil daily as a basic supplement.

The other essential fat, omega-6, can be found in fresh nuts and seeds. Eat a handful a few times a week. We only need a small amount of these two essential fats: one part omega-3 oil to one or two parts omega-6 oil.[4]

Another group of healthy oils are rich in omega-9 fatty acids. Extra virgin (first pressing) olive oil is the best source of these and makes a wonderful salad oil as well as a tasty cooking oil. It is quite stable kept at room temperature and plays a central role in one of the world's healthiest cuisines—the Mediterranean diet, with its low risk of cancer, arthritis, and stroke. (But buy domestic 100 percent pure olive oil, since so much imported oil is adulterated.) Macadamia nut oil is another high omega-9 oil.

THE SATURATED FAT SURPRISE

The savagely maligned saturated fats (SATs) in animal products and vegetables such as coconuts have now been proven both nutritionally essential and safe. These traditional fats were abundant in our diets pre-1970, when our health and weight were generally ideal. In the 1990s, it was conclusively proven that hydrogenated vegetable oils cause heart disease.

Saturated fat was officially declared innocent. A 2010 study confirmed this. It also confirmed that refined sugar is the causative factor in cardio-vascular disease.[5] Not only does saturated fat *not* cause heart disease; it is the preferred fuel of the heart, and several studies have confirmed that it is actually protective against stroke. There are many kinds of saturated fat (just as there are many kinds of *un*saturated fat). Each has a vital job in the body. Our shunning of this delicious and nutritious fat has cer-tainly played a role in the steady deterioration of our health.

Four studies, three on type 2 diabetics and one on mildly obese men and women, used a high-saturated-fat, low-carb diet. Their results: all subjects showed improvement in weight, insulin, and cholesterol levels.[6] A Harvard School of Public Health study concurred. It "found no asso-ciation between low-carbohydrate diets and increased cardiovascular risk, even when these diets were high in saturated animal fats." But these studies are really just confirming common sense. Most people all over the world have always consumed lots of saturated fat and thrived physically and emotionally. We did, too. In 1909, we consumed about 26 pounds of saturated fat per year and 9 pounds of omega-6 fat. In 1998, we consumed less than 9 pounds of saturated fat and 66 pounds of omega-6 fat! SATs are not our problem; the high omega-6 vegetable oils are—especially the hydrogenated ones.[7]

You can safely cook with SATs, because at a heat that would toxify most vegetable oils, the sturdy SATs hold up. They are uniquely resistant to heat damage and rancidity. SATs are also great for energy, converting slowly and steadily into cellular fuel as needed. This keeps our blood sugar levels rock solid, which means that our energy, mood, and vitality levels remain stable. Our cravings for carbs drop off as a result. Our obe-sity epidemic is partly due to SAT deprivation. Without SATs, food is not SATisfying, so we tend to eat too much of the carbs and vegetable oils that we do allow ourselves. Refined carbs and the commonly used vege-table oils both increase unneeded weight as well as a myriad of health problems (which I'll discuss later). Diabetics especially require all of the benefits of saturated fat to protect their glucose status and heart function, and to reduce cravings for deadly, insulin-raising sweet and starchy carbs.

Not only do we experience better endurance with saturated fat, but our immune systems are actually enhanced by it as well, in contrast to the immunity-lowering effects of low-fat foods.[8] Ghee (clarified butter) and nonhydrogenated coconut and palm oils are the fats traditionally used for cooking all over the world by people whose weights are much better than ours and who have a dramatically lower incidence of degen-erative diseases.

The crucial vitamins A, D, and E cannot be absorbed into our bodies without their carrier saturated fats, nor can calcium. For example, spinach has lots of calcium, which is not absorbed well unless it's eaten with butter (or olive oil, which also contains some SATs). In the same vein, bacon fat increases the absorption of calcium in collard greens.

Butter (or ghee) is packed with 10 vitamins, 10 minerals, 18 amino acids, and 11 kinds of fat. It's loaded with vitamin A, which it helps deliver to your eyes (night vision is absolutely dependent on an adequate vitamin A supply). Vitamin A regulates the female sex hormone progesterone, providing many mood, fertility, and other benefits. "A" also stands for "antitumor," and saturated fats such as butter assist vitamin A absorption in this life-preserving function—but too many omega-6 fats can block it.[9] Butter's butyrate, the fastest-burning of all fats, is used extensively in your brain. It serves as a base for making GABA (gamma-aminobutyric acid), your natural Valium. It can also protect you from colon cancer and is used as a medicine for precancerous colon problems.

IT'S TIME FOR CLARITY ABOUT CHOLESTEROL

Now for the even more vilified but just as vital nutrient: cholesterol. This remarkable substance is actually not a fat; it's a sterol. Most people mistake it for a fat because some animal fats contain quite a bit of it. But the human body manufactures lots more of it from a variety of foods: from plants (as cows do), from proteins, and from carbohydrates as well as fats. Why does our body make so much of it if it's so dangerous? Here are a few very good reasons:

Twenty-five percent of a healthy brain is composed of cholesterol, which protects its delicate tissues. It also protects the lining of the arteries from damage by trans-fats.

One hundred percent of the twenty-four hormones made by the adrenals are made directly from cholesterol. That means our potent stress-coping hormone cortisol and all of our sex hormones, as well as many other crucial hormones.

Ill health appears to correlate with cholesterol levels over 265. But cholesterol under 170 correlates with increased rates of suicide, violence, depression, autism, and early death! (Many statin takers complain of these adverse mood and personality changes.)[10]

THE BEST OILS FOR EVERYDAY USE

For general cooking, butter (or, even better, ghee), nonhydrogenated co-conut oil, and extra virgin olive oil are ideal choices. They have long shelf lives. (I would refrigerate once opened, unless you use them up quickly.) Moreover, ghee and coconut oil do not break down or smoke as quickly as other oils (including even olive oil) when heated. However, with all oils, it is best to cook at lower temperatures to maintain food quality and integrity. For example, set an electric wok at 250 degrees. (*Note:* Ghee is available at most health food stores and is easy to make by heating butter [preferably raw/organic] until the solids sink to the bottom, then straining them out.)

COCONUT MILK

Available fresh in some areas of the country, and canned or frozen (pref-erably without preservatives) for the rest of us, organic coconut milk is one of the most health-promoting foods on the planet. Its delicious, generous fat content causes it to look and taste like heavy cream, yet it delivers one of the most powerful antivirals, along with equally potent antifungals. It lowers harmful cholesterol levels, keeps blood sugar levels stable, digests without stress to the liver, and provides sustained energy and elevated metabolic rates. It even promotes weight loss! It is stable at high cooking temperatures and makes a delicious soup stock, as Thai-food lovers know. It can be used in any way that cream can be used; in fruit-protein smoothies it is superb and helps make a breakfast smoothie a real, sustaining meal. Coconut milk does contain protein, but not enough for a full meal, so add protein powder or cottage cheese to it for smoothies, or chicken, shrimp, beans, or other protein for soup. The ex-traordinarily healthy and beautiful people in South America cook their morning rice and beans in it.

FATS TO AVOID

Poor-quality fats and oils are the most potentially dangerous food substances in our diet. The following three categories of poor-quality oils are to be avoided.

Processed Oils of All Kinds (Even Canola!)

When a very fragile source of vegetable oil such as canola, soy, corn, or cottonseed is processed, its protective (but ugly) brown vitamin E is removed and it is exposed to heat, light, and oxygen. This processing always causes rancidity, and just bringing home the bottle and opening it continues the process of oxidation, furthering the destruction of the oil. Stale or rancid oils damage cells and encourage abnormal cell growth. Eating food containing rancid oil also destroys vitamins A, D, E, and K, and precious essential fatty acids. These cheap golden oils have also been deodorized so our noses can't discover their rancidity. The research on this is overwhelming and includes studies by the oil manufacturers themselves. Avoid all vegetable oils except organic (and domestic) extra virgin olive oil and coconut oil, which are neither fragile to begin with nor highly processed.

Hydrogenated Oils

All hydrogenated and partially hydrogenated fats and oils are dangerous. This oil is, however, the grocer's dream, because it has an almost infinite shelf life. But it's the liver's nightmare. Produced from damaged corn, soy, canola, and cottonseed oils, it is then superheated for nine hours without oxygen (it's replaced with hydrogen), until it solidifies with the help of two toxins, nickel and cadmium, making the end product lifeless. All hydrogenated fats contain highly reactive trans-fatty acids, which lead to detrimental inflammation and free-radical activity, elevated cholesterol, and arterial plaque buildup—heart disease. Because the liver metabolizes trans-fats differently than it does healthy fats, trans-fats have been implicated in liver disease and Alzheimer's, as well as infertility in women, and it is linked to the development of other degenerative diseases such as cancer and arthritis.

Check your margarine, shortening, and peanut butter for hydrogenated fats. (I'd skip them anyway because of their poor-quality vegetable oil content.) Most packaged baked goods and baking mixes contain hydrogenated fats (another good reason to avoid those foods). Avoid partially hydrogenated fats, too. Be a label cop—hydrogenated oils are still found in packaged crackers, cookies, and many other baked products.

Butter contains many beneficial oils, vitamins, and the health-promoting butyrates. If you can, choose organic butter. Remember, it's hydrogenated fats, not saturated fats, that cause heart disease. We've had the wrong facts about fats for so long that it's hard to stop avoiding saturated fat. Once you do, though, you'll remember how much better it tastes!

Fried Food

Oils in fried foods are damaged and dangerous fats. Like the hydrogenated and rancid oils they are made from, they clog our arteries and make us feel congested, tired, and sluggish. The liver is particularly hard hit by these fats. Do avoid fried foods in all forms, including french fries and chips. Because fried foods are exposed to heat for long periods of time, their fats clog the blood vessels. It's okay to stir-fry, however, because the heat is lower and the food is exposed to it for a much shorter time period. If you do fry, coconut oil and lard are safer.

CARBOHYDRATE: FRIEND AND FOE

Carbohydrates are the most efficient source of energy for all body functions. Although protein and fat can also be burned for energy, it takes more work to do it. They are stored in the body as glycogen in almost all tissues, but especially in the liver and muscles. Glycogen is a ready source of reserve energy instantly available to be metabolized into glucose, which fuels all of the body's cells. In this way, carbohydrates supply the body's immediate needs for calories to burn as energy. When you consume more calories than your body requires, the excess carbohydrates are stored as fat.

Carbohydrates come as either simple or complex. Simple carbohydrates are often called simple sugars and include table sugar (sucrose), fruit sugar (fructose), and milk sugar (lactose). Most simple carbohydrates are refined sugars or refined "white" flour-based starches, which deplete you of nutrients and health. Your body reacts to candy, cookies, sugarcoated cereals, canned fruits in syrup, ketchup, fruit drinks, and juices as if they were insulin-raising drugs. In contrast, fresh fruits are beneficial simple carbohydrates, supplying high levels of essential nutrients and fiber along with fructose.

Complex carbohydrates also consist of sugars, but the sugar molecules are made up of longer, more complex chains. Foods rich in complex carbohydrates include vegetables, legumes (beans, lentils, and peas), and whole grains. Complex carbohydrates are the ideal carbohydrates to meet the body's energy needs. They contain many nutrients and metabolize quickly. Combined with the right ratio of protein and fat, they provide sustained energy. Whether sweet or starchy, carbs are digested instantly, starting with the first chew, as your carb-digesting enzyme, amylase, goes to work on them.

VITAL VEGETABLES

These are the perfect carbohydrate source. Ideally the majority of your dietary carbohydrates will come from vegetables. At least four cups a day should do it. Veggies not only supply some carbohydrates for energy; they are the richest source of minerals in our diet. They also provide enzymes, vitamins, and some protein. Moreover, they are alkalinizing, making them an ideal counterbalance to acid-forming foods such as meat and grains.

In our clinic's many years of nutritional counseling, one simple fact has consistently proven true: People who eat the most vegetables (along with their protein and fat) do the best on our program, and become the healthiest. As an example, a study of 260,000 people found that five servings per day of vegetables (and fruits) cut stroke risk by 26 percent.[11] Scientists are now intently studying the special nutrient content of vegetables to understand why they protect health so effectively. For example, tomatoes and peas protect against prostate cancer, while phytonutrients in broccoli and cabbage help prevent colon cancer. The most intensely colorful vegetables (such as red beets, purple cabbage, yellow squash, collard greens, and spinach) contain the highest levels of nutrients, which boost the immune system and protect from degenerative disease. One of our clients who started to eat a large multi-vegetable salad and two cooked vegetables per day during Christmas break startled her classmates when she returned to graduate school, because her cheeks were so pink and her eyes so bright—from all the color and vitality supplied by her veggies.

Make sure you eat a *minimum* of four cups of vegetables daily. This may sound like a lot, but it's actually easier than it appears. For instance, a large salad containing two cups of lettuce and two cups of mixed tomatoes, bell peppers, cucumbers, and carrots at one meal, and a cup of cooked veggies such as chard, broccoli, spinach, or green beans at another will fulfill your daily vegetable requirement. Raw vegetable snacks and two to three cups of steamed or sautéed veggies with a meal (e.g., in a stir-fry) work well, too. Adding lemon and butter or a tasty sauce to the vegetables makes them even more appealing: Try curry, pesto, salsa, or salad dressing. If you can't make them yourself, buy them freshly prepared. Try a number of them until you settle on your favorites.

Homemade soup is another great way to enjoy your veggies. It's easy to make soup stock, or you can buy it; health food stores carry broths that are free of additives (like MSG and extra sodium), which you can turn into delicious soups in a matter of minutes. (See chapter twenty for recipes.)

Low-Carbohydrate Vegetables

+ Artichokes
+ Arugula
+ Asparagus
+ Bok choy (Chinese cabbage)
+ Broccoli
+ Brussels sprouts
+ Cabbage
+ Cauliflower
+ Celery
+ Chard
+ Clover sprouts
+ Cucumbers
+ Eggplant
+ Green beans
+ Green bell pepper
+ Green chilies

+ Jicama
+ Kale
+ Leeks
+ Lettuce
+ Mung bean sprouts
+ Okra
+ Onions (raw)
+ Radishes
+ Snow peas
+ Spaghetti squash
+ Spinach
+ Sunflower sprouts
+ Sweet red pepper
+ Tomatoes
+ Turnips
+ Zucchini

High-Carbohydrate Vegetables

+ Beans
+ Beets
+ Carrots
+ Celery root
+ Corn
+ Jerusalem artichokes
+ Parsnips

+ Peas
+ Red potatoes
+ Sweet potatoes
+ White potatoes
+ Winter squash
+ Yams

FEAST ON FRUIT

Fresh fruit is a delicious as well as energizing carb, and it's easy to digest. Fruit is an ideal source of quick energy, offering the extra bonus of valuable enzymes, minerals, vitamins, and fiber. Moreover, it makes a great snack food (especially when eaten with protein), requiring little or no preparation. Choose fruits you enjoy, such as apples, grapefruit, and oranges, but experiment with more exotic fruits such as pomegranates, mangoes, and kiwi.

If yeast and/or diabetes are not a problem, eat two to four raw fruits or their equivalent per day (1 apple equals 1 cup of berries). Fruit provides more digestive enzymes than any other food, because we tend to eat it raw. Fruit is also important for its minerals and vitamins (which cooking also reduces). It is a better source of fiber than grain and as alkaline as vegetables. We need to balance our protein, beans, nuts/seeds, and grains, which are somewhat acidic, with buffering alkaline fruits (and veggies). Try to eat fruit between meals or before a meal for better digestion.

BEANS

Beans are high in carbohydrates but also surprisingly high in protein, minerals, and fiber. Most beans contain 80 percent of the calcium of milk, by weight. And the calcium in milk is not the most easily absorbable for humans. Soak beans overnight and discard the original water to prevent flatulence. Try these beans and legumes:

- Adzuki beans
- Black beans
- Black-eyed peas
- Cannellini beans
- Chickpeas (garbanzo beans)
- Cranberry beans
- Flageolet beans
- Great northern beans
- Lentils*
- Lima beans
- Mung beans
- Navy beans

---

* The fastest cooking beans, lentils, can be prepared in about thirty minutes.

+ Pinto beans
+ Red beans
+ Split peas
+ *Note: Avoid soybeans* (see page 292)

CARBS TO AVOID

"CARBO-FATS"

Your body gets overwhelmed by sweet and starchy carbohydrates it can't burn off and converts them to triglycerides that clog your arteries and, eventually, store as fat. This is true even when you're overeating those carbohydrates as whole grains. The body fat that originates from eating too many carbs I call "carbo-fat."

Unless you're an athlete or a fast metabolizer, you can only burn small amounts of sweets and starches for energy. The rest, always stored as a fat called palmitic acid, accounts for much more unneeded weight gain than high-fat foods do. And carbo-fats are considered among the most damaging fats of all for the heart and entire cardiovascular system. Yet they are made from foods that we've been taught are very healthy precisely because they're so low in fat! This is the problem with MyPlate, the revised 2011 government low-fat, high-carb (but adequate protein!) diet recommendations.

SUGARS

The sugar content in foods is alarmingly high and getting higher. We eat 132 pounds of sugar a year, a huge increase from the twenty-five pounds per year we consumed in 1900. We get plenty of naturally occurring sugars in fruit (and milk), but the food industry adds refined and concentrated sugars to almost all processed foods. Sugar is often hidden on the label, disguised with other names such as corn syrup, sucrose, fructose, dextrose, and maltodextrin, among many others. And even organic sugar is still just the same druglike substance, designed to addict you. The twin form of sugar, refined (white) starch (e.g., flour) is no better.

+ Sugar is one of the most addictive substances ever invented, *four times more addictive than cocaine,* according to a 2007 study from the University of Bordeaux. It's as addictive as heroin, according to studies dating back thirty years.[12] I've referenced only a few of the many studies here. Read David Kessler's *The End of Overeating* for more.

+ Sugar depletes vital nutrient reserves, especially essential minerals and B vitamins.
+ Sugars found in junk food spoil our appetites for healthy food.
+ Sugar is the primary cause of diabetes.
+ Sugar is the preferred food of cancer cells, and so acidic and inflammatory that it promotes all illness.
+ Sugar converts quickly to stored fat.
+ In the form of fructose, particularly high fructose corn syrup (HFCS), sugar causes liver disease.
+ Overconsumption of sugar by pregnant mothers is now creating obese fetuses.
+ In 2007, the World Health Organization announced its recommendations for ending the deadly worldwide increases in obesity and degenerative disease: cut sugar consumption to 10 percent of the diet. (Ten percent was what we consumed in 1900, when there was *no* heart disease, and obesity, diabetes, and cancer were rare.)

The sugar lobby is one of the most powerful in the world. That's why this is news to you. Nancy Appleton, author of *Lick the Sugar Habit* and *Suicide by Sugar*, now lists 143(!) documented reasons sugar ruins your health on nancyappleton.com. Please memorize them!

Soda Pop Facts

Americans now drink more than twice as many soft drinks as they did in 1973. Soft drink companies produce more than 50 gallons a year for every American. The average teenage boy gulps more than 36 ounces daily. (Girls consume 75 percent as much.) This contains almost as much caffeine as 1½ (8-ounce) cups of coffee daily (not including energy drinks!).

Soda serving sizes have grown from a 6-ounce bottle in the 1950s to 64-ounce servings today. A 32-ounce serving of non-diet cola has about 27 teaspoons of sugar and 400 calories. At McDonald's, a "child"-size soft drink is now 12 ounces and a small is 16 ounces. At 7-Eleven stores, the Double Gulp is 64 ounces. Soda consumption correlates closely with ADHD incidence in boys and with diabetes in all groups because of its high fructose corn syrup (HFCS) and other sugar content (though some organic sodas are now removing HFCS).

THE OTHER THREE ESSENTIAL NUTRIENTS WE'RE UNDERCONSUMING: WATER, MINERALS, AND VITAMINS

To sustain your health, your body must have water and at least forty-five minerals and vitamins, in addition to the fat, protein, and wholesome carbohydrates I've already mentioned. Are you getting them? Gladys Block, Ph.D., at the University of California, Berkeley, summarized data from three major nationwide nutrition surveys and discovered that one of every two American women consumed inadequate amounts of almost every vitamin and mineral studied. On any four consecutive days, only 14 percent of women ate *even one* dark green vegetable. Almost 50 percent of all women avoided fruit. No wonder our risk of contracting cancer, heart disease, and stroke continues to skyrocket. Only one in five children eat the recommended five servings of fruits and vegetables daily, and nearly 25 percent of all the "vegetables" they consume are french fries.[13] Four out of five Americans believe it is all right to eat whatever they want, whenever they want it.[14] I wish this were true.

WATER

Water is more essential to life than any of the other five key nutrients. Every cell of our body requires water to carry nutrients and energy to them and to carry away toxins and metabolic waste. The human body itself is more than two-thirds water.

Today, obtaining pure drinking water is ever more challenging. Whenever we drink water with chlorine, fluoride, additives, flavorings, sweeteners, and carbonation, our overworked liver must spend time and energy to filter and remove the additives. Only then can we use the water that is contained in the drink. In contrast, pure water requires no special processing by the body. It can be absorbed and used right away as soon as it touches our lips.

Choices in Drinking Water. Despite claims from regional water-treatment officials, tap water isn't a very good source of drinking water anymore, because it contains large amounts of chlorine to kill the bacteria and protozoa in it. Chlorine is toxic, especially to the kidneys, liver, and heart, and it depletes the body of vitamin E and other vital nutrients. Carbonated water is much too high in phosphorus (which can leach calcium from the body) to drink more than occasionally. Bottled springwater is a good choice when it is low in TDS (total dissolved solids; i.e., sludge). Higher-quality bottled waters print their TDS in parts per million (ppm) on their labels. Look for brands that have TDS ratings below 100 ppm.

It's okay to drink distilled water, but only occasionally. It's good for detoxifying the body, but unlike springwater or purified water, it is lifeless, so don't drink it regularly. Reverse-osmosis filtered water has been treated with a combination of two filtration systems plus ultraviolet light. Carbon-block filtration units, which can attach to your faucet or are part of a water pitcher, remove chlorine and other harmful chemicals. But make sure to change your filters regularly, as once they are full they will begin to recirculate waste back into your drinking water. Buying your own water filter is cheaper, more convenient, and safer for you and the environment than using plastic containers. *Note:* Chloramine and fluoride may be impossible to filter out unless the water is filtered using reverse osmosis or distilled, which removes beneficial minerals. (For bathing, the San Francisco Public Utilities Commission recommends 1,000 milligrams of powdered vitamin C in your bathtub to break down chloramine.) Spring and well water may also contain contaminants.

MINERALS

Minerals buffer acids, which makes this nutrient category crucial, as it balances out the mild acids in protein and fat and helps neutralize the unhealthy acids from drugs such as sugar and caffeine. But that's only the beginning! There are twenty-two minerals that we know of that are vital to health. Leading health authorities tell us that more than three out of four Americans are deficient in one or more minerals.[15] Without minerals, the foods we eat and the vitamins we take do little or no good, because our body can't make use of them. Although the body can manufacture a few vitamins, it cannot manufacture a single mineral. Minerals must be supplied through foods.

Despite the importance of minerals, calcium is the only one whose function (in bone building) is widely known and accepted. Clearly, the remaining minerals need a better publicist! Every cell of every living organism requires minerals for proper function and structure. Minerals act as catalysts for many biological reactions, including muscle response, nerve transmissions, digestion, energy production, growth, and healing.

Minerals are present in a wide variety of foods, but they are most richly supplied by vegetables, fruits, and legumes. (See page 279 ["Vital Vegetables" in this chapter] for more.) Of course, this assumes these foods are grown in mineral-rich soils, which is often not the case. Therefore, a balanced multiple-mineral supplement can fill in certain inevitable deficiencies. Seaweed and unprocessed salt can, too.

VITAMINS

Vitamins are absolutely essential to life. Their discovery in 1910 was one of the most important scientific achievements of the twentieth century. Vitamins promote growth, health, and life itself as well as regulate the metabolism and assist the biochemical processes that release energy from digested food. Vitamins are considered micronutrients because we need relatively small amounts of them as compared to the macronutrients (protein, carbohydrates, fat, and water).

With a few exceptions, vitamins must be supplied daily in our diets or as supplements, because our bodies cannot synthesize them. The vitamin content of food can vary greatly depending upon where it was grown, when it was harvested, and how it has been stored and processed. Vitamin content is highest when food is fresh and minimal when heat is applied. For example, heating food in a microwave destroys significant vitamin content.

A lack of one or more vitamins can cause a variety of deficiency symptoms and health problems, interfering with many physical and mental processes and how the body utilizes other nutrients as well. Because vitamins are essential to the body's energy production, when we're low in them we feel fatigued or lethargic. But much worse effects show up if deficiencies continue. A terrible vitamin B_3 (niacin) deficiency syndrome called pellagra killed ten thousand Americans in the South after 1915 and sent thousands of others to mental institutions. Until this mysterious scourge prompted an investigation, we'd had no idea such consequences could result from this single nutrient deficiency. The cause? A period of severe poverty forced many Southerners to a high-carb (mostly corn) diet. Corn contains virtually no tryptophan. Tryptophan, besides providing antidepressant serotonin and sleep-promoting melatonin, is also a primary source of vitamin B_3.

There are thirteen recognized vitamins: The fat-soluble ones include A, D, E, and K; the water-soluble vitamins are C and B complex (thiamine, riboflavin, niacin, pantothenic acid, B_6, B_{12}, biotin, and folic acid). Additionally, choline and inositol are two water-soluble members of the B complex family. Fat-soluble vitamins can be stored in the liver and the body's fatty tissue. However, we need to take in water-soluble vitamins daily because our bodies cannot store them and they will be excreted in one to four days.

HEALTHY EATING TIPS

EAT ORGANIC, RANGE-FED, AND FRESH AND WILD WHENEVER YOU CAN

Sales of organic food have increased more than 2,500 percent since 1990.[16] Supermarket sales now account for more than 50 percent of all organic produce sold in the United States. It's everywhere! While more costly than nonorganic food, the prices are going downward, and organic fruits and vegetables are not only richer in nutrients; they are devoid of pesticides and other chemical residues. And they taste better! The same can be said of meat and poultry raised outside and fish swimming free.

COOKED OR RAW? THE ENZYME QUESTION

The best convenience, or "fast," food is uncooked fresh ripe fruits and some vegetables. Foods containing high levels of fragile vitamins and digestive enzymes are best consumed in the raw state. This group includes most ripe fruits and some vegetables, like avocados. Unripe fruits, many vegetables, and most grains, nuts, seeds, and beans contain enzymes that can negatively impact digestion. With these foods, ripening, soaking, sprouting, and/or cooking enhances nutrient absorption and provides a higher nutritional value. Examples of these foods include carrots, tomatoes, and potatoes, all having higher digestibility of proteins and starches after cooking.

Supplemental digestive enzymes can be very helpful for all of those in recovery from dieting and eating disorders. Since your body can tolerate raw vegetables, have lots of them. It's best to include *both* raw and cooked veggies in your meals, but find what works for you—and your lifestyle. It seems to work best to eat more raw foods in the warmer months and more cooked in the cooler months. Optimally, half of the vegetables you eat will be raw, assuming you digest them well. So don't overlook the raw veggies, as they supply many nutrients that cooked vegetables do not. But if you find you feel hungry or unsatisfied after eating only raw foods with protein, it's a sign that the next time you should add more cooked vegetables to the meal. This small addition will usually leave you feeling more satisfied and fulfilled.

CONSIDER EATING FOR YOUR BLOOD TYPE

If you don't know what your blood type is, order a blood-type test through a physician (it costs about twenty dollars), donate to a blood bank, or order a home test kit online (e.g., craigmedical.com or 4yourtype.com). Each of us is biochemically unique; food I thrive on may make you sick, or vice versa. Your blood type offers a key to some of the secrets of your individual health, disease, and longevity. What your ancestors ate in the past still has a direct bearing on your present health, as you have genetically inherited their digestive strengths and weaknesses along with their blood types.

If your blood type is O—the oldest, the original blood type—you'll probably thrive on a "caveman" diet: meat, fish, vegetables, nuts, seeds, and fruit. It is almost impossible for an O type to be a successful vegetarian. Milk products, beans, and grains, especially wheat, present significant digestive problems for type O's. Animal protein seems to be particularly essential to people with blood type O (you'll need 20 to 40 grams at each meal, depending on your body size, metabolism, and activity level).

If your blood type is A, you can usually handle ancient grains such as rice and corn better than type O's, as your ancestors were the original agrarians—planting crops for food. Legumes (beans, peas, and lentils) are even better. Type A's often do best avoiding milk products and the more recently introduced wheat, rye, barley, and oats, especially if weight loss is an issue. Our clinic has found that most A's need animal protein and do well on poultry and fish. Though they often need hydrochloric acid supplements to digest red meat well (they're often deficient), meat benefits them.

If your blood type is B, you are the only blood type that seems to thrive on milk products, as your more recent ancestors regularly consumed and adapted to the raw, unprocessed (and more digestible) version.

A widely varied diet including meat and fish is best for B types, though they don't seem to be able to digest chicken and the gluten-containing grains very well.

If your blood type is AB, you may have inherited the strengths and weaknesses of both types A and B. Your immune system is probably strong and you can adapt to a variety of different foods, but you don't need as much animal protein (meat) as type B and may also have trouble digesting chicken. AB's may have a better tolerance for dairy and gluten than some other blood types (but they're so rare that we haven't seen enough to be sure).

FOOD COMBINING

Some nutritionists have set up elaborate rules concerning food combining; that is, what foods should or should not be eaten together. For some people with sensitive digestive tracts, it can be helpful to follow the protocol of proper combining. For others it doesn't seem to matter much at all. If you have a sensitive digestive system, you'll usually feel better when you eat fruit first or alone, eat vegetables and fat with anything, and avoid eating protein with starchy food.

GET ENOUGH FIBER

Diets high in fiber help lower cholesterol levels and reduce the risk of heart disease. Fiber has also been shown to prevent colon and other cancers. In general, populations that consume high-fiber diets have fewer hospital stays and less disease. Make fiber a part of all your meals. Fiber, or "roughage," is found almost exclusively in plant foods—vegetables, fruits, legumes, whole grains, nuts, and seeds. Beans, lentils, peas, corn, prunes, blackberries, raspberries, and blueberries are exceptionally rich in fiber. Avoid wheat and oat bran fiber if you are gluten intolerant. Remember that processed foods lack fiber, and cooking vegetables and fruit to the point of being mushy destroys much of their fiber.

Fiber has other benefits, too: It binds with toxins and excess hormones and waste and helps neutralize them before they cause bodily damage. It also adds bulk to the stool, which assists in maintaining regular bowel function. Without enough fiber, you can experience constipation, which is a contributing factor in many diseases. (*Caution:* If you have a digestive disorder, consult with your physician before embarking on a high-fiber diet.)

FOODS AND FOOD ADDITIVES TO AVOID

PESTICIDES AND ESTROGEN-PROMOTING CHEMICAL ADDITIVES (BUY ORGANIC!)

Seventy of the three hundred pesticides used on U.S. crops are known to be probable human carcinogens. The following produce evidences the highest levels of pesticide residues: strawberries, bell peppers, spinach, cherries (United States), celery, apples, lettuce, pears, potatoes, nectarines, and grapes (Chilean). Rinsing produce does not remove many pesticides. Farm workers and farm families have high cancer rates.

ASPARTAME (NUTRASWEET) AND OTHER SWEETENERS

Aspartame is two hundred times sweeter than sugar. It increases the appetite in general and the desire for sweets in particular. In some people, it is highly addictive. Incredibly, aspartame accounts for 75 percent of all nondrug complaints to the FDA, including for headache, fatigue, mood problems, and much more. (See chapter two and *Sweet Deception* by Joseph Mercola, D.O.) Aspartame use is associated with both overweight and diabetes. Avoid other sweeteners, too. Saccharin is associated with cancer and agave is contaminated and sweeter than sugar. Use this book to eliminate your interest in sweetened foods of any kind! (And read more on this in chapter two.)

CAFFEINATED BEVERAGES

Coffee, black tea, and colas are powerful stimulants that can overstress the body in many ways. They diminish sleep quality and deplete nutrients such as vitamin B_1, biotin, inositol, vitamin C, calcium, potassium, and zinc. Caffeine also increases thirst and appetite; overstimulates and weakens the kidneys, pancreas, liver, stomach, intestines, heart, nervous system, and glands (especially the adrenals); and over-acidifies the body's pH (a factor in premature aging). Coffee is laced with pesticides and free-radical-producing hydrocarbons that weaken cell membranes. Studies show individuals who drink the most coffee often suffer chronic depression, insomnia, gout (now epidemic), arrhythmia, high cholesterol, bone thinning, infertility, and fibrocystic problems. What's more, a small amount of coffee can set off those negative effects. Decaf coffee contains a small amount of caffeine as well as all the pesticides and hydrocarbons, and it's closely associated with rheumatoid arthritis. (Read *Caffeine Blues*, by Stephen Cherniske, for more.)

CARBONATED BEVERAGES

In the carbonation process, phosphorous levels in beverages increase significantly. If you regularly drink soda, you will upset the mineral balance in your body. If your body doesn't have enough calcium to buffer higher phosphorus intake, it will "borrow," or leach, calcium wherever it can be found—from muscles and bones. The net result can be a gradual weakening of bone structure, contributing to osteoporosis. Furthermore, HFCS content in carbonated sodas is proving to be lethal, and diet sodas with aspartame or other artificial sweeteners aren't much better. On the other hand, natural carbonation is fine (e.g., mineral water, which you can make yourself with Sodastream).

PROCESSED MEATS

These include bologna, salami, hot dogs, most sausages, and smoked meats and fish. The problem with processed meats is that they are very high in nitrates and nitrites, which form potentially carcinogenic by-products. Frequent consumption is also linked with diabetes. Most are now available nitrite- and nitrate-free, so choose these whenever possible.

MONOSODIUM GLUTAMATE (MSG)

This flavor enhancer is responsible for countless headaches in diners at Chinese eateries. The phenomenon is so common that it's been given the name CRHS (Chinese restaurant headache syndrome). No wonder so many people have negative reactions to it: glutamate is a neurotoxin that destroys brain cells in laboratory animals and potentially in humans. Check food labels; it shows up in a lot of unexpected places. Check with waiters, too. They can order your meal to be made without MSG.

Microwave Cooking: Zap and Be Zapped

In our fast-paced society, the microwave oven is an incredible convenience. Unfortunately, there are some health risks associated with its use. German studies show microwaving of food is associated with a drop in hemoglobin and lymphocyte levels in the blood and a significant rise in white blood cell counts. An increase in white blood cells is an immune response that usually means the body is fighting some type of infection or inflammation. Some researchers feel that heavy reliance on microwaved food may be linked to a significant increase in autoimmune disorders. Moreover, the microwave kills almost all enzymes present in food. Because enzymes are biochemical catalysts that contain the life force of food—the key to all life processes—the loss of enzymes is a real problem. Some people report feeling more tired and lethargic after eating microwaved food. So use your microwave to reheat or defrost, or even cook, food only occasionally; don't rely on it. It is far better to dirty a pot and cook on the stove.

Be a label reader. It's a primary means of survival. Just because a substance is allowed in stores does not mean it is safe or nutritious.

SOY CAUTION

The evidence on soy is disturbing. Soy has proven to be a thyroid suppressor and a hormone dysregulator. (See chapter four for more on the thyroid and soy.) And despite all the fanfare about soy being a miracle food for menopausal women, there are actually very few documented benefits of soy phytoestrogens (called isoflavones), according to a 2006 review study by Oregon State University.[17] In fact, soy's well-established estrogenic effects are associated with obesity and diabetes as well as elevated rates of breast cancer. Pregnant and nursing mothers, and infants, particularly, should be soy-free.[18]

Soy is also notoriously hard to digest because it is composed of extremely long chains of protein that have to be "cut up" into small pieces by the stomach. Tempeh, soy sauce, and miso digest more easily because of fermentation, but they contain high levels of the estrogenic compounds genistein and daidzein, which have been implicated in tumor and cancer promotion. Soy formula, soy milk, soy protein powders, and other soy protein isolates not only promote obesity and diabetes, but not being fermented, they can be irritating to the digestive tract, and all can disrupt thyroid function. As of May 1999, the U.S. soy industry website (centralsoya.com, "Soy protein content for animal feed") was showing pigs whose intestines had been hopelessly ulcerated by soy feed and advising farmers to strictly limit the amount of soy fed to piglets. The Web site has since been dismantled, but similar damage is documented elsewhere.[19]

Those of you who are vegetarian may be especially shocked and upset by this—I was. But one of my clients recently said that she was relieved because she'd never really enjoyed the taste of soy, but had forced herself to eat it anyway, because it was "healthy." Fortunately, beans other than soy are high in protein, more benign, and easier to digest. (See the delicious Falafel Patties recipe in chapter twenty.)

VEGETARIANISM—CAUTION

The Vegetarian and Vegan Plates

Vegetarian eaters will have a different plate. They must consume a higher proportion of carbohydrates because their protein sources, such as beans and grains, are also higher in carbs than meat, fish, and poultry. Nuts, seeds, eggs, and cheese are almost carb-less, but not all vegetarians eat eggs and cheese, and they shouldn't overdo nuts or seeds, because of their tendency to go rancid and their high omega-6 content. Cooked beans contain about 15 grams of protein per cup (and approximately 45 grams of carbs), but high-carb fruits, vegetables, and grains contain very little protein. So if you are vegan (and eat absolutely no animal products) it will be almost impossible for you to maintain your protein-carb balance. Please watch very carefully to see that you get enough protein to keep yourself free of cravings and health problems.

Vegetarian diets have become trendy for the first time in the history of the world (outside of a few places in the Far East). Spiritual and ethical considerations are more influential now and very persuasive. What I am concerned about, though, is the increasingly common misconception that a vegetarian diet is a healthy diet. In fact, many people sacrifice their health on vegetarian diets, particularly on the all-too-common fast-food version. Keep in mind that humans were free of degenerative disease until the twentieth century. And almost no peoples were vegetarian.

If you are eating plenty of vegetables, beans, fruit, eggs, and cheese, you may be healthier than most meat eaters. Unfortunately, most vegetarians today rely more on low-protein grains, starches, sweets, and excessive omega-6 fat than they do on legumes and vegetables. This cancels any health benefits of vegetarianism. Others rely on higher-protein dairy products and too often choose low-fat versions or run into trouble with allergies (milk is one of the five top food allergens). Many also have difficulty digesting carbs made from whole wheat (or white) flour, and these high-starch foods, like highly sweetened foods, often provide the body with more stress than nutrition. Moreover, wheat, rye, barley, and possibly oats contain a chemical called phytate, which blocks the absorption of minerals such as calcium. The gluten in these grains often causes allergic and/or addictive reactions. (See chapter five.)

We have not had much success with vegans, who eat no eggs or milk products. They tend to end up sneaking junk food, overeating dates (especially those who eat only raw food), or trying to rely permanently on nutrient supplements (which I don't recommend).

Some A blood types may do better on a nutrient-rich vegetarian diet. But many do not. If you are an O blood type—the original Paleolithic type—you will definitely not do well as a vegetarian; you will certainly need to at least eat fish and eggs.

Your own body's unique responses to foods are by far your best guides. A recent client came in with his 12-year-old daughter. The whole family was on an adequate-calorie vegan diet, but the daughter had developed a seizure disorder, and her formerly athletic father was weak and pale—two symptoms many of our vegetarian clients complain of on admission. Both father and daughter revived when animal protein was reintroduced, and the whole family's health and energy improved. The literature on seizure disorders among children is replete with evidence that inadequate protein is the primary cause. Carefully monitor your mental and physical health. Be sure to eat enough protein at every meal (at least 20 grams, or 3 to 4 ounces, per meal; a cup of black beans or 3 eggs, for example). As a vegetarian, you also need to take supplements that supply iron, zinc, B$_{12}$, and L-carnitine, and if you're menstruating, pregnant, or breastfeeding you will need iron and folic acid supplements as well.

Because their diets, at best, tend to be high in carbohydrates, vegetarians really do need to eliminate refined sweets and starches *altogether*. Make grain the side dish of your meals, with vegetables and beans, cheese, and nuts as your central focus. If you can tolerate eggs and dairy products, you can use them to increase your protein and vitamin B$_{12}$ intake.

CONCLUSION OF THE NUTRITIONAL SURVIVAL GUIDE

Come back to this chapter as a reference as often as you need to. I truly wish that healthy eating were made easy for us all. I know that this chapter will help you to keep fighting for the food you need to survive and thrive. To further bolster your nutritional skills, I've suggested a group of specially selected books.

Readings

Sally Fallon with Mary G. Enig, Ph.D., *Nourishing Traditions: The Cookbook That Challenges Politically Correct Nutrition and the Diet Dictocrats*, 2nd Edition (Washington, DC: NewTrends Publishing, 2001).

Ann Louise Gittleman, Ph.D., CNS, *Get the Sugar Out: 501 Simple Ways to Cut the Sugar Out of Any Diet*, 2nd Edition (New York: Three Rivers Press, 2008).

Mark Hyman, M.D., *Ultrametabolism: The Simple Plan for Automatic Weight Loss* (New York: Atria Books, 2008).

David A. Kessler, M.D., *The End of Overeating: Taking Control of the Insatiable American Appetite* (New York: Rodale Books, 2009).

Nina Planck, *Real Food: What to Eat and Why* (New York: Bloomsbury, 2007).

Michael Pollan, *Food Rules: An Eater's Manual* (New York: Penguin Books, 2009).

Uffe Ravnskov, M.D., Ph.D., *Fat and Cholesterol Are Good for You* (Sweden: GB Publishing, 2009).

Julia Ross, "Fat Is Not the Enemy: A New Perspective on the Pros and Cons of Oily Foods," *Price-Pottenger Journal* 33, no. 3. Available at dietcure.com.

NINETEEN

Shopping for Supplies for Your Master Plan and Planning Your Meals

By this time you know what foods and supplements you'll need for your individualized Master Plan. Now it's time to go shopping. The object of this chapter is to give you suggestions on where to find these foods and supplements and how to develop new eating, cooking, and grocery-shopping habits. Many of us are away from home for ten or more hours a day, so we need quick and easy suggestions for how to eat well every day, no matter how busy we are or where we are—at a friend's house, dining out, or on an airplane. I'm confident that you'll find it easier than you think to stick to your Master Eating Plan even when you're pressed for time or the choices on the menu are limited. There's so much wonderful food out there that you can enjoy that I know you won't miss the foods you're giving up. And if you're concerned about the costs of buying food and supplements, please don't be. You are worth it. Many supplements are needed only short-term. And think of all the money you'll be saving on chocolate!

MASTER PLAN COSTS

All of these supplements and organic foods may seem expensive to you, but put it in perspective. How much have you paid over the years for diet programs, prepackaged diet foods, or foods to binge on or to satisfy cravings? Have you had health problems due to your thyroid, adrenal, or hormone imbalances, or due to an eating disorder that made you dig into your pocket? How much time have you lost from work because you didn't feel well enough to go in?

Some of the foods I recommend will cost more than the counterparts that you used to buy before starting your Master Plan. For example, organic produce usually costs more than conventional produce. But think of it as a type of health insurance—a "nutrition insurance" against future costs of poor health. Besides stopping cravings and enabling you to maintain your body's natural weight, properly balanced body chemistry can prevent cancer, heart attacks, and other debilitating or fatal diseases. This isn't another diet we are talking about. The Diet Cure is a holistic program that will allow you to be healthy and vital for the rest of your life. You deserve that.

Besides the savings from avoiding the negative effects of eating poorly, you will often save money by buying fresh items and cooking them yourself over buying the processed equivalent. For example, potatoes are very inexpensive when bought in the produce section, but those frozen hash browns, french fries, and Tater Tots more than triple the price per pound.

EMPHASIZE EATING MORE VEGGIES

What do vegetarians, nutritionists, doctors, the Food and Drug Administration, and the average person have in common? We all know we should be eating more fresh veggies. I know you have heard this before, but it can't be said enough: there just is no better source for many of the things your body needs than lots of fresh vegetables. As you explore this style of eating you will find variations of some of your old favorites and many entirely new dishes that will become favorites. It's an adventure! Prepare and expect to enjoy it.

WHICH FOODS SHOULD YOU BUY?

Produce that is grown organically instead of conventionally draws a broader range of nutrients from the richer soil it is grown in. Just as junk food is made from refined sugar and flour that have been stripped of nutrients, conventional farming uses fertilizers that are refined until they contain only the minimum nutrients necessary to produce a saleable crop. In contrast, organically grown food contains the complete range of nutrients available from whole, organic compost, natural fertilizers such as manure, and mineral sources like kelp. Just as refined foods will eventually cause depletion of nutrients in a person, refined fertilizers result in foods with nutrient deficiencies.

In an ideal world, we would eat only fresh, raw, organic produce and naturally raised meat, poultry, and fish, and we would never touch sugar or refined carbohydrates. Lack of available sources of these preferred foods, lack of time, and price limit our ability to reach this ideal. The following suggestions are to help you work with these limitations in the real world.

Also, select foods rich in color; they are highest in nutrients. Choose intensely orange carrots over pale ones, emerald green spinach over light green, and ruby red tomatoes and strawberries over pink ones.

Food Value Continuum

Most Food Value:	Fresh, organic, naturally raised, home cooked
Next Best:	Fresh, conventionally raised produce and meat; frozen organic
Okay Sometimes:	Frozen, canned, dried
Avoid at All Times:	Processed, prepackaged, sugary, doughy, fried, junk, and most fast food

---

SO WHERE DO I FIND THESE FANTASTIC FOODS AND MY MASTER PLAN SUPPLEMENTS?

IN YOUR GARDEN

Though organic produce has made great inroads in many areas, the best source is still your own garden. Growing your own leafy lettuce, mesclun, carrots, tomatoes, cucumbers, peas, or other veggies is both delicious and rewarding. You have the benefit of knowing the nutrient history of what you are eating. You also benefit from the short amount of time elapsed from garden to plate. If you don't have the space for a big garden, try growing some vegetables in pots on your patio or balcony. Some vegetables, like the patio tomato, are especially bred for growing in pots. An herb garden takes up little room but will save you a lot of money—just snip off what you need to use. Depending on the space and time you have available, you can add other crops to your garden. Chatting with the clerk at the nursery or reading seed packages (which describe the size of the plants and the amount of space they need) will give you an idea of what is practical in your circumstances.

AT THE FARMERS' MARKET

Shop your local farmers' market, if one is available to you. These are organized by farmers in a given area to give them an opportunity to sell direct to the public. They are usually held weekly and vary considerably in size. The produce is usually much fresher than the produce you find at your supermarket. Grocery store fruits and veggies may have been stored in a central warehouse for days, or even weeks, before being shipped to your local grocer. Farmers' markets often sell produce that was picked that very morning. Organic produce is more common at farmers' markets, too. You may be lucky enough to live near one of the growing number of CSAs (community supported agriculture). You pay a monthly fee or "invest" in the year's crops at the beginning of the season and receive your "dividends" each week in the form of truly farm-fresh produce. Find your nearest CSA at csacenter.org. Prices vary. Deals can be made.

SHOPPING ON THE PERIMETER OF
THE SUPERMARKET

Avoid the center aisles of the supermarket, which are usually filled with highly processed foods—mixes, packaged foods, canned goods, and frozen foods. These foods typically have nutrients processed out and sugar and saturated fat processed in. Instead, shop around the edges of the store, where you'll find the produce section, the meat section, and the dairy section. Hold your breath through the bakery section. The perimeter of the store is where you will usually find the foods needed to fulfill your Master Plan: fresh vegetables, fruit, meat, poultry, seafood, bulk grains, bulk beans, nutritional grains, eggs, and milk products.

Recent years have seen the development and growth of markets specializing in healthy foods. These stores carry more organic vegetables, raw or lightly processed foods, naturally raised meats and poultry, and bulk foods such as flour, nuts, and beans than your traditional supermarket. They are larger than health food stores and stock many more products. See the Resources section at the end of the chapter for some of these markets that might have branches in your area. They can be a boon to those of us who shop for fresh, organic produce, range-fed meat, a wide array of food supplements, and special foods for allergy sufferers. But remember, just because it's from Whole Foods doesn't mean it's healthy. Read labels!

AT YOUR HEALTH FOOD STORE

Health food stores are often a good source of beans, nuts, seeds, grains, gluten-free bread and pasta, yogurt, tempeh, cheese, tortillas, polenta, organic pasta sauce, and salsa. They may also have a selection of fresh, organic produce. Many carry frozen meats and poultry raised without chemicals, or they may have fresh meats, depending on their size. But remember, just because a food is found in a health food store does not necessarily mean it's healthy. Use the same vigilance that you would shopping anywhere else. Not-so-healthy "health" foods include cereals and cookies sweetened with organic sugar, concentrated fruit juice, or agave, which can be found in abundance in most health food stores. These intense carbohydrates can create cravings and deplete nutrition, just as any other sweetened goodies can.

Your health food store will have most of the nutritional supplements your Master Plan calls for, and it may be able to order any that it doesn't stock. When you buy supplements at your health food store, you have a better chance of finding people to consult with personally. They can guide you to the products available in your area that contain the particular nutrients you need for your Master Plan. Consult with them, but be sure you do not compromise your needed nutrients when making a product decision. Check that you will be getting each nutrient in the strength suggested on your plan. You may need to go to more than one source to get all the nutritional supplements you require. See the Resources section at the end of this chapter for health food stores that might have branches in your area. Most of the supplements sold in these stores are high quality. The NOW brand tends to be the best buy.

ONLINE AND MAIL ORDER SUPPLEMENT SOURCES

Supplements can be purchased at discounts of 20 to 40 percent online or by mail order. Some of the larger companies that take orders by mail, phone, and/or website are listed in the Resources section for this chapter. Some of these companies have people answering their phones who can help fill your particular supplement needs. Most websites post information on the potencies and uses for particular supplements.

MORE TIPS FOR PURCHASING MASTER PLAN FOODS AND SUPPLEMENTS

BUYING FISH

In today's world, the most healthy choice of fish is often wild-caught frozen, especially if you live inland. So-called "fresh" fish in most supermarkets is anything but fresh. When choosing a whole fish, press the skin; if the depression remains, it's not fresh. The eyes should be clear, not frosty; the gills red and bright, not turning yellow. The nose knows, so follow it; if it smells very fishy, choose frozen instead. Most frozen fish today is "fresh-frozen" soon after it is caught.

BUYING SPICES

Add your favorite spices to a variety of foods to enhance both flavor and food value. Spices can make a boring meal interesting. Experiment: borrow a bit from a friend if you don't want to plunk down four dollars on an entire bottle, or buy in small quantities from a store that sells herbs and spices from bulk containers. It's better to buy spices in small amounts anyway, as they go bad long before you'll use up a big container. Throw them out when they no longer have a strong smell. Maintaining an herb garden is a great way to ensure you'll always have plenty of fresh herbs on hand, and a great way to save money.

BUYING SUPPLEMENTS

The cost of nutritional supplements will vary depending on your particular Master Plan and where you buy. In 2011, my clients paid an average of $250 retail when beginning elaborate protocols for correcting seven or eight of the eight imbalances. These initially purchased supplements run out over varying periods of time. The cost range for supplements for a twelve-week program at the Recovery Systems Clinic is $500 to $1,000 retail. This may sound like a lot of money, but remember that the clinic prices are not discounted (you can shop around), and you will only be taking the complete Master Plan nutritional supplements for a limited time. Once your body has repaired itself enough to maintain balance through a healthy diet, you will be taking only the basic supplements. Comparison shopping can result in substantial savings.

READ THE LIST OF INGREDIENTS

Wherever you shop, make sure all foods and supplements that you buy are free of hidden sugar and any foods you are intolerant of or allergic to. (See chapter five for information on food intolerance.) Read labels' ingredients lists carefully; ingredients differ from product to product. For example, soy sauce is usually made with wheat in addition to soy, but there are a few brands made without wheat. One brand may have soy sauces with different ingredients under two different labels, one containing wheat and the other not. The only way to be sure of what you are getting is to read the ingredients list on each product. It's quite educational!

When buying supplements, pay attention to dosages. Also, always check expiration dates.

STAPLES OF THE DIET CURE PLAN

Many of the foods I recommend may not yet be staples in your household. The following are items I like to keep on hand.

FRUITS AND VEGGIES

These fruits and vegetables can be kept for longer periods than others, so they're good to keep on hand.

✦ Apples
✦ Carrots
✦ Celery
✦ Garlic
✦ Onions
✦ Oranges
✦ Potatoes
✦ Tomatoes

PANTRY ITEMS

✦ Spaghetti (marinara) sauce. Look for organic brands with no added sugar.
✦ Extra virgin olive oil. Worth the extra price for its extra nutrients. Look for organic and domestic, since imported oils are often adulterated.

+ Organic coconut milk (canned or dehydrated).
+ Pasta. Whole wheat is fine if you aren't gluten-intolerant, but rice, corn, quinoa, bean, and others are also good choices.
+ Bragg Liquid Aminos. A soy sauce–like product, but with twice the protein (amino acids) and half the sodium of soy sauce (and no wheat).
+ Hummus. A Middle Eastern spread/dip made from garbanzo beans, sesame, garlic, lemon juice, and spices. I add fresh parsley and extra lemon juice before dipping.
+ Baba ghanouj. A Middle Eastern eggplant-based spread.
+ Corn tortillas. One hundred percent whole corn flatbread, preferably organic (non-GMO). Keep refrigerated or frozen.

GLUTEN-FREE BAKING AND BREAD-MAKING ESSENTIALS

You may want to start making your own bread and other baked goods, especially if you are gluten intolerant. (See recipe on page 340.) If so, you will find the following useful:

+ Garbanzo bean flour (also called chickpea, gram, or chana flour)
+ Brown rice flour
+ Quinoa flour
+ White buckwheat groats (blend quickly into fresh flour)
+ Baking powder. Try Rumford, which is free of aluminum (excess aluminum builds up in the brain and is a suspect in Alzheimer's disease), or make your own: 1 part baking soda to 2 parts cream of tartar.
+ Baking soda
+ Xanthan gum (helps give baked goods a consistency similar to gluten-containing products)
+ Dry yeast

WHAT TO EAT

EASY PROTEIN

Here are some hints for adding protein to your meals without excessive effort.

Your Master Plan for the Diet Cure

✦ Roasting a chicken (or a turkey breast or thigh) will provide enough protein for your whole family in one meal, or for future quick, left-over meals. See chapter twenty for recipes. Crock-Pots make it *soooo* easy and yummy.

✦ You'll also find recipes for Easy Baked Protein, which can be used with poultry, fish, or meats, to help add variety to your meals.

✦ Keep canned beans on hand (be sure there are no sweeteners listed in the ingredients; just beans, water, and salt) or soak and cook a big batch ahead to freeze or have on hand for a few days. After soaking, discard water to help prevent flatulence. Cook in fresh water below the boiling point to enhance digestibility. A slow cooker or pressure cooker is ideal for preparing all sorts of beans. Freeze in serving-size packets. Use beans in your vegetable salads, or add them to soups, chili, and stews. If beans give you gas, try one of the commercial enzyme products such as Beano. When using canned beans, drain and rinse them to reduce sodium and improve digestibility. (People with blood type O tend not to tolerate beans well.)

SNACKING

Nuts and Seeds. For protein, healthy fats, and plenty of other nutrients, these are a sure bet. The original fast food, nuts and seeds don't require cooking or any complicated preparation. Just pop them in your mouth and chew. Remember that raw nuts and seeds contain many nutrients and enzymes that are lost during roasting. Trail mixes of nuts, seeds, and coconut flakes (with little or no dried fruit) are only slightly more complicated to prepare, or they can be bought already mixed. Avoid rancid (un-fresh) grains, seeds, and nuts. Eating such foods depletes the body of protective antioxidant (anti–free radical and anticancer) nutrients such as vitamin C, essential fatty acids, and especially vitamin E, the body's primary fat-soluble antioxidant. Try to buy nuts and seeds in nitrogen-sealed packages (they are sold this way in many health food stores) to get them at their freshest. Discard any broken or misshapen nuts and seeds before eating; if they aren't rancid yet, they will turn rancid more quickly. Keep these foods under refrigeration once opened, and use them up promptly. Discard them at the first sign of rancidity. Walnuts, in particular, go rancid within a month after shelling unless refrigerated or frozen. Aflatoxin, a toxic mold, which grows on these foods (especially peanuts), has been directly linked to cancer. Have a handful portion two or three times a week with veggies or a piece of fruit as a snack. (Minimize trail mix because of the dried fruit.)

Fresh Fruit and Veggies. Keep lots of these on hand. Raw veggies or fresh fruit alone may suffice, or combine them with a hard-boiled egg, cheese, nuts, seeds, hummus, or baba ghanouj.

Sliced Roasted Turkey or Beef. Avoid the processed lunch meat varieties with additives and nitrates. Wrap slices around carrot sticks or slices of avocado, bell pepper, green onion, or a combo.

Cheesy Snacks (if you tolerate milk products). Try cottage cheese with either fruit or veggies, or your favorite cheese and a piece of fruit, or feta pressed into celery sticks.

Protein Powder. A necessity for blended drinks as snacks or, occasionally, quick meals when there isn't time to cook. If you have intolerances or allergies, read the label. Some contain wheat, oat, or milk products, especially whey. I recommend the pea or rice. Beware of chocolate, sugar, and other sweeteners. Twelve grams of protein per tablespoon is ideal (with little or no carb content). Make an extra-large breakfast smoothie and take part of it to work for a snack.

FOODS FOR SPECIAL NEEDS

Gluten Intolerant? If you are allergic to the gluten-containing grains— wheat, rye, barley, and oats—gluten-free (GF) bread and pasta are available at health food stores, natural food chains, and, increasingly, at supermarkets. But most GF bread is made from highly refined or sweetened ingredients. I freeze Food for Life's black or red rice breads for the occasional toasted sandwich. Look for products such as Tinkyada's organic brown rice pasta, which is made from stone-ground brown rice flour and water, nothing else. One gluten-free pasta line, Pastato, is derived largely from potatoes. Ancient Harvest makes corn and quinoa spaghetti and veggie curls. Try 100 percent buckwheat soba noodles. Pastariso and Ener-G make rice spaghetti, lasagna, and other noodles that defy the wheat eater to distinguish them from the usual products. Yam or bean-thread pasta is available in many markets, in the section with other Asian foods.

You can also make your own gluten-free bread. I have included one of my favorite bread recipes in chapter twenty for the kind of bread that can be easily made in your bread machine.

See the Readings section in this chapter for cookbooks with specific recipes for making your own gluten-free yeast breads and pasta from scratch. Many of these cookbooks have bread recipes formulated to be made in your bread machine.

Corn or rice tortillas are delicious to use instead of bread or flour tortillas.

Polenta (regular, quick, or ready-made) is good as a hot cereal or pasta replacement.

Rice is also gluten-free. Choose brown basmati rice, as regular brown rice tends to go rancid rapidly during storage.

Quinoa flakes cook up like quick oatmeal, have a nutty flavor, and are gluten-free.

Cider vinegar, wine vinegar, or balsamic vinegar (watch for lead; see page 196) replace and improve on distilled vinegar.

Mayonnaise must be made by you, since jarred brands are made with processed vegetable oils, even though they may be made without grain-based vinegars. See recipe, page 331, or keep searching for pure olive oil mayo or aioli.

Condiments, such as mayonnaise, ketchup, relish, and others are a special problem, because most contain sugar and vinegar and most commercial vinegar is made from wheat. Stay away from any prepared condiment listing vinegar or distilled vinegar as an ingredient. A little hunting will turn up gluten-free condiments such as Bragg Liquid Aminos, San-J, Eden, Soken, or Chun King soy sauce, or any miso without wheat or barley.* Look for mustards made with cider or wine vinegar instead of distilled. When you avoid these foods because of the vinegar, you get the added benefit of skipping the refined sugar many of them contain. Bragg makes the only pure olive oil salad dressing around.

---

* These brands have some varieties containing wheat; check the ingredients list.

Time-Saving Tips to Get More Veggies into Your Diet

✦ Use a very sharp knife to chop vegetables. It makes the job easier and gives you more control over the final product. Food processors are fine, although I find that the extra setup and cleanup time offset any time saved in preparing the vegetables. Though veggies are most nutritious when eaten soon after being cut, you can chop them ahead of time, if necessary. Be sure to refrigerate them and use them within two to three days.

✦ Prepare a large salad, full of a variety of raw vegetables and different types of lettuce, and store it in an airtight plastic container to use for a few days in a row. Use romaine, red leaf, green leaf, or fancy mixed greens, like mesclun, because iceberg lettuce is not nutritious (and is hard to digest, too). Keep in mind when counting your daily 4 to 6 cups of vegetables that lettuce only counts as half a serving (that is, 1 cup of lettuce really only counts as ½ cup of vegetables) because of its bulk and relatively low nutritive value. Make sure your salad is chock-full of other vegetables.

✦ Bake potatoes or yams, several at a time, then use them as needed for quick snacks or soups, or sliced and sautéed as side dishes.

✦ Make large quantities of vegetable soup or stew, and freeze 2-cup portions for future use.

✦ Steam vegetables in a stainless steel steamer or a steaming basket.

✦ Stir-fry vegetables by putting 1 teaspoon to 1 tablespoon extra virgin olive oil in a cast-iron skillet or wok. Heat the skillet over medium heat and add vegetables, stirring until tender but still crisp. You may use beef, chicken, or vegetable broth for additional liquid and flavor.

✦ Steam-sauté veggies in a sauté pan, with a small amount of water or stock and Bragg Liquid Aminos. Heat to boiling, then remove from heat, cover, and let stand 15 to 20 minutes. You'll love the great flavor! Or sauté vegetables in water only and add 1 teaspoon to 1 tablespoon of coconut oil or extra virgin olive oil after cooking.

✦ Buy vegetarian or vegetable cookbooks for ideas. (See the Resources section for this chapter for some suggestions.)

✦ Make your own sprouts. Clean the seeds thoroughly first! When prepared properly, sprouts are a wonderfully rich source of enzymes, vitamins, and nutrients. Unfortunately, most store-bought alfalfa sprouts are not healthy to eat. Since 1995, U.S. health officials have traced thirty outbreaks of salmonella and *E. coli* to sprouts. The FDA has issued an advisory suggesting sprouts be avoided by the elderly, the very young, and anyone with a compromised immune system.[1] Usually, if sprouts have gone bad you can see a yellowish discoloration at the root ends. This yellow color indicates the presence of a fungus known as damping-off. Do not eat this type of sprout. Instead, grow them at home yourself, and eat them a day or two after sprouting occurs, before the fungus ever appears. It's helpful to add a few drops of hydrogen peroxide or grapefruit seed extract to the water when watering the sprouts to discourage the damping-off reaction.

Lactose Intolerant? Lactose-free milk is available at supermarkets. Milk with acidophilus to reduce lactose is also available at many stores.

Some people who are lactose intolerant can eat goat's or sheep's milk products. Cheeses made from these milks can be less allergenic. Pecorino and French feta are traditionally made with sheep's milk, but check the ingredients list on the package to be sure. Markets, delis, health food stores, and specialty stores such as Trader Joe's (see the Resources section for this chapter) are carrying an increasing variety of both kinds of cheese and yogurt.

Trying to Raise Your Serotonin Levels? Keep foods in your pantry that are high in serotonin or serotonin-raising tryptophan: any high-protein food, especially turkey, as well as pumpkin, bananas, and sunflower, sesame, and pumpkin seeds.

On the Anti-Yeast Diet? Bragg Liquid Aminos may be substituted for soy sauce on the yeast diet. When fighting yeast, increase the veggies you eat while you are limiting fruit. Have some celery, carrots, or other veggies prepared, ready to be eaten raw when you want a snack.

BE PREPARED FOR EATING ON THE GO

Eating on the go is one of the biggest sabotagers of a healthy eating plan. Plan ahead for meals away from home. Prepare salads and vegetables, and pack them in a small cooler with a refreezable ice container in the lid.

You should also make sure you always have a can opener with you; you never know when you'll be stuck somewhere and the only healthy food choice is a can of salmon. I also suggest you bring bottled water rather than relying on tap water to get your eight glasses a day. An insulated water bottle carrier is not only convenient, but can prevent the plastic bottle from overheating and leaching hormonelike chemicals into your water.

EATING AT RESTAURANTS

Restaurants present a challenge when you are following the Diet Cure plan. Instead of ingredient lists, you are faced with menu descriptions that provide more temptation than information. Your first strategy is simple and direct. Simply say to your server, "I need your help. I'm on a restricted diet, and can't have any [milk products; wheat, oats, rye, or barley; or whatever]" or "I'm trying to avoid too many carbohydrates, so could I have half the amount of rice and twice the amount of the side vegetable?" Most of the people who wait tables are happy to serve your needs. More and more, restaurant staffs are familiar with various diet restrictions and happy to help you make appropriate choices. Tell them your restrictions up front, then repeat them when giving your order, to be certain it's understood.

Be assertive about asking questions: "Is there sugar in the soup?" "Are there milk products in that dressing?" "Is the [entrée] breaded or floured?" "Can I get that broiled instead of fried?" "Does the house dressing use distilled or wine vinegar?" As your experience grows you will learn the specific questions that have to be asked in your particular case. Don't be embarrassed or intimidated. Getting the information you need may mean a trip or two to the kitchen for your server, but you are paying for this meal, you are expected to give a tip for the service you are requesting, and we are talking about *your* health!

Even after you have asked for general help in avoiding dishes that contain foods off-limits, explained the restrictions, and asked your questions, you still need to be careful. If you don't ask enough *specific* questions, you may be confronted with flour thickening in the clam chowder, croutons on your salad, or sugar in the Chinese food. The struggle to keep the bread off your table can become comical. If, after all your efforts, your dinner arrives with unacceptable ingredients, send it back. You and your health are worth it.

BROWSING THE MENU

Breakfast is probably the easiest meal of the day to have in a restaurant and still keep to your program. Eggs are great (even according to the American Heart Association!). You can get in one of your vegetable servings by choosing an omelet with spinach, zucchini, or other vegetable offerings. The high sodium, sugars, and nitrates and nitrites of ham (and most contains gluten), bacon, and sausage rule them out as regular fare. Juice concentrates the sugar of the fruit and is too sweet, but whole fruit is fine, or order vegetable or tomato juice with lemon to squeeze in it. You are probably steering clear of coffee and black tea because of the caffeine, but many restaurants now offer herb teas, or you can bring your own tea bags and just order hot water.

Any of the eggs and omelets listed on the menu with potatoes on the side are fine, but scrambled may contain milk or cheese unless you specify. If toast, biscuits, or a muffin are included with the entrée, ask if they will substitute potatoes or fruit. If you are gluten intolerant, you can bring a slice of your own gluten-free bread and ask them to toast it. Most restaurants will oblige.

At lunchtime, concentrate on the salads, especially those with meat or poultry, such as one with grilled chicken, or a chef's salad or a Cobb salad. If you are avoiding lactose you will, of course, omit cheese from the salad. It will still be a very satisfying meal. All of these salads should contain some protein and mixed vegetables along with whatever lettuce is used as the base. Ask for olive oil and wine vinegar to make your own dressing, or travel with Bragg nice pure olive oil dressing (or your own homemade). Chicken soup (with rice, not noodles, if you are gluten intolerant), bean or pea soup, vegetable or vegetable-beef soup, or turkey or chicken with vegetables have a good protein-to-carb ratio and are often gluten-, sugar-, and milk-free.

If you are gluten intolerant, skip the sandwich section on the menu or ask them to hold the bread and serve between lettuce leaves; if not, sandwiches heavy on the protein filling can be a good choice. Most restaurants offer whole-grain bread. But if you need yours gluten-free, you might bring your own bread to be made into a sandwich. Skip the pasta and dessert sections unless the pasta is whole grain (which you'll find in some health food restaurants) and the dessert is a lovely fresh fruit plate, which most restaurants can provide on request.

Entrées that are broiled, grilled, steamed, sautéed, roasted, or stir-fried are more likely to be healthy and gluten-free than fried offerings, which are often floured or breaded. Ask your waitperson to check with the kitchen if you need to avoid gluten, because some fish, poultry, and meats are floured before being sautéed, stewed, or roasted. Avoid deep-fried entrées, which are almost always coated with wheat-flour batter and cooked at carcinogen-creating high temperatures.

Because alcohol is like a super-carb, you'll need to keep your intake low and be sure to drink only when eating a protein-rich meal. Even the nonalcoholic beer and wine are high in empty carbs and typically contain some alcohol. Watch for grain-based booze if you're gluten intolerant.

Anticipating Allergy Problems You Could Have

When you consider:	You might ask the server to check:
Soup	Whether it is thickened with wheat flour or contains any pasta, has cheese, sugar, cream, or milk added, or has cheese on top.
Salad	Whether it has any croutons on it and if the dressing has distilled vinegar; if it has any cheese in it and if the dressing has milk products or sugar; if it contains mostly iceberg lettuce or better quality lettuces with other vegetables; and how big it is (you may want to order a large instead of a side salad).
Gravies/sauces	Whether it is thickened with wheat flour; if it contains sugar; if it is made with milk or cream.
Entrées	Whether the meat/fish/poultry is floured before cooking, has breading or batter on it, or is deep-fried; if it has any cheese (Parmesan is common); and how large the portion size is (ideally, it will take up one quarter or more of your plate).

The highly refined and processed foods that are so prevalent in American diets and are the source of so many of our food-related problems are largely missing from the diets in other countries. This makes ethnic or foreign restaurants promising choices when you want to eat out and stay with your plan. Comparing Diet Cure elements and culinary features shows us why.

CHINESE AND OTHER ASIAN CUISINES

I recommend steaming and stir-frying as preferred cooking methods. Chinese cooking features these methods in a high percentage of its recipes. Chinese restaurants can be found nearly everywhere and feature many different entrées with steamed or stir-fried vegetables, chicken or fish, and various spice combinations. You will probably want to steer clear of things like sweet and sour pork because it combines a particularly fatty meat with concentrated sweeteners, but there will be plenty of dishes featuring a variety of meats, seafood, and lightly cooked veggies for you to try.

Be sure to try some of the Chinese soups. Look for hot and sour soup, which is rich, spicy, and practically a meal in itself.

A few words of caution for the gluten intolerant regarding Chinese restaurants: Most of them use a soy sauce in the cooking and on the table that is made from wheat and can give you a problem. The wrappers on many foods—dim sum, spring rolls, wonton, and others—are also made from wheat. I have found the gluten-avoidance problems outweigh the benefits and have sought out other Asian cuisines in which small changes in ingredients result in big increases in interesting choices.

Thai, Cambodian, Vietnamese, and other Southeast Asian cuisines usually share the attributes of their Chinese cousins—lean meats, fresh veggies lightly cooked, and emphasis on steaming and quick stir-frying, for example. As an added bonus, Thai and Vietnamese restaurants usually have many gluten-free items on the menu; they tend to emphasize rice over wheat in their meals. For example, often the noodles are made from rice and are therefore gluten-free; ditto the spring roll wrappers. But remember, you'll still have to watch out for sugar in everything and for wheat in the soy sauce (you may want to bring your own). Milk is rare in Asian cuisines. Japanese, Chinese, Thai, and Vietnamese food seldom contain any milk products, making these restaurants' menus easy to choose from when avoiding milk.

One thing to beware of when eating Chinese food is monosodium glutamate (MSG). MSG, used heavily in Chinese food in the past, causes "Chinese restaurant headache syndrome," because many people are intolerant of it. Today, many Chinese restaurants forego the MSG, but some still use it. Ask. You may have to request that they leave it out.

MEXICAN FOOD

This is a good choice for eating out while sticking to the Diet Cure. It is especially easy to find in cities in the western United States, where Mexican restaurants and taquerias are prevalent.

Everybody's favorite appetizer in a Mexican restaurant is guacamole and chips. The good news is that the guacamole is fine, especially if it is made fresh at the table. The bad news is the deep-fried chips are on the "nonfood" list. Use the guacamole as a condiment on your entrée or bring a few of your own baked chips by Guiltless Gourmet.

The standard side dishes for entrées in Mexican restaurants are beans and rice. Just ask them to hold the rice to cut down on the carbs. Large salads with lettuce, veggies, and grilled chicken are found in most of these restaurants. Tortilla bowls that salads are sometimes served in are almost always made of deep-fried flour tortillas. Ask them to hold the tortilla bowl and serve your salad in a dish instead.

If you are avoiding gluten, get corn instead of flour tortillas, but ask, since wheat is sometimes added to corn tortillas now. Most flavored tortillas (spinach, tomato, and others) are made from refined wheat flour. Order a burrito on a plate without the wheat tortilla wrapper, to be eaten with a fork. Ask if they will substitute beans for the tortilla. Some burritos use whole wheat tortillas or soft corn tortillas. Enchiladas are traditionally made with corn tortillas, but they are sometimes made using wheat tortillas, and enchilada sauce can contain flour thickening, so ask if you are gluten intolerant.

You might also want to try tamales, which consist of meat (usually pork or chicken) or cheese wrapped in a cornmeal dough and steamed inside a corn husk wrapper. Add some salsa and guacamole. Fajitas are now fashionable in almost every Mexican restaurant and represent an excellent choice. Beef, prawns, or chicken are grilled and then served with warm tortillas (preferably corn), grilled veggies, salsa, guacamole, and sometimes other condiments.

If you are lactose intolerant, cheese will be your main concern when you eat Mexican food, because it is found in many dishes. It is usually a topping and easy for the kitchen to omit. It will sometimes be included in dishes such as burritos automatically, so it is best to ask.

ITALIAN FOOD

You won't have any trouble eating at an Italian restaurant, unless you don't like Italian food! After all, this is a Mediterranean cuisine using the right oils and lots of veggies. What's not to like? Well, they often feature marvelous Italian bread and pasta dishes that are out of balance, with too much starch. So you'll have to leave some on the plate if you have it "as is," and concentrate on other Italian delights. Consider the usual terrific salads made with a wide variety of greens, ripe red tomatoes, a little zesty onion, and a dressing based on extra virgin olive oil. Or how about a serving of roasted potatoes and some lightly sautéed herbed veggies with a nice piece of chicken or fish? Or polenta, a delicious cornmeal dish formed into firm cakes, may accompany your entrée. Deep-fried items are practically unheard of in Italian cooking, and real minestrone soup contains no pasta!

There will almost certainly be salmon on the menu, which you should consider ordering. Roasted chicken with rosemary and garlic is another frequent offering on Italian menus.

There are also wonderful vegetable dishes that appear as appetizers, such as baked eggplant with tomato, herbs, Gruyère or goat cheese, pesto, and a light tomato sauce; or portobello mushrooms stuffed (make sure there aren't any bread crumbs, if you are gluten intolerant) and baked. Keep your proportions in mind and you won't have any trouble finding ways to assemble a flavorful and satisfying meal.

Choices for the gluten and milk intolerant are, of course, much more limited in a cuisine built around wheat pasta and featuring lots of cheese, but you can always order meat, chicken, or fish, ask for a vegetable appetizer as an entrée, or order a salad (omit the croutons and grated Parmesan cheese). Most Italian restaurants will be happy to substitute polenta for pasta as a side dish, but the milk sensitive should check to be sure it contains no cheese. Stay alert: cheese in the polenta is something the waiter is apt to forget, even after you have told him of your allergy problem and quizzed him about other dishes. It's you who will suffer the discomfort (or worse) if a mistake is made, so always ask the extra question.

BUFFETS AND SALAD BARS

The variety of choices on a buffet or salad bar make them especially good places for eating lunch or dinner out. Try the roast meats, some vegetables, and a large salad composed of as many different vegetables as possible. If you don't have your own salad dressing with you, your best bet is simply oil and vinegar that you put on yourself. Large buffets will often have a fish entrée or two, which can be good choices. Chicken is fine unless it is deep-fried. Remember the balance between protein and carbohydrates and the "palm-size" guide to protein serving size. Let the veggies outnumber the starches about three to one. Choose lots of raw veggies, skipping the mayonnaise-laden potato and macaroni salads (the mayo almost certainly contains distilled vinegar anyway, plus damaged oils and sugar). Top a baked potato with salsa, cheese, sour cream, or butter (if you tolerate milk well), chopped broccoli, and/or chopped green onion. Vegetable, bean, or split pea soups or chili are a good combination with salad for a different meal and are often gluten- and milk-free.

THE FAST-FOOD GAUNTLET

Sometimes you just can't avoid fast-food places. The birthday boy simply *must* go to Chuck E. Cheese's. Soccer practice runs late and everybody ends up at Burger King. Here you are in deep-fried sodium heaven, so now what about your individualized Master Plan? Do you say, "What the heck," and order up a bacon double cheeseburger, jumbo fries, and a chocolate shake? Before we go there, let's consider some options.

If you have had some notice, you can pack something from home to take along. This is obviously the best alternative if it is available. You will have complete control over the meal. If you are the victim of a surprise attack, your best bet is to find out what the salad offerings are. Some of the pizza restaurant chains have a salad bar, where a better-than-fair meal can be assembled. If there is no salad offering and everything in sight is deep-fried, sodium soaked, or worse, then all you can do is limit the damage. But McDonald's offers three salads with grilled chicken and a few other workable items. Wendy's has better salads, heavy on the romaine, plus baked potatoes and of course grilled chicken sandwiches (again, discard half the bread). Taco Bell has a lot of beans, cheese, guacamole, some salad within the fajitas, and several entrée salads. (Hold the fried tortilla chips.) Best of all, Baja Fresh has bowls and salads high in protein and loaded with vegetables. They now have stores in more than fifteen states, where everything is made fresh—no frozen food and no microwaves. Avoid their salad dressings. Fast-food restaurants won't have olive oil on the side, or even vinegar or lemon, so bring your own dressing or forgo it altogether. Mexican salads, with their salsa, avocado, and cheese, taste fine without dressing. And you're not going to be eating there often, right?

If you have intolerances, avoid the poisons. If you are gluten intolerant, tell the people at Burger King that "your way" means "no bun." If milk is a problem, have them make your pizza without cheese. (I know it sounds odd, but lots of pizza in Italy—and New York City—is sold this way.) Just do the best you can. One meal will not be fatal to either you or your Diet Cure plan.

EATING AT THE HOMES OF FAMILY OR FRIENDS

Most of the problems you might face while dining in other people's homes can be addressed by simply and politely controlling your own portions. As we have seen earlier, foods on the Diet Cure plan are mainly the foods everybody eats; it is the proportion of meat to vegetable to starch that is different. See chapter twenty for more help on visualizing proportions. Keep the ratios in mind and focus on the protein and vegetables. Most people will admire you if you say you're seriously low carb.

If you are dealing with allergies and intolerances, your host or hostess would much rather hear your dietary needs ahead of time, before you sit down to eat the meal he or she has carefully prepared. Your host certainly doesn't want you to feel that you are not getting enough to eat because you are avoiding something he has cooked, or that you might chance hurting your health by eating something you shouldn't just to please him. Give examples to make it clear what you are saying. For example, if you are gluten intolerant, you could say, "That means no bread, flour, or pasta for me. I can have rice and corn, but wheat, oats, rye, and barley are out." Then offer to bring a dish of your own, if your special needs would inconvenience him or her. But if your host would be discomfited by your needs or you're at a work function of complete rigidity, eat heartily *before* you go. Don't try to wait till afterward to eat. Your blood sugar will drop, you'll feel edgy, and you'll end up in the dessert.

Obviously, the best way to ensure that you stick to your Diet Cure plan is to prepare your own meals from fresh ingredients. While that's not always possible, in the next chapter you'll see that it's a lot easier to do than you might think.

Readings

Janet Bailey, *Keeping Food Fresh: How to Choose and Store Everything You Eat* (New York: HarperPerennial, 1989).

Mark Bittman, *How to Cook Everything: 2,000 Simple Recipes for Great Food—Completely Revised 10th-Anniversary Edition* (Hoboken, NJ: Wiley, 2008).

Andrea Chesman, *Serving Up the Harvest: Celebrating the Goodness of Fresh Vegetables* (North Adams, MA: Storey Publishing, 2007).

——, *The Roasted Vegetable: How to Roast Everything from Artichokes to Zucchini for Big, Bold Flavors in Pasta, Pizza, Risotto, Side Dishes, Couscous, Dips, Sandwiches, and Salads* (Boston: Harvard Common Press, 2011).

Barbara Cousins, *Cooking Without: Recipes Free from Added Gluten, Sugar, Dairy Products, Yeast, Salt, and Saturated Fat* (Northampton, England: Thorsons Publishing, 1997).

Phyllis Z. Goldberg, *How to Tolerate Lactose Intolerance: Recipes and a Guide for Eating Well Without Dairy Products* (Springfield, IL: Charles C. Thomas Publisher, 1998).

Bette Hagman, *The Gluten-Free Gourmet: Living Well Without Wheat*, Revised Edition (New York: Henry Holt, 2000).

——, *The Gluten-Free Gourmet Cooks Fast and Healthy: Wheat-Free Recipes with Less Fuss and Less Fat* (New York: Henry Holt, 2000).

——, *More from the Gluten-Free Gourmet: Delicious Dining Without Wheat*, 2nd Edition (New York: Henry Holt, 2000).

Beth Kidder, *The Milk-Free Kitchen: Living Well Without Dairy Products* (New York: Henry Holt, 1991).

Joanne Stepaniak, *The Ultimate Uncheese Cookbook: Delicious Dairy-Free Cheeses and Classic "Uncheese" Dishes* (Summertown, TN: Book Publishing Co., 2003).

Jane Zukin, *Dairy-Free Cookbook: Over 250 Recipes for People with Lactose Intolerance or Milk Allergy*, 2nd Edition (New York: Clarkson Potter, 1998).

Resources

LOCAL SUPPLEMENT RESOURCES

Nearby health food stores and pharmacies carry many supplements. Walmart stores (and walmart.com) do, too. Trader Joe's and (less so) Costco also supply supplements, and many supermarkets are increasing their supplement offerings.

The Vitamin Shoppe
vitaminshoppe.com; (866) 293-3367
The Vitamin Shoppe has four hundred stores, phone shopping, online shopping, and twenty thousand products available at up to a 40 percent discount.

GNC (General Nutrition Centers)

gnc.com

GNC has more than four thousand stores in all fifty states and forty-eight foreign countries. Their website includes a convenient search engine that will locate stores by distance from your home. It also allows you to shop online. Their offerings are more limited than other suppliers', but it may be the only store available in some areas.

ONLINE AND PHONE SUPPLEMENT RESOURCES

Use these suggestions, listed in order of my staff's preference, to comparison shop; or start with the top shop, which has everything listed in this book, and explore options when you start feeling feisty.

Diet Cure Online

dietcure.com; (800) 733-9293, Monday–Friday, 9:00 A.M.–5:00 P.M. MST

This is my clinic's order line, which has all of the supplements recommended in *The Diet Cure*.

Swanson Health Products

swansonvitamins.com; (800) 824-4491

Swanson provides a huge variety of products at very reasonable prices. In business since 1969, live people answer their phones!

Vitacost

vitacost.com; (800) 381-0759

More than thirty-five thousand supplements of top brands at prices that are 33 to 70 percent less than retail, and a thirty-day money-back guarantee on all products returned for any reason.

iHerb

iherb.com

More than six hundred brands and twenty thousand products on this computer-friendly site. No phone orders.

Vitamin Express

vitaminexpress.com

A family-owned company offering discounted prices since 1982, along with great service, health information, and enthusiasm for *The Diet Cure*.

FOOD RESOURCES

Farmers' markets: USDA Agricultural Marketing Service

apps.ams.usda.gov/FarmersMarkets/

AMS works to maintain a current listing of farmers' markets throughout the United States. Find the one closest to you by using their maps and/or search criteria.

Community Supported Agriculture
csacenter.org
Locate a CSA farm near you by ZIP Code, state, or farm name, using this national database provided by Wilson College's Robyn Van En Center.

Whole Foods Market
wholefoods.com
Whole Foods Market has stores in more than thirty states. It also sells supplements and herbs, so this can be one-stop-shopping heaven. But check contents before you buy. There's so much sugar in many of the products. Organic sugar is still addictive and void of nutrients! The gluten-free foods are very sweet and full of nonfat dried milk. Much of the produce is not organic. See the website for the location closest to you, but watch the prices; it's not referred to as "Whole Paycheck" for nothing.

More conventional supermarkets, such as Trader Joe's, are now carrying organic food and supplements (and online sources of supplements have even better prices). Haggle at farmers' markets if you find their prices too high (which is an unfortunate trend).

The Gluten-Free Mall
glutenfreemall.com
Offering online shopping for those on gluten-free diets since 1998, the Gluten-Free Mall may have the best prices and selection of gluten-free, wheat-free, casein-free, and other allergy-related health foods and special dietary products on the Internet. (Watch for sweeteners and high-starch items, as you should anytime you shop for gluten-free.)

TWENTY

Menus, Meal Ideas, and Recipes

MEAL IDEAS

BREAKFAST: DON'T LEAVE HOME WITHOUT IT

If you want to eliminate cravings, breakfast is the most crucial meal for you. Too many people grab a quick muffin or bagel and coffee on the way to work, starting the cycle of craving sweets and starches that leads to blood sugar instability and more craving. Start your day right, with a nutritious breakfast. Here are some suggestions. (See also specific recipes later in this chapter.)

Smoothies. Smoothies, or fruity blender drinks, are delicious and easy-to-digest meals in a glass. They can be a terrific balanced protein-carbohydrate-fat beverage. Use milk, yogurt, or coconut milk (not fruit juice or rice milk, because of the high sugar content), then blend in whole fruit. For protein, add nuts or seeds and protein powder.

Fresh fruit is best, but frozen fruit can be added all year round and is excellent in smoothies. Totally frozen smoothies may be too cold for your body to handle, especially in the cooler months of the year or first thing in the morning. (You don't want to freeze your kidneys!)

Other Quick and Delicious Breakfast Ideas
  ✦ Have a bowl of cottage cheese (1 cup) with sliced fresh fruit and a few almonds or sunflower seeds.

✦ Make a base of ½ cup rice or a corn tortilla (heat in a skillet with a few drops of water and the lid on). Top with some of the following:

  ✦ leftover turkey or chicken, with tomato, avocado, onion, and lettuce
  ✦ hummus (garbanzo bean spread/dip)
  ✦ crumbled hard-boiled egg

✦ Cream of Rice cereal, or soft, hot polenta with a dash of cinnamon or nutmeg, plus any or all of the following sources of protein:

  ✦ protein powder and/or nutritional yeast
  ✦ raw nuts or seeds
  ✦ coconut milk, seed or nut milk (see recipe on page 327)
  ✦ protein powder, yogurt, or cottage cheese (unless, of course, you're lactose intolerant), or an egg (stir in just before removing the cereal from heat, so the egg will cook)

✦ Two or three eggs (including the yolk) with one of the following:

  ✦ polenta and tomato sauce.
  ✦ vegetables, scrambled with the eggs (you can use leftovers or frozen mixed vegetables, if needed, to make this faster). Sauté 1 to 5 cups (measured when raw) zucchini, tomatoes, onion, or other veggies, using extra virgin olive oil or butter (with a little broth or water, if needed). Then add 3 eggs and scramble. If you need more carbs, add potatoes or whole grain toast.

LUNCH IDEAS

Lunches you make yourself are a sure way to get the foods you want to eat while sticking to your Master Plan. If you have a refrigerator available where you work, store an assortment of raw veggies, some cooked poultry or meat (not lunch meat), cooked beans, and salad dressing to be assembled into a large salad; or bring a large mixed-vegetable salad with protein from home and store it until lunch. Even if you don't have refrigeration available, you can bring your lunch to work, school, or any other outing in one of the insulated containers made for that purpose. Alternately, you could bring soup in a wide-mouthed Thermos bottle.

SNACKS

Snacks are an important part of the Diet Cure Master Plan. You should not go more than four to five hours without food. Snacks can tide you over between meals. Also, snacking gives you an opportunity to work foods you might not otherwise eat, such as fruit, into your day. Carry around your own healthy snacks, so you don't get stuck with convenience-store fare.

Try these healthy snacks for when you just want a bite of something:

✦ A piece of fruit, with nuts or cheese.
✦ A handful of sunflower or pumpkin seeds, raw almonds, cashews, or other nuts.
✦ Carrots, celery, or other fresh vegetables with hummus, bean dip, or nut butter.
✦ Plain, low-fat yogurt or cottage cheese with ½ cup berries or sliced fruit of your choice.
✦ Vegetable sticks. Aside from carrots and celery, you can snack on red pepper strips, broccoli and cauliflower florets, cucumber and zucchini circles, jicama slices, or cherry tomatoes. Wrap them in thinly sliced turkey or beef.

DINNER IDEAS

You've come home tired after a typically hectic day at work, or your afternoon has been full of running errands and cleaning up after the kids, or your energy just isn't high enough to cook a big meal. Yet dinner is traditionally the biggest meal of the day, and maybe the only one you eat together with your family. The following dinner suggestions are easy to prepare, nourishing, and tasty, while staying with the proportions of the ideal meal.

You could make baked fish or chicken and a baked potato or yam in the same oven, plus two or more cups of steamed veggies, coleslaw with oil-and-vinegar dressing, or cherry tomato and cucumber salad. Or stir-fry lots of veggies with shrimp, chicken, meat, or, occasionally, tempeh chunks, with ginger, garlic, and soy sauce to taste, while your brown basmati rice cooks. Or sauté or bake duck legs, prawns, or another favorite protein (without breading) and serve on baked spaghetti squash or whole grain pasta (rice, corn, or quinoa for the gluten intolerant) with pesto or marinara sauce; complete this meal with a large salad with olives, onions, peppers, and cucumbers.

Preparing Your Meals: Recipes and Menus

Here's what's coming up in this section.

✦ **General Help for Getting More Protein and Vegetables into Your Meals**
   ♦ Slow Cookers
   ♦ Select-a-Salad—an easy-to-follow chart for a salad to go with a meal, or one to be an entire meal
   ♦ Construct-a-Sandwich—steps to making a Diet Cure sandwich
   ♦ Delicious Vegetable Protein; Soup; and Pasta, Polenta, and Rice Suggestions
   ♦ Toppings for Vegetables
✦ **Specific Recipes for Breakfast, Lunch, and Dinner**

All are gluten-free and milk-product-free (or optional).

✦ **Sample Menus for Two Weeks**

The recipes are separated by meal type, but don't let that limit you. Go ahead and have Joe's Special for breakfast, or Egg-and-Vegetable Frittata for Dinner, or even a smoothie for a quick lunch on the run. Leftovers make an easy-to-fix meal or snack. Cook in large batches, providing "planned-overs" to have the next day.

SLOW COOKERS

Slow cookers (e.g., Crock-Pots) are back and we love them, especially the ones with timers that turn down to "warm" once the food is cooked. Put meat and vegetables in the pot in the morning, set the timer, and supper is ready when you get home in the evening. Just add a salad and enjoy. The chicken recipe on page 332 is my favorite! Also try cooking duck legs on low in a slow cooker for six hours. They come out tender, confit-style. Throw them in a hot skillet before serving, if you like your duck crispy.

SELECT-A-SALAD

Salads are a great way to enjoy all your food groups and get the nutrients you need. They're also easy to make, lovely to look at, and delicious when made fresh. Use the following chart for hundreds of salad variations.

For a complete-meal salad: Select items from lists 1, 2, 3, 4, and 5 and combine for a salad that is a satisfying meal.

For a side salad to go along with a protein entrée: Select from lists 1, 2, 5, and if there's no other starchy carb in the meal, 3.

1 2 cups or more from this list	2 1 cup or more from this list	3 Total of ½ cup from this list	4 ¾ cup or more from this list	5 2 tbs. from this list
✦ green or red leaf lettuce ✦ spinach ✦ romaine lettuce ✦ arugula ✦ mesclun ✦ other mixed greens ✦ cabbage ✦ *or* omit this list and use 1 more cup from list 2	✦ raw broccoli or cauliflower ✦ steamed broccoli, asparagus, green beans, or cauliflower ✦ tomatoes ✦ cucumber ✦ bell peppers ✦ avocado ✦ carrot, sliced or grated	✦ green peas ✦ black-eyed peas; lima, kidney, garbanzo, cannellini, black, or pinto beans ✦ corn, rice, or other cooked grains ✦ cooked potatoes or sweet potatoes	✦ roast beef, chicken, or turkey ✦ ¼ cup nuts and/or seeds ✦ cottage cheese ✦ ¼ cup feta cheese ✦ ½ cup beans or peas	✦ vinaigrette ✦ Vegetarian Caesar Salad Dressing (see recipe on page 330) ✦ other salad dressing with good oils and no sugar

CONSTRUCT-A-SANDWICH

1. Start with rice toast or other wholegrain bread served open-faced.
2. Add hamburger or tuna, chicken, or turkey salad.
3. Top with quality lettuce.
4. Stack on raw veggies (for example, onions, tomatoes, carrots, celery, cucumber, red bell peppers).
5. Enjoy!

DELICIOUS VEGETABLE-PROTEIN SUGGESTIONS

✦ Bean-, nut-, and/or rice-stuffed vegetables (zucchini, squash, tomatoes, bell peppers, or some other). Be sure to count your protein grams to be sure you get enough.

✦ Vegetable stew or soup (see recipe on page 333) served with a palm-size piece of meat, or grated parmesan cheese stirred into the soup.

✦ Steamed, raw, or roasted vegetables topped with melted cheese.

✦ Egg and Vegetable Frittata (see recipe on page 328).

✦ Stir-fry veggies and 3 to 4 ounces of meat, poultry, fish, or shrimp.

✦ Shish kebob.

SOUP SUGGESTIONS

✦ Split pea (with curry powder), Lentil (with tomato), Black Bean (add Mexican seasoning).

✦ Vegetable: Use mixed vegetables, or feature a single vegetable (leek, onion, peas, spinach, watercress).

✦ Chicken or turkey and rice or potatoes with other vegetables (see Easy Turkey or Chicken Soup recipe, on page 333).

✦ Minestrone without pasta—the traditional way!

✦ Vegetarian Stock: Blend cooked garbanzo beans with lemon zest and cumin; add Bragg Liquid Aminos and water to taste. Use as a stock for cooking green veggies (snow peas, snap peas, summer squash, and others).

PASTA, POLENTA, AND RICE SUGGESTIONS

✦ Soft polenta (or warmed leftover or store-bought polenta, sliced) with vegetables, tomato sauce, and meat, fish, or chicken

✦ Pasta with vegetables, tomato sauce, and feta cheese

Note: Do not use white flour pasta. Try corn, rice, bean thread, yam, or quinoa pasta, 100 percent buckwheat soba (12 percent protein), or others made with whole wheat flour (if you tolerate it well).

TOPPINGS FOR VEGETABLES

If you aren't used to eating a lot of vegetables, you have a lot to discover about easy preparation methods that give veggies a new twist. Try these for a treat.

- Olive oil. Good on everything.
- Tomato sauce with sheep or goat feta and/or pumpkin seeds. Good with steamed zucchini or other squash.
- Butter and lemon juice. Wonderful with broccoli or asparagus.
- Fresh herbs. Try dill on carrots, or mint with peas.
- Garlic. Spinach or other greens are delicious sautéed until tender in a little olive oil with minced or crushed garlic.
- Almond, cashew, or sesame butter. Make it into a sauce by blending it with a little water—great on green beans.
- Mustard or horseradish sauce. Mix powdered mustard or horseradish with a little water and oil. Either is good with broccoli or asparagus, especially when served with beef.
- Yogurt with fresh herbs, salt, pepper, and garlic. Delicious mixed with green beans, broccoli, and onion.
- Avocado dressing. This can be made quickly in a bowl. Mash an avocado with a fork. Add about 2 tbs. olive oil or ¼ cup yogurt, a little garlic salt, pepper, herbs (cilantro or parsley is good), and lemon juice to taste. A thinner dressing can be made by adding more yogurt and/or using a blender.
- Bragg Liquid Aminos and pepper.
- Bragg Liquid Aminos and lemon juice.
- Homemade oil-based salad dressing. Quickly makes brussels sprouts, broccoli, cauliflower, or green beans something special.

Breakfast

PROTEIN SMOOTHIE

As a base, choose one of the following:
    8 ounces of whole-fat cow's or goat's milk, yogurt or kefir
        (unsweetened), or 4 ounces of coconut milk (plus water, if
        more liquid is needed)
Pour into blender.

Add:

   ½ banana (or ½ cup pumpkin, sweet potato, or winter squash)
      and other fresh fruit, such as ½ cup berries or a peach
   2 tablespoons pea, rice, or whey protein powder (20–30 grams
      protein)
Plus any or all of the following:
   1 teaspoon to 1 tablespoon nutritional yeast
   Some leafy greens, like chard, spinach, or beet tops
   2 tablespoons flaxseeds

Blend well. Drink and enjoy!

Note: Do not use milk, yogurt, or whey if you have milk intolerance. Limit protein powder to once a day.

SEED OR NUT MILK

A half cup of seeds will usually make 2 cups of seed milk, which will keep two to three days in the refrigerator.

½ cup sunflower seeds, pumpkin seeds, pine nuts, filberts, and/or
   almonds
2 cups water

Soak the seeds or nuts overnight in enough water to cover them.

Drain off soaking water and put nuts or seeds in blender with enough fresh, cold water to cover. Blend into a cream. Add water to the blender until the milk is a texture that you like. If you like an ultrasmooth consistency, strain the seeds, add more fresh water, and blend again.

NUT MILK SHAKE

This occasional variation is especially good for building up your serotonin level, and the pumpkin is a good alternative to fruit.

Liquid base of 1 to 2 cups seed or nut milk (see recipe above);
   or 2 tablespoons raw tahini; or ¼ cup soaked seeds blended in
   ½ to ¾ cup water; or 3 tablespoons coconut milk (frozen in ice
   cube trays if you like cold smoothies)
Into this base add:
   ½ banana (yellow, not overripe, frozen or fresh)
   ½ cup fruit (such as frozen or fresh berries or apple) or
      cooked or canned pumpkin (if fruit is too sweet for you)

2 tablespoons protein powder
Nutmeg, cinnamon, cloves, fresh ginger, or other spices
**   to taste**

Place ingredients in a blender and blend until the shake reaches a desired consistency. Add water or ice to create a texture you like.

QUICK HOT CEREAL

¹/₃ cup quinoa flakes (or polenta, or blender-ground cooked
**   [leftover] brown/red/wild rice)**
1 cup water
Pinch of salt

Add quinoa to boiling water. Return to boil and cook 90 seconds, stirring often. Makes 1 cup, which is one serving. You can flavor your hot cereal with tahini, chopped almonds, protein powder, cinnamon, ground flaxseeds, or butter.

Note: Make a double batch; leftover cereal can be heated the next day by adding a little water or milk.

FRUIT BOWL

Place in blender:
**   2 pieces of fruit (e.g., ½ large banana or 1 cup berries or**
**   papaya)**
**   ¹/₃ cup nuts or seeds soaked overnight**
**   2 tablespoons protein powder**
**   Your favorite spice (e.g., cinnamon, nutmeg)**
**   Just enough water to blend into a creamy sauce (start with a**
**   couple of tablespoons)**

Blend half the fruit with all other ingredients until it is as smooth as you like, adding more water if mixture is still too thick to suit you. Pour it over the remaining fruit cut into cubes and placed in a bowl.

EGG AND VEGETABLE FRITTATA

¼ red onion, chopped
1 cup kale or ½ cup other vegetables, chopped

2 teaspoons butter or ghee
3 whole eggs, well beaten
2 tablespoons crumbled sheep's or goat's milk feta (if tolerated)

Sauté onions and vegetables in the butter in a small ovenproof skillet. (If using leftovers, add them when onions are translucent.) Add the eggs and the cheese, and cook without stirring, tilting the skillet while lifting the edge of the cooked egg with a spatula, allowing uncooked egg to flow underneath. When no more uncooked egg will flow, put under a broiler until top begins to brown, 1 to 2 minutes.

Lunch or Dinner

See page 324 for the Select-a-Salad section (which I'll refer to frequently as Side Salad or Complete Meal Salad) and many other lunch and dinner suggestions.

PROTEIN SALAD

Place your Protein Salad on top of a Side Salad, on a piece of bread with lettuce and tomato, or on half a red bell pepper or avocado.

Salmon, chicken, turkey, or egg salad: Chop 3 to 4 ounces or 3 boiled eggs and mix with:
1 to 2 tablespoons mayonnaise (preferably your own, from the recipe on page 331)
1 teaspoon mustard
2–4 tablespoons mashed avocado
Any of the following, chopped: red onion, scallion, parsley, pine nuts, red bell pepper, cilantro, basil, or other herbs

Alternate ingredient suggestions:
✦ Sheep feta, walnuts, and canned organic cannellini beans
✦ Garbanzos, goat cheese, mint, and pine nuts
✦ White beans, sage, goat gouda, and roasted peppers

VEGETARIAN CAESAR SALAD DRESSING

This dressing can be stored in the fridge in an airtight container for about a week. (Top with grated Parmesan cheese, if you tolerate it.)

In a blender, purée the following ingredients:
  1 cup olive oil
  1 teaspoon Dijon mustard
  2 teaspoons brewer's yeast
  1 teaspoon capers
  2 teaspoons water
  1 teaspoon vegan Worcestershire sauce
  ½ cup lemon juice (about 2–3 lemons)

SESAME TAHINI SAUCE OR DRESSING

Make this thick (½ cup water) for a sauce for Falafel Patties, page 336; or thin for a salad dressing on tomatoes, cucumbers, red onion, grated carrot, and/or beets with arugula and/or chopped romaine.

¾ cup tahini (sesame butter), well mixed
2 cloves garlic, crushed
¼ cup lemon juice
Salt to taste
½–1 cup water, as needed (more for dressing, less for sauce)

Stir or purée in a food processor. Add mint and/or any other fresh herbs you like.

AVOCADO DRESSING

Juice of 2 fresh limes
3 small avocados
1 clove garlic
2 scallions, chopped
½ cup water
1 jalapeño pepper, seeded
1 tablespoon fresh cilantro
Salt and pepper

Purée the ingredients in a blender or food processor. Season with salt and pepper, and serve on your favorite salad.

PERFECT BLENDER MAYONNAISE

MAKES ABOUT 1¼ CUPS

Combine in a blender jar:
    1 large egg
    1 tablespoon apple cider vinegar
    ½ teaspoon salt
    ¼ teaspoon dry mustard
    1 cup extra virgin olive oil
    1 tablespoon lemon juice

Combine first 4 ingredients in a blender jar, cover, and blend 5 seconds. With blender running on the *slowest speed*, add ½ cup extra virgin olive oil in the thinnest steam you can, aiming for halfway between the side of the jar and the vortex in the middle. Add the lemon juice. Gradually add ½ cup more olive oil until blended. If the oil stops moving into the center, stop the blender and break the surface tension using a spatula, or turn the blender off and on again. Store for up to four weeks in a tightly covered jar in the refrigerator.

RED QUINOA TABOULI

SERVES 3 TO 4

After trying this, you, too, will say, "This recipe's a keeper!"

2 cups water
1 cup red quinoa (white will do if you can't find red)
3 firm ripe tomatoes, chopped (2 cups)
1 cucumber, peeled and chopped (1 cup)
2 tablespoons fresh mint, minced
1½ cups parsley, chopped
1 cup scallions, chopped
1 can garbanzos, drained and rinsed
½ cup fresh lemon juice
½ cup extra virgin olive oil
Salt to taste

Place the water and quinoa in a 1-quart saucepan. Bring to a boil. Reduce heat to a simmer, cover, and cook for 10–15 minutes or until all water has been absorbed. Cool slightly before adding to vegetables.

While the quinoa is cooking, finely chop the tomatoes, cucumber, mint, parsley, and scallions. Put into a large bowl with the garbanzos, and add lemon juice and olive oil.

Stir in cooked quinoa and salt. Mix well. Refrigerate for 8–24 hours to blend flavors.

CAJUN-RUBBED CHICKEN ROASTED IN A SLOW COOKER

SERVES 4

An easy recipe for tender, spicy, fall-off-the-bone chicken! (Even easier if you substitute 3–4 tablespoons Cajun's Choice or other brand creole seasoning for the first 8 ingredients.) This recipe is also good with chicken or turkey thighs.

2 teaspoons salt
2 teaspoons paprika
1 teaspoon cayenne pepper
1 teaspoon onion powder
1 teaspoon thyme
1 teaspoon white pepper
½ teaspoon garlic powder
½ teaspoon black pepper
1 large roasting chicken (or 6 chicken or 2 turkey thighs)

In a small bowl, combine the spices. (Skip if you are using prepared seasoning.)

Remove any giblets from the chicken, rinse, and pat dry. Rub spice mixture all over the chicken, inside and outside. Place chicken in slow cooker pot and cook on low 4–6 hours.

The juices can be used to make gravy: Skim the fat off the drippings and place them in a skillet. (You should have 3–4 tablespoons.) While heating the fat, add about ¼ cup of garbanzo flour and stir with a wire whisk until the flour is thoroughly blended in. Cook a minute or two over medium heat; add the remaining juices, while stirring, and cook until bubbly and thickened.

EASY TURKEY OR CHICKEN SOUP

SERVES 4

This one-pot meal is ready in about 30 minutes from start to finish, and the kale provides essential omega-3 fatty acids.

1 tablespoon olive oil
1 pound boneless turkey or chicken breast,
    cut in ½-inch cubes
2 medium carrots, sliced
2 stalks celery, sliced
1 medium onion, chopped
4 cups natural chicken stock
1½ teaspoons Italian herbs
1 bay leaf
2 cloves garlic, minced (or ½ teaspoon
    granulated garlic)
2 medium potatoes, diced
1 bunch kale or chard (stems removed and chopped fine)
Salt and pepper to taste

Heat the oil in a large pot over medium heat, then add the poultry, carrots, celery, and onion. Sauté, stirring frequently, until turkey or chicken is no longer pink. Add the stock, herbs, bay leaf, garlic, potatoes, and kale. Bring to a simmer. Turn heat to low, cover, and simmer until the vegetables are tender (about 10 minutes). Add salt and pepper to taste. Remove the bay leaf before serving.

Variations: **You now have a basic recipe for a soup or the beginning of a stew. You can add any other vegetables you like and simply adjust the liquid for desired thickness.**

If you would like to add more starch, this will thicken the soup and make it more like a stew. Add one of the following:
✦ ½ cup split peas
✦ ½ cup buckwheat
✦ ½ cup rice noodles
✦ ½ cup lentils

Add 2 extra cups of water with added starch.

For **Dahl-Style Indian Stew**, omit Italian herbs and add with stock:

✦ ½ cup lentils
✦ 2 teaspoons curry powder
✦ Fresh chilies to taste
✦ 1 stalk lemongrass, chopped into big pieces and sautéed (used to flavor, but not eaten)

Add the following with the kale:

✦ ¼ cup cilantro, chopped
✦ 1 can coconut milk (or light coconut milk)

Substitute sausage for the chicken and add split peas for another hearty stew.

CORN CHOWDER WITH VEGETABLES AND SHRIMP OR FISH

SERVES 6

1 tablespoon butter
1 onion, chopped
2 stalks celery, chopped
1 large yellow bell pepper, chopped
1 pound new potatoes, diced
1½ quarts vegetable or chicken stock
Kernels cut from 6 ears of corn (or 6 cups frozen corn)
1 tablespoon chopped fresh basil
1 tablespoon chopped fresh thyme
1½ pounds cooked shrimp (about 30 shrimp per pound is a good size)
2 cups milk (optional; or substitute 2 extra cups stock or canned tomatoes)

In a large stockpot melt the butter and add onion, celery, pepper, and potatoes. Sauté on medium heat for about 5 minutes. Add the stock. Lower the heat and simmer until the vegetables are tender. Add the corn, herbs, shrimp, and milk, and heat through.

Variation: For Fish Chowder, omit shrimp and instead use 1½ pounds fish cut in small pieces and sautéed. Add to chowder along with herbs, corn, and milk, and heat through.

CLASSIC POT ROAST

1 medium onion, sliced into rings
2 pounds beef roast (chuck or rump, thawed or frozen)
½ teaspoon salt
½ teaspoon black pepper
2 cloves garlic, pressed
4–6 medium red potatoes, cut in quarters
2 cups baby carrots (or regular carrots, cut in 1-inch slices)
1 cup sliced celery
½ cup red wine or beef broth
3 tablespoons gluten-free Worcestershire sauce (optional)

Place the sliced onion in the bottom of a slow cooker (Crock-Pot). Add meat and seasonings. Toss in the potatoes, carrots, and celery. Pour wine (or beef broth) and Worcestershire on top. Cover and cook on low for about 6 hours if meat is thawed or 8 hours if frozen.

EASY BAKED PROTEIN
(FISH, POULTRY, OR MEAT)

1. Squeeze **Bragg Liquid Aminos** on both sides of the **protein (fish, poultry, or meat)**.
2. Cover the bottom of a baking dish with **balsamic vinegar, fresh lemon juice, fresh orange juice,** or **wine**.
3. Place cuts of fish, poultry, or meat in baking dish and turn them to coat both sides (some drier cuts of meat will need **1 tablespoon extra virgin olive oil**).
4. Sprinkle the protein with **one or two herbs or spices: oregano, parsley, cilantro, thyme, dill, basil, rosemary, garlic or onion powder, cumin, curry,** etc. Parsley, onion powder, and garlic powder can be used by themselves or in combination with one or more other herbs or spices. Thyme, marjoram, oregano, and rosemary go well together (they are the basis of the Italian seasoning sold in stores). Curry and dill seem to be best on their

own. Cilantro and cumin make a nice combination. Look on spice or herb labels; they often suggest companion spices.

5. Bake at 400 degrees for 20 to 30 minutes (time depends on the type and thickness of the protein).

FALAFEL PATTIES

MAKES 6 PATTIES
(10 GRAMS PROTEIN EACH)

I cup (about ½ pound) dried chickpeas (garbanzos)
3 cups water
½ cup quinoa flakes
½ cup boiling water
I red onion, cut into 6 pieces
¼ bunch parsley, chopped finely
I–2 cloves garlic, minced or pressed
2 tablespoons nutritional yeast
I teaspoon ground cumin
I teaspoon ground coriander
I teaspoon salt
Dash cayenne
I–2 tablespoons extra virgin olive oil

Soak the chickpeas in 3 cups water overnight. (They will almost triple in volume.) Drain the water off the chickpeas. Grind them in your food processor until finely ground. Place ground chickpeas in a medium-size bowl.

Place quinoa flakes in a small bowl and pour the boiling water over them.

Place the red onion pieces in the food processor and process until they are finely grated. Place the onion in the bowl with the chickpeas.

Place the parsley and garlic in the bowl with the chickpeas. Add the quinoa (which will have soaked up the water by now) to the chickpeas along with the nutritional yeast, cumin, coriander, salt, and cayenne. Mix thoroughly.

Heat the oil in a skillet over medium heat. Form the mixture into patties (a scant ⅔ cup per patty) and sauté for three minutes on each side or until evenly browned.

Note: These can be made with canned chickpeas, but the patties will be soft and fall apart easily. If you like, substitute two 14-ounce cans of chickpeas, drained and rinsed, for the dried chickpeas and 3 cups water, and eliminate the salt.

STEAMED SALMON

SERVES I

1 slice lemon
1 bay leaf (optional)
4 to 5 ounces salmon fillet

Put the lemon slice and bay leaf (if using) in a pot. Put a stainless steel steamer basket in the pot and add water to come up to, but not cover, the bottom of the basket. Bring the water to a simmer over medium heat. Place the salmon fillet in the basket and cover the pot with a lid. Steam the salmon just until it looks pink and no longer red inside when flaked with a fork (check after about 5 minutes). Serve with lemon, salt, and pepper to taste. Can also be served with Roasted Red Bell Pepper Butter (page 340) or dill mayo (1 tablespoon Perfect Blender Mayonnaise [page 331] blended with ½ teaspoon dried or minced fresh dill). Remove bay leaf before serving.

JOE'S SPECIAL

SERVES 4

Gluten-free and milk-free, Joe's Special is a nutritious standby for a quick meal.

4 ounces (1 cup) fresh mushrooms, sliced
1 onion, finely chopped
2 tablespoons butter
1 pound lean ground meat (turkey or beef)
1 bunch spinach, cleaned and chopped (other greens, such as kale, can be substituted, but will take longer to cook)
1 teaspoon garlic (2 cloves, minced)
Salt and pepper
6 eggs, beaten

Sauté sliced mushrooms and onion in the butter until lightly browned, then add ground meat and cook until it has browned. Stir in the spinach, garlic, salt, and pepper. When spinach has cooked down, pour in the eggs and stir, scrambled-egg style, until done and lightly set. Turn over once with a spatula and cook a minute or so longer. Serve very hot.

ZUCCHINI WITH CHERRY TOMATOES

SERVES 2

2 teaspoons olive oil
4 cups sliced zucchini (about 6 zucchini)
4 ounces mushrooms, sliced
2 to 3 cloves garlic, minced
8 ounces cherry tomatoes, halved
Salt and pepper to taste

Heat olive oil in a heavy pan or skillet on medium heat. Sauté zucchini, mushrooms, and garlic until zucchini are just tender. Add the cherry tomatoes, and salt and pepper to taste. Heat just until the cherry tomatoes are warm, and serve.

PAN-SEARED GREENS

SERVES 1–2

I tablespoon olive oil
I teaspoon garlic (2 cloves, minced)
4 cups of any of the following, chopped (listed in approximately the
  order of time they take to cook, from fastest to slowest):
    Spinach
    Bok choy
    Chard
    Purple cabbage
    Kale
    Collard greens
Salt to taste

Heat the oil in a large cast-iron skillet or pan until hot. Add the garlic and greens to the oil and sauté, tossing until wilted. Add little sprinkles of water to keep the greens from burning, until they are cooked through. Add salt, if needed.

OVEN-ROASTED OR GRILLED VEGETABLES

SERVES 2–3

2 cups high-carbohydrate vegetables along with 2 cups low-
carbohydrate vegetables, sliced.
Here are some suggestions:

High	Low
Jerusalem artichoke	Leeks
Onions	Carrots
Winter Squash	Turnips
Parsnips	Kohlrabi
Yams	Eggplant
	Brussels sprouts
	Asparagus
	Summer Squash or zucchini

2 tablespoons olive oil
Salt to taste
1 teaspoon garlic (2 cloves, minced)
2 teaspoons chopped rosemary

Preheat oven to 400 degrees, or heat grill to medium-high. Toss the vegetables with the oil, salt, garlic, and rosemary, and place them in a baking sheet or on the grill.

Roasting: Toss the veggies once and remove from the oven when tender and browned on edges (30–45 minutes, depending on density).

Grilling: 4–10 minutes (4 minutes for asparagus).

CREAMY POLENTA

6 cups water
2 cups polenta
Salt and pepper
2 tablespoons butter, Roasted Red Bell Pepper Butter (see page 340),
or olive oil

Bring the water to boil in a large pot and slowly stir in the polenta. Lower heat and cook, stirring almost constantly, until polenta forms a very thick mass, 20–30 minutes. Add salt and pepper to taste. Stir in olive oil or Bell Pepper Butter if desired. You can put the leftover polenta in an oiled loaf pan, cover, and put in the refrigerator. When it's cool, slices can be cut and warmed in a lightly oiled or buttered pan for a few minutes, then served with breakfast or dinner.

ROASTED RED BELL PEPPER BUTTER

Use this butter wherever you would use plain butter, from polenta or hot cereal to baked potatoes or vegetables. You can also toss it into rice or with rice noodles. Roasted bell peppers can be bought in jars at Trader Joe's or other stores.

1 cup roasted red bell peppers
½ pound (2 cubes or 1 cup) butter, softened
Squeeze of lemon (optional)

Purée the peppers with the butter and lemon in a food processor or blender at lowest speed until smooth. Place in a container and refrigerate. It will become firm when cold.

HIGH-PROTEIN YEAST BREAD

Made in a bread machine (like a Breadman), this has a hearty, moist texture and good flavor. This gluten-free, grass-grain-free bread holds together well for sandwiches, if lightly toasted. Have all ingredients at room temperature.

Place dry ingredients in a large bowl and stir together (a wire whisk works well):
1½ cups buckwheat flour (finely ground in blender from white—not roasted—buckwheat groats)
½ cup garbanzo bean flour
1½ cups quinoa flour
¼ cup arrowroot
2 teaspoons xanthan gum
2 teaspoons salt
1 tablespoon garlic granules
1 tablespoon dry yeast granules

Place wet ingredients in a bowl or blender jar and blend together:
2 eggs
¼ cup (½ stick) melted butter (or ¼ cup oil if dairy intolerant)

I cup water
I cup apple juice

Put wet and dry ingredients into bread machine container, according to manufacturer's directions. Set machine to Basic-Rapid setting (approximately 2 hours) and push Start. Using a spatula, scrape the sides of the pan to mix all ingredients. Close lid and let machine do the rest.

SAMPLE MENUS

Here are sample meals for two weeks to help you implement the Daily Food Guide (page 266). We're saving you time and effort by building in leftovers. Don't forget to add snacks.

WEEK ONE

DAY 1

Breakfast
1 orange, sliced with ½ cup blueberries
Egg and Vegetable Frittata (page 328)

Lunch
Complete Meal Salad (Select-a-Salad, page 324)

Dinner
4 to 5 ounces of baked chicken thighs (Easy Baked Protein, page 335)
    with lemon and rosemary
1 cup brown basmati rice with 1 tablespoon butter
1 cup steamed asparagus with butter and lemon
1 cup cherry tomato halves and cucumber slices with pitted Kalamata
    olives

DAY 2

Breakfast
Protein Smoothie (page 326)

Lunch
Mexican (leftover) chicken salad, tostada, or taco, with ½ cup beans,
    ½ avocado, lettuce, and/or finely sliced purple cabbage with chopped
    cilantro, and fresh salsa or fresh tomato, lemon or lime juice, and ha-
    banero sauce. (Optional: Steamed or baked-until-crisp tortilla.)

Dinner

Top ½ cup Creamy Polenta (page 339) with at least 1 cup vegetables (sautéed onions, bell peppers, and mushrooms with garlic in 1 table-spoon olive oil would be good); 4 to 6 ounces leftover chicken from Day 1; and ½ cup commercial marinara sauce
Side salad (Select-a-Salad, page 324)

DAY 3

Breakfast

½ cup leftover Creamy Polenta (page 339) with protein powder (con-taining 10–15 grams protein) and ½ cup chopped apples, peaches, or berries; a dash of cinnamon or nutmeg; and coconut or cow's milk to moisten as desired
2 links turkey or pork sausage

Lunch

Complete Meal Salad (Select-a-Salad, page 324)

Dinner

2 Falafel Patties (page 336) with ¼ cup Tahini Sauce (page 330)
Pan-Seared Greens (4 cups raw) (page 338)
Leftover basmati rice (½ cup)

DAY 4

Breakfast

½ grapefruit or ½ small melon
3 eggs, scrambled, boiled, or poached
1 piece of buttered whole grain toast or a corn tortilla

Lunch

Leftover Falafel Patties crumbled on top of a Side Salad (Select-a-Salad, page 324) with an extra serving from column 3

Dinner

1 beef or turkey burger with avocado (or cheese) slices
3 cups Oven-Roasted Vegetables (page 339)
Side Salad (Select-a-Salad, page 324)

DAY 5

Breakfast

Fruit Bowl (page 328—no other nuts or seeds today)

Lunch

Made-ahead Easy Chicken Soup (page 333)
Cherry tomatoes and bell pepper slices

Dinner

5- to 7-ounce steak or 2–3 lamb chops (with bone), cooked in a skillet or broiled
2 cups steamed broccoli with lemon and butter
Buttered corn on the cob

DAY 6

Breakfast

½ cup sliced fresh fruit
3 scrambled eggs, avocado, and salsa wrapped in 1–2 corn tortillas

Lunch

Complete Meal Salad (Select-a-Salad, page 324) with ½ cup beans plus any other option from column 4

Dinner

Joe's Special (page 337) over ½ cup rice or 2 oz (measure when dry) whole grain pasta (make enough for leftovers)
Raw cherry tomatoes, celery, and carrot sticks

DAY 7

Breakfast

Leftover Joe's Special

Lunch

Open-faced roast beef sandwich, with tomato, lettuce and onion
1 cup cucumber slices and bell pepper sticks

Dinner

Steamed Salmon (page 337) with dill mayo
Pan-Seared Greens (page 338)
1 cup Red Quinoa Tabouli (page 331)

WEEK TWO

DAY 1

Breakfast

1 cup chopped vegetables (chard, green onions, red peppers, or others) sautéed until just tender, then add 3 eggs and scramble until cooked to your liking (with 1 oz. feta cheese, if tolerated)

1–2 corn tortillas with 1 teaspoon butter or avocado slices

Plug in the slow cooker and do Cajun-Rubbed Chicken (page 332) for dinner.

Lunch

Leftover salmon and Red Quinoa Tabouli

Dinner

Cajun-Rubbed Chicken (page 332)

Side Salad (Select-a-Salad, page 324) with a carb from column 3

DAY 2

Breakfast

Nut Milk Shake (page 327; no more nuts or seeds today)

Lunch

Construct-a-Sandwich (page 324) with leftover chicken, tomato, lettuce, and ½ avocado

1½ cups raw veggies (celery, cherry tomatoes, carrots, cucumber, or some other)

Dinner

4 to 6 ounces Easy Baked Fish (page 335) brushed with garlic, olive oil, lemon juice, and soy sauce (gluten-free or Bragg Liquid Aminos), and 5 halved olives

2 cups Zucchini with Cherry Tomatoes (page 338)

1 cup baked sweet potato or yam (bake extra for leftovers) with 2 teaspoons butter

DAY 3

Breakfast

1 orange, sliced, or ½ grapefruit

3 scrambled eggs with ½ cup leftover sweet potatoes (sautéed in butter or coconut oil)

Plug in slow cooker and prepare Classic Pot Roast (page 335) for dinner.

Lunch
Complete Meal Salad (Select-a-Salad, page 324)

Dinner
Classic Pot Roast (page 335)
2 cups Grilled Vegetables (page 339), choose low-carb varieties
2 cups romaine with Vegetarian Caesar Salad Dressing (page 330)

DAY 4

Breakfast
½ cup Quick Hot Cereal (page 328) with ½ cup berries, 1 ounce walnuts, and 2 tablespoons protein powder or nutritional yeast, plus ¼ cup coconut milk

Lunch
2 leftover pot roast tacos (warm and shred meat and top with lettuce, ½ avocado, and salsa on 2 corn tortillas)
1½ cups raw veggies (carrots, celery, jicama)

Dinner
Egg and Vegetable Frittata, adding thinly sliced potatoes (page 328)
Side Salad (Select-a-Salad, page 324)

DAY 5

Breakfast
½ cup tropical fruit
2 scrambled, poached, or boiled eggs
2 pieces of thick bacon

Lunch
Complete Meal Salad (Select-a-Salad, page 324)

Dinner
Easy Turkey Soup (page 333; make enough for leftovers)
1 cup cherry tomatoes and other raw veggies

DAY 6

Breakfast
Protein Smoothie (page 326) made with blueberries and persimmon

Lunch
Large bowl of leftover Easy Turkey Soup
Nut crackers

Dinner
Stir-fry 3 to 5 cups veggies and 4 to 5 ounces scallop chunks with ginger, garlic, and soy sauce to taste
½ cup basmati rice with butter and curry powder
½ cup fresh fruit salad with 2 tablespoons coconut milk and mint

DAY 7

Breakfast
½ small melon
3 eggs, scrambled, topped with avocado (or cheese)

Lunch
Complete Meal Salad (Select-a-Salad, page 324)

Dinner
Corn Chowder with Vegetables and Shrimp (or variation, page 324)
Side Salad (Select-a-Salad, page 324), choosing ½ cup beans from column B

Readings and Online Resources

Mark Hyman, M.D., *The Ultrametabolism Cookbook: 200 Delicious Recipes That Will Turn On Your Fat-Burning DNA* (New York: Scribner, 2007).

Rebecca Katz with Mat Edelson, *One Bite at a Time: Nourishing Recipes for Cancer Survivors and Their Friends*, 2nd Edition (Berkeley, CA: Celestial Arts, 2008).

Shari Lieberman, Ph.D., CNS, FACN, with Linda Segall, *The Gluten Connection: How Gluten Sensitivity May Be Sabotaging Your Health—And What You Can Do to Take Control Now* (New York: Rodale Books, 2007).

Stephanie O'Dea, *Make It Fast, Cook It Slow: The Big Book of Everyday Slow Cooking* (New York: Hyperion, 2009). Based on her blog "A Year of Slow Cooking," crockpot365.blogspot.com.

Paleo Diet Lifestyle, paleodietlifestyle.com. Amazing Paleo recipes without re- fined foods or grains. (One of my staff's favorites: Kale Chips.)

Kay Sheppard, *Absolutely Abstinent! Recipes for Recovery* (Palm Bay, FL: kay- sheppard.com, 2005). An O.A.-supportive book from a world expert on food-addiction recovery.

Note: See gluten- and dairy-free resources at the end of chapter thirteen (about allergies) and chapter nineteen (about shopping).

TWENTY-ONE

Essential Support

Exercise, Relaxation, Counseling, Testing, and Health Care Resources

While supplements and the right foods are, as you have seen, the core of the Diet Cure, I'd like you to have all the additional support you need to make your cure as complete as possible:

- For a lifetime cure, exercise and relaxation are a must. And I think that what I have to say about these topics may surprise you.
- Counseling will be essential for some of you and just plain helpful for others.
- Without the help of certain holistic health professionals, some of you will not be able to pull off important features of your cure, such as getting blood or saliva tests or prescriptions.
- You and your physician may well need to know where to get special tests and how to contact compounding pharmacies to fill prescriptions tailored to you.

FINDING SUSTENANCE IN EXERCISE

Close your eyes. You're in a lovely, long meadow leading to some low curving hills near the ocean. Do you feel like walking along the trail, running across the field, sitting on a bench enjoying the view, riding a bike, or taking a nap in the high grass and flowers nearby?

Did you think about which choices would burn the most calories? If you did, then try again after taking several deep breaths. This time imagine you will burn just as many calories no matter which choice you make. So you can choose what you honestly want to do or not do.

I asked these questions of Kim in a family session that took place early in her recovery from bulimia and not long after an abortion. Kim kept saying, "I've got to exercise hard every day. I've just been going for walks, and it's not enough." (She'd been a star athlete in college.) Then I asked her what she would do if she could do anything she wanted, anywhere. She smiled for the first time in the session and said, "I'd go to the south of France. And I'd lie on the beach and just go into the water to cool off every once in a while. And I'd have a dog with me." Her answer revealed how much she needed rest and comfort above everything else at that point in her life.

Exercise can be invigorating, strengthening, and *fun*. Healthy bodies naturally like, or even love, to get out there. But are you, like so many people who come to the Recovery Systems Clinic, feeling guilty and lazy because you don't exercise enough? Please don't.

I actually should be the one feeling guilty, because I used to chide clients who were not exercising, or who were not exercising up to our standards. Eventually, I realized something that I should have suspected from the start. In the San Francisco Bay Area—probably anywhere in California—everyone knows how to exercise and why to exercise, and feels lots of pressure to do so, particularly if they are not thin. The main reason my clients weren't exercising was because they didn't have the energy. Later, when we had treated their imbalances and solved that problem, they were delighted to be able to get moving. If you are too tired to exercise, you probably need to read about adrenal and thyroid burnout in chapters three and four. Another possibility is that foods such as wheat and sugar are literally dragging you down (see chapter five).

If you hate exercise, I'll bet money that your body is being sapped of its natural vitality by dieting or some other physical drain. If you want to exercise, and love it when you do, but you just can't find the time, you may not have an energy problem, but you may have both a time problem *and* an energy problem!

You can always walk out the front door and circle the block three times. If you think exercise means a big production of dragging yourself to a crowded gym and sweating it out on a stationary bike as you stare at a wall, then no wonder you are avoiding exercising. Exercise can, and should, be pleasant. Enjoy the outdoors as you walk, bike, hike, or ski. Make going to the gym a social event—have an exercise partner. Work out on a mini-trampoline or a NordicTrack at home in front of your favorite television show, use an aerobics video, or dance in your living room to your favorite music. When exercise is a pleasure, it's easier to find the time for it.

EXERCISE ADDICTED?

Do you get depressed or anxious, or both, if you can't exercise hard almost daily? See chapter one on how amino acids can permanently elevate your mood so that you can exercise for strengthening, stress reduction, and good health, not for keeping yourself sane. I want you to be able to break your leg and not fret even though you won't be exercising for a while.

Kari was a prime example of an exercise addict. She was training for a triathlon when she came to our clinic. She'd always been a jock, but her exercise regimen had never been so obsessive. She had just cracked her pelvis, but kept on training, so her therapist sent her to us. Kari was afraid to stop overtraining because she was an addictive carbo-loader. Like many athletes, she ate lots of starch: pasta, cereal, granola, pasta, bagels, and pasta. She was so addicted that she could not cut her carbs to match a reduced exercise program.

On the amino acids, she lost her carb cravings and quit overexercising with no anxiety. For the first time, Kari began to realize how much time she had wasted on excessive exercise. She began to date more, read, write letters, and rethink her career. Blessed with this new insight into herself, she was happier than she'd been in years. When she went back to exercise, her performance was better, even without the constant workouts.

YOUR EXERCISE MAY BE TOO STRESSFUL FOR YOU

Many clients who come to us are too tired to exercise, but they force themselves to anyway. Usually they feel worse afterward: more tired, drained, sometimes emotionally down, too. They usually turn out to have exhausted adrenal glands (see chapters three and eleven for information on remedying stress exhaustion). One of our clients (a fitness trainer!) finally started losing weight when she cut her own workouts in half. Chronic stress and weight loss are not compatible.

CREATING YOUR EXERCISE PLAN

Think of it this way: Imagine you've been given a darling pony that means the world to you and your family, but it's a lot of work. It needs regular feedings. And it needs to be exercised a lot; otherwise it gets depressed, sluggish, weak, and sick. You love it, so you take care of it. Well, I want you to take the same kind of loving care of your body.

There are three important facets to exercise: strengthening, stretching, and maintaining heart function with steady movement. Getting exercise of some kind at least four times a week seems to correlate best with staying healthy long-term. So make it your goal to exercise four times a week until you sweat a bit for fifteen to twenty minutes (or more) at a session. It may take a while to reach that goal, so be patient with yourself.

What kind of exercise animal are you? Are you a pony that needs to run and stretch its neck? A fish that lives to swim? A dancing dolphin? A stretching, meditative cat? Are you more of a stallion than a pony, with a capacity and need for really arduous exercise? One way to identify your best personal exercise style is to look at your blood type. O blood types can, and usually love to, exercise hard. A blood types seem to do better with gentler, shorter workouts, like yoga and walking. B blood types are somewhere between O and A, doing well in a variety of types of exercise. AB types are so rare that I'm not sure about how they tend.

At the very least you can usually walk, preferably outside (or inside—hit your local shopping mall, then enjoy a few shops or a movie). Walking is a great exercise because it's always available, and you can walk any distance you like. Add a block a week or month. Add hills when you can, or stairs. Try to walk away from traffic and off pavement as much as you can. And get good shoes with cushioning and traction so that you can walk anywhere in comfort.

Other exercises that have been shown to benefit people of all ages are simple stretches and home weight lifting. Nancy began lifting five-pound dumbbells because she used to get backaches carrying groceries or anything heavy (she played electric guitar in a band and every time she carried her sixty-pound amplifier she'd pull a muscle). It was easy to do in front of the TV, and the best reward was that by keeping this up, she never, ever pulls muscles in her upper body now.

Stretch classes (such as tai chi and gentle yoga or gentler Pilates) or videos can teach you to do the simple stretching that will keep you physically relaxed and protect you from damaging yourself with stiff, pulled muscles. It doesn't take long to do—just a few minutes a day. This is surprisingly helpful even for those who've had serious injuries.

FINDING SUSTENENANCE IN
REST AND RELAXATION

I'm going to give you some specific suggestions about relaxation in this chapter, but there may not be anything on my list that you haven't already thought about or even done. The problem is that it's so hard for most of us to find the *time* to relax. We seem to be running out of time. In surveys about what people would most like to have more of, time is now valued over money. So here you have very little time and I'm already suggesting that you take more time to eat and prepare food, take supplements, get exercise, and find a health professional.

Let me explain. I'm not just advocating relaxation to make you feel extra-good for a little while. I'm imploring you to make the time to relax because I think that it can save your life and make your Diet Cure a bigger success. If you need a Diet Cure, you have been under more than the usual external stresses from work, family, friends, financial problems, pollution, traffic, and a host of other problems. You've also been under *internal* stresses from not enough food or too much toxic food (or both), from an eating disorder or an addiction, from food allergies or yeast overgrowth. These are all serious and usually long-term assaults. Meanwhile, you can rarely take time to relax and you may have been too anxious and mentally obsessive to have been able to relax effectively. So many of us are. That's why the very first chapter of this book is about how to revamp your own mood (and craving) chemistry. And it's why I wrote a second book, *The Mood Cure*.

Now you can be free of internal stressors by identifying them and going after them with supplements, good foods, and whatever other strategies you'll need, so it's time to make the time for relaxation.

RELAXATION: WHAT IS RELAXING TO *YOU*?

Techniques that will provide sustaining rest in a hectic world:

✦ Close your eyes and rest during the day, even if just for five or ten minutes.
✦ Take breaks at work—just clear your mind with a short walk, or lie down. Get out and get some air, particularly if you work in an office building with closed windows.
✦ Don't let more than four or five hours go by without consuming protein-containing meals, which will provide you with energy. In between have snacks.

+ Get plenty of rest, eight hours of sleep a night (although some people require slightly more or less—listen to your body), and try to get to bed by three hours after sunset for optimum health.
+ Eat within one hour of waking up.
+ Use hot water bottles or microwaveable pillows on tense or chilled spots on your body. You'll be surprised at how relaxed you get. Let the bottle conform to your body—don't overfill it. Put another one at your feet, if they are cold. (You may become addicted to this luxury.)
+ Take long hot baths with relaxing essential oils such as lavender.
+ Take vacations. Choose destinations that don't require too much air flight or any tight scheduling. Take long weekends off and go away, especially if you are burned out; recharging is the only remedy. The adrenal support supplements can help a lot, but they are not enough without extended rest.
+ Meditate and pray. These practices can be tremendously regenerative. There are many resources available on how to meditate and pray.
+ Walk. Walks, especially in nature, are very relaxing. Appreciate your surroundings, whether it's the scent of pine as you walk through the woods or the myriad faces you see while walking in the city.
+ Work in a garden. For many people, gardening is regenerating, bringing one back in touch with nature, the earth, and the seasons.
+ Practice stretching, yoga, and tai chi. Try classes that are slow and sensual, not athletic.
+ Get massages. There are several types of massages available. A masseuse can concentrate on your neck, shoulders, back, or feet, or can work on your full body for an hour or two.
+ Indulge in body pampering. Get a facial or a manicure. At first it might seem uncomfortable having someone fuss over you, but you'll get used to it quickly!
+ Listen to relaxation CDs. Progressive relaxation CDs step you through the process of relaxing every part of your body, or send you on a guided fantasy to relaxing places.
+ Sing or play a musical instrument. Forget about sounding perfect; have fun with it.
+ Listen to music. For some, quiet music such as New Age or traditional Japanese is relaxing, while for others, listening to rock-and-roll oldies or lyrical classical pieces does the trick.

What Is It That Really Needs to Rest, and How Can You Rest It Most Effectively?

There is only one part of you that sallies forth to meet all of life's challenges on your behalf: your adrenal glands.

The adrenals were designed for the simple life. Like the rest of the body, the adrenals haven't changed much in a hundred thousand years. They were designed to kick in and provide adrenaline to keep you going in times of famine and danger (such as during the hunt or warfare). But a hundred thousand years ago, there were long periods of R&R naturally. No one had to work at making time for it. When it was dark, they went to sleep. When it was light, they woke up. Their winters were very long, restful months when they couldn't do much but sleep. In other words, the adrenals had to perform their emergency services only occasionally and they could regularly do nothing. Not anymore. Especially if you have inherited weak adrenals that wear out easily, modern times are an adrenal nightmare.

If you just can't relax and seem to be permanently wired and stressed out, and the relaxation techniques here don't help, please turn to chapter three and read the adrenal exhaustion section, if you haven't already.

FINDING A COUNSELOR

At our clinic, we always make sure that whoever comes in gets whatever counseling and education they need along with their nutritional therapy. I learned the value of individual, group, and family counseling many years ago when I became a counselor myself. I have never gotten over the thrill of seeing my clients balanced out emotionally as well as nutritionally. You may have already had years of counseling, or have no problems that you really need to talk about. But please consider counseling if any emotional problems do continue to affect you. For example, maybe you now realize you want to quit hating and obsessing about your body; if so, look for a counselor who is experienced in women's issues and/or eating disorders. Ask if she has a group. Interview your prospective counselor. Will she support your working with this book? Is she aware that there's a physical basis for many psychological problems? Does she understand that lack of discipline is not the issue if you have a weight or overeating problem? Do you like her? Can she stand up to you without being intimidating? You must find a counselor if you have an eating disorder or an addiction to a drug or alcohol, or to a behavior (see chapter eighteen). Please explore twelve-step programs, such as Overeaters Anonymous, Alcoholics Anonymous, and Gamblers Anonymous. Just go. Decide later if it helps.

Some people need therapy for issues beyond simple (though crucial) body-image reeducation and diet-mentality deprogramming. Sexual abuse may have deeply affected your body image. I have had two clients who had to stop our program because they weren't emotionally ready to lose weight. When they did and began to receive sexual attention, they felt vulnerable, powerless, and frightened. They needed to stop and do some therapy first. Most of my other clients have been able to follow the Diet Cure and do their psychotherapy at the same time, quite successfully.

I have had a few clients who found that once they were in biochemical balance, issues that had been repressed came up and they needed therapy. When you are no longer eating foods that numb and distort your feelings, when you can think about something besides food and your body, you may become aware of issues within yourself and in your relationships that need some attention. You'll need a counselor to discuss your new feelings with. A side benefit of getting physically healthy is that it becomes more possible to be emotionally healthy, too.

One of my clients was sent to us by her therapist, who had been unable to help her with her depression and anger. After a few weeks on the program, she discovered that she did not hate her job or her mother-in-law after all. Her brain chemistry deficiencies had produced negative feelings that had no real basis. When her negativity was neutralized by amino acids, she discovered she was actually a contented person with a pretty good life. Several marriages have been saved by this same process, "Oh, I do like him. It was me after all!" these women say.

I like to see chronic dieters get counseling, because they have a tendency to undereat no matter what, and that sabotages any weight loss they might actually need and the benefits of their total program. With a counselor, they can look at the old patterns and work their way out of them. But again, the counseling must not compete with the nutritional program. They're both important. Sometimes a counselor can help you to find the time to set up your new life—how to eat, buy, and prepare food; exercise; relax; and still work and have a family and social life, without more stress.

Ask family and friends for referrals, or look in your Yellow Pages or online for local options. Try searching for "counseling," "marriage and family therapists," "psychologists," "psychotherapists," or "eating disorders."

FINDING THE RIGHT
HEALTH PROFESSIONALS

As early as 1997, there were 243 million more visits made to holistic health practitioners than to conventional primary care physicians.[1] We are spending more than 30 billion dollars a year out-of-pocket for holistic health care[2], and more insurance policies are now covering holistic practitioners. I would like to see you find your own holistic health practitioner, one who agrees with the general approach of the Diet Cure, is experienced with helping people correct the eight key imbalances, and can order tests and prescribe medications if you need them. The only practitioners that I know of who can do all of this in every state are holistic M.D.'s and D.O.'s (doctors of osteopathy). N.D.'s (naturopathic physicians) are currently licensed in fifteen states, including California.

Holistic health practitioners focus on the whole person: the physical, mental, emotional, and spiritual aspects of the individual. Ideally, the relationship with a practitioner involves cooperation and respect for a patient's wisdom and knowledge of him- or herself. You will want your practitioner to consider both conventional and complementary therapies when making a treatment plan. Always ask how toxic or risky the treatment is, what the side effects are, and whether there are treatments available that have fewer adverse effects.

THE DIFFERENCES AMONG VARIOUS
HEALTH PROFESSIONALS

Ordering Tests. Most health professionals can order urine, stool, and saliva tests, or skin-prick testing. M.D.'s, D.O.'s, acupuncturists, and some N.D.'s can order blood testing. But keep in mind that often doctors are financially punished for ordering too many tests, hence their reluctance. Ask your doctor to be up front with you about why she doesn't want to order particular tests. Argue your points and she'll often compromise. Perhaps you can pay for some of them out of pocket by ordering via the Internet or through a practitioner that belongs to a lab cooperative (for half-price testing). Both Quest Diagnostics and LabCorp have co-ops.

Advising You on Nutrition. Whether you consult your local health food store expert or a private nutritionist, acupuncturist, chiropractor, naturopath, D.O., or M.D., ask what their nutritional experience and approach is. They are all potentially good candidates, but you'll need to ask good questions. (In some parts of the country, you'll be lucky to find any holistic practitioners at all, unfortunately.)

Providing Medication. Holistic M.D.'s and D.O.'s are the only health practitioners who can order any test in any state and prescribe medications as well as advise you nutritionally. Find one if you possibly can. Or, if you really like your chiropractor or acupuncturist, ask him or her to help you get whatever medical services you need, beyond what he or she can do. Most will have a working relationship with a cooperative M.D. or D.O.

HOW DO YOU KNOW WHAT KIND OF HOLISTIC PRACTITIONER YOU SHOULD SEE?

Within different holistic specialties are many schools of thought. Ask potential practitioners how they would treat your condition and you'll probably get different answers from each one. To keep it simple, show them *The Diet Cure* and see if they are open to the recommendations in it.

Holistic Medical Doctor (M.D.). A medical doctor has four years of graduate training and specializes in a particular area of medicine. Endocrinologists, for example, specialize in disorders of the thyroid and other glands, but are not usually holistic. Until recently, medical doctors have received very little training in nutrition. A holistic medical doctor typically takes additional training from a certified school; for example, of naturopathy or functional medicine. Many doctors research holistic medical treatments on their own and through various conferences or workshops, but don't have a formal certification in holistic medicine. The American Holistic Medical Association requires its members to be state certified in holistic medicine.

Doctors of Osteopathic Medicine (D.O.). An osteopath has medical training but is also trained to correct structural problems in the body with adjustment techniques that predate chiropractic. This is an old and highly respected form of treatment in Europe. Some are more nutritionally and holistically oriented than medical doctors, but many are not.

Licensed Naturopathic Physician (N.D.). A naturopath attends a four-year graduate-level naturopathic medical school and is educated in all of the same basic sciences as an M.D. Naturopaths also study holistic and nontoxic approaches to health with a strong emphasis on disease prevention and optimizing wellness. Even though they are not medical doctors, they are licensed in at least fifteen states and practice with many of the same freedoms. You can do a search for a naturopathic physician in your state at naturopathic.org.

Unlicensed Naturopathic Physician (N.D.). A naturopathic degree can also be obtained from correspondence courses. Students who complete a correspondence course are not eligible to sit for the naturopathic exam, required by states that offer licensure. Most states do not license naturopaths at this time. Even though unlicensed, these naturopaths can be helpful regarding your nutritional and health needs.

Chiropractor (D.C.). A chiropractor practices spinal manipulation and structural adjustments. There are many schools of thought within the chiropractic profession. "Straight chiropractic" practices structural adjustments exclusively, while others include holistic modalities in the practices. Some "network" chiropractors hardly touch the body at all. Most chiropractors have some nutritional expertise, and chiropractic is usually covered by insurance. Some states allow chiropractors to order blood and other tests; others do not. You will have to ask what tests they can order for you. They cannot prescribe medication.

Acupuncturist (L.A.c.). Acupuncture has more than a twenty-five-hundred-year history. It uses thin needles that penetrate the skin to stimulate energy and healing systems in the body. Acupuncturists also use Chinese herbs and sometimes supplements, depending on their orientation. Typically, American-educated acupuncturists will incorporate the use of nutritional supplements and other treatment options, while traditional Chinese acupuncturists use only herbs along with their needles. Acupuncturists are generally licensed for diagnostic and treatment procedures pertaining to "Oriental medicine" only. In some states they can order Western biomedical clinical tests, but in others they cannot. Insurance often covers acupuncture. Acupuncturists cannot prescribe medication. (Only the acupuncture methods developed in Japan and France directly treat the thyroid.)

Nutritionist (R.D., C.N.S., C.N., N.C., C.N.C., or C.C.N.). Be cautious about registered dietitians (R.D.), who have an undergraduate degree and have taken American Dietetic Association–approved course work in dietetics with an additional six- or twelve-month internship in a hospital. Most dietitians believe you can get what nutrients you need from the food you eat (including fried and processed food) and often do not approve of the use of supplements. Certified nutritionists have different approaches, which usually include the use of nutritional supplements. Their training and certification varies. There are many holistically oriented nutritional training programs. Many use my books as texts. You will need to ask the nutritionists you interview what their experience is. Our nutritionists are all supporters of the traditional eating concept (see westonaprice.org).

After employing many R.D.'s in the six years before founding my clinic, I finally found a certified nutritionist, and the real success of our work began. We do not usually find R.D.'s helpful because they are only now beginning to update their profession regarding the use of nutritional supplements. (Even worse, they are the ones responsible for hospital food!) But they are starting to learn from the research confirming the effectiveness of nutritional supplementation (and from their work with AIDS patients) how beneficial a wide range of supplements can be.

Still, certified nutritionists aren't perfect either. Find out if they have received any formal training in the use of supplements. Avoid nutritionists who are enthusiastic about fasting or have any other very narrow eating philosophy that does not match the philosophy of *The Diet Cure*. For example, do they advocate low-fat, low-calorie, or strictly vegetarian diets? Ask what their approach to your imbalances is and which nutrients they use. Be sure that they have been counseling people for a while, and try to get a reference (as you should for all practitioners).

HOW TO FIND A HOLISTIC PRACTITIONER
IN YOUR AREA

If you want to find a good holistic practitioner whom you can work with, start asking for referrals from friends, family, or colleagues. The next best source is a search online or in the Yellow Pages for "holistic" or "alternative medical practitioners," or the type of practitioner you need: medical doctor, acupuncture, chiropractic doctor, to name a few. You may have to look for key words in the practitioners' ads, like *holistic, alternative, nutrition, complementary, integrative, wellness, prevention, nontraditional, natural,* and *food allergy.* In ads or brochures, holistic practitioners might say that they treat the whole person (body, mind, and spirit), that they believe in patient education, that they include you as part of the treatment team, and that they trust your knowledge and wisdom about your own body.

You can visit your local health food store bulletin board or ask the store manager how to find a holistic practitioner in your area or to recommend one to you. To find a health food store online, you can use sites such as Google, Yelp, or Citysearch, or in the Yellow Pages look under "health and diet foods products" or "health foods."

There are also many resources on the Internet for finding health practitioners in your area. Most professional organizations offer referrals by phone, on the Web, or through a referral directory. Remember that practitioners usually pay to be listed or are members of that association, so the lists do not include every practitioner in your area. If you don't have access to a computer, libraries will allow you access.

The following resources will lead you to books and holistic practitioners, testing, and pharmacists.

RESOURCES

The following list includes holistic professional organizations and health-related consumer organizations to contact for practitioner referrals in your area.

FIND HOLISTIC MEDICAL HELP (M.D.'S AND D.O.'S)

American College for Advancement in Medicine
acamnet.org; (800) 532-3688

American Holistic Medical Association (AHMA)
holisticmedicine.org; (216) 292-6644

International College of Integrative Medicine (ICIM)
icimed.com; (419) 358-0273

International Society for Orthomolecular Medicine
http://orthomed.org/isom/isom.html; centre@orthomed.org

CHIROPRACTORS

American Chiropractic Association
acatoday.org; (800) 986-4636

HOMEOPATHS

National Center for Homeopathy
homeopathic.org

ACUPUNCTURISTS

Acufinder.com acupuncture referral service
acufinder.com

American Association of Acupuncture and Oriental Medicine
aaaomonline.org; (866) 455-7999

MISCELLANEOUS HOLISTIC PRACTITIONERS

American Holistic Health Association
ahha.org; (714) 779-6152

NATUROPATHIC PHYSICIANS (N.D.'S)

American Association of Naturopathic Physicians (AANP)
naturopathic.org; (866) 538-2267

NUTRITIONISTS

International and American Associations of Clinical Nutritionists (IAACN)
iaacn.org; (972) 407-9089

National Association of Nutrition Professionals (NANP)
nanp.org; (800) 342-8037

Nutritional Therapy Association
nutritionaltherapy.com; (800) 918-9798

LAB TESTING

You can order some saliva and other tests yourself through these resources, or you can ask your health practitioner to order them for you. All can provide adrenal, reproductive hormone, and melatonin testing. Most provide additional tests as well. We find conventional testing labs (e.g., Lab Corp, Quest) for vitamin D (25OHD), thyroid and sex hormones, cholesterol, and many other markers very helpful.

Note: I do not recommend urinary neurotransmitter testing to determine which amino acids to take. *Instead*, use the much more reliable and less expensive research-based self-diagnosis chart on pages 122-123, and if desired, confirming blood platelet testing at Health Diagnostics (or plasma testing at conventional labs).

BioHealth Laboratory (4- and 5-sample saliva testing for adrenal cortisol and 16-sample female sex hormone tests)
biodia.com; (800) 570-2000

Doctor's Data, Inc. (fatty acid-red blood cell lining-analysis and urine testing for mercury, lead, and other toxic metals)
doctorsdata.com; (800) 323-2784

Genova Diagnostics (-sample salivary sex hormone and plasma amino acid testing, as well as testing for fatty acids and intestinal yeast and bacteria. Insurance often covers their testing.)

Health Diagnostics and Research Institute (accurate blood-platelet neurotransmitter tests, sensitive urinary thyroid measures, pyroluria, fatty acid testing, and much more)

Metametrix Clinical Laboratory (accurate and comprehensive stool testing)
metametrix.com; (800) 221-4640

ZRT Laboratory (saliva testing for cortisol and single sex hormones, blood spot for thyroid, Vitamin D and sex hormone testing, and urine iodine testing)
zrtlab.com; (866) 600-1636
These ZRT tests may be ordered directly through the Canary Club website, canaryclub.org.

COMPOUNDING PHARMACISTS

There are many excellent compounders in the United States and beyond. They work primarily with licensed M.D.'s, D.O.'s, and N.D.'s from any state.

International Academy of Compounding Pharmacists (IACP)
iacprx.org; (800) 927-4227

Professional Compounding Centers of America (PCCA)
pccarx.com

Women's International Pharmacy
womensinternational.com; (800) 279-5708

ALLERGY TESTING AND TREATMENT

EnteroLab (stool testing, may be ordered without a physician)
enterolab.com; (972) 686-6869

Immuno Laboratories (blood)
immunolabs.com; (800) 231-9197
Note: This is the lab we use most often.

Nambudripad's Allergy Elimination Techniques
naet.com; (714) 523-8900

READINGS

Many of these books are available from Gürze Books at bulimia.com

EXERCISE

Miriam E. Nelson, Ph.D., with Sarah Wernick, Ph.D., *Strong Women Stay Young* (New York: Bantam Books, 2005).
Pauline Powers, M.D., and Ron Thompson, Ph.D., *The Exercise Balance: What's Too Much, What's Too Little, and What's Just Right for You!* (Carlsbad, CA: Gürze Books, 2007).

OVEREATERS ANONYMOUS

Caroline Adams Miller, *My Name Is Caroline* (Los Angeles: iUniverse, 2000).
Kay Sheppard, M.A., *Food Addiction: The Body Knows*, Revised Edition (Deerfield Beach, FL: HCI Books, 1993).

——, *From the First Bite: A Complete Guide to Recovery from Food Addiction* (Deerfield Beach, FL: HCI Books, 2000).

RELAXATION

Martha Davis, Ph.D., Elizabeth Robbins Eshelman, M.S.W., and Matthew McKay, Ph.D., *The Relaxation and Stress Reduction Workbook*, 6th Edition (Oakland, CA: New Harbinger, 2008).

Contacting Julia Ross and the Recovery Systems Clinic

Recovery Systems Clinic
147 Lomita Drive, Suite D
Mill Valley, CA 94941-1451
(415) 383-3611
recoversysclinic@gmail.com
recoverysystemsclinic.com

TWENTY-TWO

Your Master Plan in Action

The Diet Cure from Day One to Week Twelve

Now that you have worked your way through the book, you're ready to put all that you've learned into action. Read this chapter now and plan to read it again as you move through this process. In this final chapter I'm going to tell you everything we typically tell our clients as they go through their twelve-week programs. After that point, they usually don't need much from us, though they may be working on long-term projects such as major weight changes or thyroid medication adjustments. By then they have determined just what foods and supplements work for them. They are well established in their new way of eating—and feeling. They've often forgotten, until we remind them, how overpowering their food cravings and negative moods used to be. I'd like to see you develop the same amnesia.

Let's look at what you need to do before you start your Master Plan.

✦ Review the Quick Symptom Questionnaire. Even a few yes answers, if they indicate significant symptoms, may need to be explored, either now or later, if the symptoms continue. Each of the first eight chapters contains a much more complete list of symptoms than the Quick Symptom Questionnaire so that you can do more exploring if any of the imbalances are in question.

✦ Study pertinent chapters in Parts I and II, and all the chapters in Part III.

✦ Think through and plan your first week of meals (at home and out).

✦ Get the nonfoods and druglike foods out of the house.

✦ Buy your supplies of supplements and food.

✦ Organize your supplements, so that you will be equipped all day. Set your cell phone alarm to remind you about taking supplements, if you'll tend to forget. Get a vitamin-organizing system that will work for you. Buy several daily pill boxes and fill them all up once a week to make your life simpler.

✦ Take your time. Don't get overwhelmed. If you are due for PMS or your period, wait until afterward to begin the full eating-changes program. You can start taking your supplements immediately, though. If you've been misled before about quick cures and you're afraid you're being misled again, in just twenty-four to forty-eight hours you will definitely notice a change.

✦ Optional: If needed, set up an appointment with a health professional for ordering tests. Start interviewing counselors, if necessary, or wait until you see how you feel after Week Two. Many people never need testing or other professional help.

WEEK ONE: DETOX WEEK

DAYS ONE TO FOUR

In your first day or two your food cravings should disappear (unless you start during PMS, which I don't recommend). You should lose your food cravings entirely by Day Five, at the latest. If they have not decreased dramatically by Day Two, gradually increase the amounts of the supplements that are intended to reduce your cravings. The aminos, especially L-glutamine, 5-HTP, and DLPA (or DPA) are the usual helpers here. Open an L-glutamine capsule under your tongue if you get a sudden carb craving; this often works within five minutes. If you eat for an energy lift and really need your caffeine, try some extra L-tyrosine.

If you forget to take your supplements at any point, or do not eat as planned (for example, if you don't get protein at all three meals), you can expect your cravings to return briefly. But bumps like this should quickly smooth out and you'll be craving-free again. What does it mean to lose your cravings? It means you'll be indifferent to old favorites; that you wouldn't even cross the room to get formerly irresistible foods; that you might have brief thoughts about old eating habits, but that you really won't care to act on them. The old food fantasies will really be gone. Our clients call us during their first week in our program, to give progress or problem check-ins. I love hearing about these calls, because I get such happy reports. Typically, clients say, "I didn't believe you when you told me that I was going to stop wanting chocolate in twenty-four hours, but it's true! I really don't care about it now. I'm really satisfied without it. I can't believe it! Amazing! It's a miracle!"

Troubleshooting Note

If you are doing everything right and you still have cravings, turn to page 98 and take the long questionnaire to make sure that you don't have a yeast overgrowth, if you haven't already done so.

Even our problem calls are rarely real stumpers. Usually the trouble is easily resolved by increasing the amounts of amino acids to completely eliminate any cravings that may be hanging on. The other minor problem that comes up occasionally is loose bowels, usually caused by too much magnesium. If you should suddenly get loose bowels, just cut back on any supplement that contains magnesium until it stops. More rarely, loose bowels are a short-term detox symptom that does not feel debilitating or draining, but more like a good cleaning out.

You may lose your appetite or even get a bit nauseated in your first four days on the Diet Cure. One of our food-addicted clients, a 50-year-old psychotherapist, told me during her check-in on Day Two that until now she'd never *not* wanted to eat before in her life. If any nausea continues past two days, it may be that the supplements are bothering you. (If you take your with-meal supplements without food, the same thing can happen.) Very rarely, the aminos cause an overly acidic feeling. If they do, try them with a bit of vegetables or fruit, which are naturally antacids. Or take them with meals if necessary. If it continues, stop and consult a practitioner (could you have an ulcer?). In the first two to four days some people feel tired, though you may already be so tired that you won't notice. The other top detox symptom is headache. If you are prone to migraines you may get one in the first few days of your detox. At least a quarter of our clients who are migraine sufferers do. But it may be the last migraine you ever have!

To treat these symptoms, feel free to take whatever over-the-counter painkillers you need during this week. Alka-Seltzer Gold is a helpful antidote to detox discomfort, which is largely due to your system becoming very acidic. Two tablets of Alka-Seltzer (Gold only) will deacidify you, as will baths with 3 cups of Epsom salts. One thousand milligrams of powdered vitamin C, or ascorbate, in a medium-size glass of water may be even better. But the truth is that we seldom get any complaints at all. Certainly by Day Five, you should feel very good.

Troubleshooting Note

Please do not ever use the fact that the supplements have relieved you of food cravings as an opportunity to undereat. Even if you feel guilty about a final binge the night before Day One, eat something with protein in it for breakfast on your first day and again at lunch and dinner. Unless you really are too nauseated to eat for a day or two, eat well at least three times per day from the start to make sure you get the benefits of the Diet Cure right away. A smoothie with protein powder as a temporary lunch or dinner meal will do if you feel queasy in detox, until you get a healthy appetite in a few days. *But undereating is our enemy.* It will cause the cravings to come back and keep your weight static. If you aren't used to eating breakfast, a big omelet may be unappetizing. In that case, make the breakfast Protein Smoothie on page 326. It will go down easily and keep you happy until lunch. If you have trouble even swallowing a smoothie in the morning, you're probably still drinking coffee when you wake up. Caffeine kills your appetite, so it will have to go. If you are tapering off of caffeine, wait until after your smoothie to have a cup of decaf (which has a little caffeine but much less than regular coffee). Even decaf can disrupt your blood sugar and appetite. Get off it as soon as you can. It's easy with the amino L-tyrosine!

Possible Temporary Detox Symptoms
+ Headache (may be severe only if you have a history of migraine)
+ Loss of appetite
+ Low energy

The Food-Mood Log

Every day, pay attention to how you feel and how food, or the lack of it, changes how you feel emotionally (e.g., stressed or irritable) as well as physically (e.g., bloated, tired, craving sweets). Do this for several months, until listening to your body and mood becomes second nature. After that, just use your log at the end of any problem days to help you figure out what went wrong. Think back: Did the problem actually start a few days or weeks before, for example, with a trip out of town during which you started eating foods that unbalanced you?

By keeping the food-mood log, you will discover much interesting nutritional information about your own body and its likes and dislikes. Your body must be the final authority in choosing what is right for you. The process of recovery is really the process of establishing a relationship with your body, free of the damaging foods and drugs (like caffeine) that have alienated you from yourself.

In any relationship the most important element is communication. True communication is the ability to listen and to respond. Your food-mood log will help you reestablish real communication with your body. In my experience, any cravings occur primarily because true nutritional needs are not being met, although external stresses can play a part, too. Please keep this log until your body is mostly functioning without problems. I like calling this record a log, because it's essential to the process of successfully navigating your body and brain into safe waters.

In your food-mood log, record the following information:

+ All food and beverage intake, and approximate time of intake. Note whether you ate the recommended amounts of protein and vegetables and the protein/carb ratio. Did you skimp or skip any meal? Any sugar or caffeine?
+ Any supplement that you did *not* take according to your plan. This includes any supplement that you took more of or less of, or that you took with food when you should have taken it without (and vice versa). Note the time you should have taken the supplement.
+ Do you have any cravings? For what and at what time of day?

+ How you felt throughout the day, emotionally and physically (bloated, depressed, energetic, cheerful, constipated, or some other).
+ How you slept the night before.
+ Your temperature. (You only need to do this if you're checking your thyroid, and then you only need to do it three days a month during your period if you're premenopausal.)
+ Your exercise time and intensity. Record how you felt before and after you exercised.

Possible Mild Emotional Reactions During Detox

+ Grief, loss (of old food friends, habits)
+ Deprivation or envy of "normal" eaters (this typically indicates cravings and that more aminos are needed)

Check In with Yourself. It is crucial that you monitor yourself closely. Try to check in with a buddy daily during the first week of your program, too. Keep the food-mood log!

REACTIONS OF FAMILY AND FRIENDS

You can expect mostly interest and support in your Diet Cure efforts. Maybe you can launch your Diet Cure plan along with some friends or relatives to keep each other motivated, share ideas and meals, and have fun with it. Check in with each other often (daily during Week One).

Some friends and family members may not support this effort. The changes involved may be threatening to them. Have they been eating buddies for years? Sharing a latte every morning? Their initial negativity often passes or improves as they see that you really transform. If not, you'll need to detach from them for a while, at least until you are firmly on your own feet and know how to handle the temptations that they represent. Don't let them make you feel like a prude because you've stopped eating junk food.

If you live with someone, ideally he or she would share the benefits of the Diet Cure with you. See if you can help him design a supplement plan for himself to make it easy for him, too, to give up junk food. If he won't, I hope that he will at least agree to keep junk food out of the house and eat it elsewhere, and that you won't be expected to make both his food and yours, too.

LOSING WEIGHT

In the first week, it is not unusual to lose more weight than you ever do again at any one time. If you are giving up foods you've been allergic to, you'll probably lose water weight—up to ten pounds of it. One of the doctors who consults with us was on a very healthy diet and exercised regularly, but could not get rid of twelve pounds of mysterious weight. At my suggestion she went off gluten-containing grains and lost it all, most of it in Week One.

Men have the faster weight loss, because once free of burdensome foods, their higher testosterone levels and greater muscle mass burn calories like crazy. One of our favorite clients practically disappeared in the first three weeks on the Diet Cure, and he was eating plenty of food.

Women usually lose slowly and steadily. This is best, as they avoid the health consequences of quick weight loss and it ensures that the weight stays off. Usually they also lose their obsession with weight loss and are so thankful to be free of compulsive eating, mood swings, and fatigue that they move along serenely. If you continue to fret about not losing weight fast enough, you'll need to do two things: reread chapter two, and try taking a serotonin booster such as 5-HTP, L-tryptophan, and/or St. John's wort. Low-serotonin states breed negativity, worry, obsessiveness, and low self-esteem. (See chapters one and nine.)

Food-Mood Log

DATE	TIME	FOOD, DRINK, OR DRUGS CONSUMED	TIME	SUPPLEMENTS TAKEN AT WRONG TIME OR DOSAGE OR NOT TAKEN AT ALL	TIME	CRAVINGS; PHYSICAL, MENTAL, EMOTIONAL SYMPTOMS; DAY OF CYCLE TEMERATURE; EXERCISE

What if you stop overeating and start feeling on an even keel emotionally, but do not lose weight? Ask yourself:

1. Am I gaining weight? In more than twenty-five years, we've had only three people continue to gain weight. For all those who have been gaining for years, no gain is weight loss! Especially considering that most of them eat more calories than they'd ever allowed themselves before (except when bingeing). For some, until the thyroid is corrected, weight loss is slow.
2. Am I eating enough to speed up my metabolism (more than 2,100 calories)?
3. Am I looking and feeling better in my clothes? Many people who begin to lose fat build muscle at the same time. Muscle, being heavier than fat, can keep you at the same weight, but it changes your body a lot. Sometimes your dress size will change, but not your weight. (That's one of the many reasons I hate the scale.) In one such case, a woman wore her old, baggy jeans to the office to demonstrate this point to us.
4. Am I eating enough protein in relation to carbohydrates?
5. Is my metabolic rate too slow for me to lose weight? Your thyroid is in charge here. It probably needs help if diet and exercise don't budge your weight, or if you're too tired to exercise.

The adrenals and thyroid usually work together—or fail to work together—to keep your metabolism active. Follow the directions in chapters eleven and twelve for correcting one or both of these imbalances, if your answers to the first three questions here are yes.

Please don't get frustrated and jump into a low-cal diet if your weight loss is slow. Slow is safe. You now have the opportunity to find out why it is slow! If you have low thyroid function, you will need to spend a few months of your life attending to it, because it is serious. Restoring these glands to full function will benefit you for the rest of your life, far beyond (but including) any weight considerations.

WEEK TWO

Are you stuck in a rut, eating the same foods because it was all so new, unfamiliar, and intimidating at first that you just picked a few dishes that you liked and kept repeating them? If so, you're probably sick of them. That's why I've included lots of quick and tasty food ideas in chapters nineteen and twenty. Take the time to use these chapters. Talk the problem over with friends. Find solutions, because you can't afford to get bored. Get food delivered. Hire a cook. There are lots of good cooks doing made-to-order meals to go now. Pick up freshly made food at places you've researched. Be sure that you are taking enough supplements—boredom is sometimes craving in disguise ("I'm so bored with this food, I think I'll just go back to the old food"). Check your food diary. Have you been eating enough? Are you, in particular, taking enough amino acids? Some people forget them when things start improving. Or do you have an adrenal or thyroid problem making you too tired to prepare or plan appealing food? If so, read chapters eleven and twelve and take action.

Don't forget: This is a diet *cure*, not a diet! You may have gone into "diet mode" without even realizing it when you started this program, undereating and expecting just another short-term weight loss at best. No! Relax. Eat well. You won't have to white-knuckle your way to eventual surrender this time. Don't fear that dreaded "permanent maintenance" phase. The hard part will be to keep eating and eating *well*, not trying to count and minimize calories.

Try to forget about calories, fat grams, and pounds. Please stop weighing yourself. I have seen more binges triggered by weigh-ins than any other single cause. Now that you are free from cravings for the kinds of foods that put on unneeded weight, why would you gain weight? The foods that you are eating are safe and healthy, not binge foods. Remember, the more safe foods you eat, the better off you are, because your metabolism responds to freedom from sweets and other junk foods and steady doses of plentiful *and* nutritious food.

You may think, "It's so much food. I'll never be able to eat that many vegetables." Just keep working at it. Don't get overwhelmed; you'll get the hang of it.

SLIPS

If you do find yourself eating sweets or other nonfoods, you'll probably find it's surprisingly hard to binge on them. But if you do it often enough, you'll unbalance yourself again and be back where you started. But please do *not* go into the usual broken-diet/self-blame/oh-what-the-hell-eat-more-junk routine. Either outer pressure or inner imbalances, or both, are at fault, not your intentions. Instead, look at what actually happened. Did you miss lunch and then have to go to a cocktail party with hors d'oeuvres? Fatal. Did you have too light a breakfast and then go out to lunch at a restaurant that brought bread to your table? Fatal. (Don't be a wimp. Make the server take it away!) Skipping or undereating really is the most common problem, so be clear—you have to think through your day ahead of time to be sure you can get enough of the right foods at least three times a day. Did you experience emotional upset or stress? A terrible week at work, a marital problem, or the revisiting of a childhood trauma can set off a need for druglike foods. Your amino doses may need a boost. Counseling and Overeaters Anonymous can both provide support and better techniques for handling these kinds of upsets if they continue to sabotage you.

WEEK THREE

TEST RESULTS ARE BACK

If any results are abnormal, it's time to add new supplements or medications to your Master Plan, depending on what needs correction. Take this book to your session to compare its suggestions with whatever your practitioner's suggestions might be. Be sure to review and mark the pertinent sections in the book, or copy them for your practitioner. This will make your discussion and planning really productive. If your practitioner cannot prescribe medication and I have indicated that you might need it, make copies of your test results to take to an M.D. who can prescribe. I hope you're either already seeing an M.D. or D.O. or you will be referred to a holistic M.D. with whom your practitioner has been able to collaborate on prior cases.

WEEK FOUR

Mild afternoon or evening cravings sometimes start to crop up around this period. You may be forgetting the crucial midafternoon aminos. Set an alarm! This could get out of hand. If you are not eating enough food at your three-plus meals, the supplements won't protect you from cravings. These kinds of cravings are inevitable when you undereat. Even if they're turning you toward eating the wrong foods, their basic message, "Eat more," is right on. As soon as you add more protein and/or fat and/or whole-food carbs to your meals, any yen for sweets will disappear again. One of our clients said she was eating "so well" that she couldn't understand why the same foods she'd been eating successfully for two and a half weeks weren't still "working." It turns out that when she said "eating so well" she meant "*under*eating so well." She had dieted so often that she only had two ways of eating: undereating and overeating. She had cut back too far on carbs. This is a common mistake. I suggested she eat more generous portions of all three kinds of foods (protein, fats, and carbs). It worked right away, with no weight gain.

If you are skimping on carbs, add a potato with butter or olive oil, or some brown and wild rice pilaf to your salad with chicken breast or to your steamed veggies with broiled salmon steak. Sometimes just adding oil and lemon juice or vinegar makes all the difference, allowing you to feel full and satisfied. Fats will often turn off your appetite at just the right point, the point of real satisfaction. Your body can't be satisfied without a certain amount of fat, protein, and healthy carbs.

WEEKS FIVE THROUGH SIX
GOING OUT TO DINNER

Frank was a tall, friendly man who owned a local restaurant. He was a recovering alcoholic who had become a compulsive eater in sobriety. He came to us miserable from eating too many pastries and other goodies from his own restaurant for too long. He responded beautifully on the supplements, dropping some weight right away (as men, with their higher testosterone and muscle mass, tend to do). But the date finally arrived to go to a long-scheduled business banquet. He called the caterer ahead and found that the main course would work for him (chicken breast stuffed with spinach and mushrooms, rice pilaf, and sautéed vegetables with a side salad). He began to look forward to the evening, until he arrived and was seated within reaching distance of the dessert buffet! He broke out into a cold sweat, knowing that he was doomed to reach over all night long, as he had done so often before, and wreck his successful new program. Ten minutes later, he realized that he'd forgotten that he was sitting next to all those desserts. It turned out not to be a real problem for him at all, because he had naturally become immune to dessert. He just wasn't interested anymore.

While it's important to keep trigger foods out of your home entirely (if possible), you, too, should be able to manage well around former temptations when you are out to dinner after the first month, if you take precautions. Ask ahead about the menu, and bring food or eat something before you go, so that you won't get hungry and eat something that will throw you off. Discuss your strategy with your hostess or host, if you can, so that she will understand when you don't eat her best recipe lasagna or black forest cake. If your hostess entices you, saying, "You've got to try this, it's so good," or, "It's my birthday, you've got to have at least a tiny piece," just say, "Oh, I wish I could," and quickly change the subject.

The hardest thing tends to be your own inner nostalgia about going to occasions where everyone is expected to have a good time by eating and drinking. A longtime successful OA member once told me something I've never forgotten: "My feeling is, I don't *have* to eat that stuff anymore, not 'I don't *get* to.' I feel relieved, not deprived."

Consider this: You've already tasted just about every interesting food that you're going to avoid now. It's not like you've never had any. I think you'll find you won't miss it once you start eating the foods that make you feel terrific.

Why not quit dieting by just eating whatever you want? I don't advocate the feminist approach that Geneen Roth and others have developed to end dieting through free eating of any and all foods. For people who are still relatively well balanced, that approach can be great. But for the many people whose biochemistries have been seriously unbalanced by dieting and other problems, this approach can be dangerous. One of our clients developed some minor food cravings five years after using our clinic's nutritional techniques to stop a twenty-year problem with compulsive eating and major depression. She had gone back to college, where she was inspired by her feminist instructors. She decided, rather than revisit us to figure out why she was having these cravings, that she'd just try to end them by giving in to them (though it had never worked in the past). She came to us a year and 125 pounds later, still bingeing. This is a story I've heard many times.

PLAN, PLAN, PLAN

Just like you can't leave the house without the right clothes on, don't leave the table without the right food. Whatever you do, please don't leave the table after *any* meal without your protein. I can offer you a deal: Go ahead and eat a high-carb dessert occasionally, as long as you get a "dessert" of extra protein, too. A side of chicken breast with your crème brûlée, anyone? Be sure not to leave lunch or dinner without considering how you're going to get your four cups of vegetables that day. If you don't get some vegetables at lunch, you'll need to plan on a big salad or a medium salad and some cooked veggies at dinner, or you can have a huge helping of steamed veggies with lemon butter for a fast, easy, and yummy solution to your veggie needs. Don't go to bed without your veggies. But if you have some days when you can't get them all, don't be too hard on yourself. Just be sure to get them the next day. Do not go into a long low-veggie slump.

WEEKENDS, OR LONGER, AWAY

If you plan to eat out at every meal because you're going away, you'll need to be prepared. In California we have no problem getting the foods we need in restaurants because there is so much fresh food available, but in other areas it may be more difficult to customize your orders. Breakfast is always easiest: fresh fruit, eggs, omelets, potatoes. Many restaurants have "light" menus for all meals, with cottage cheese and tomatoes, breadless sandwiches, and other appropriate selections. Do not go hungry trying to keep to the Diet Cure. If you plan to make at least some of your own meals on a trip, take a cooler. They come in all sizes, with ice packs. Pack some protein powder and make your own smoothies by stirring it into some plain yogurt to pour on a fruit plate.

Do Not Forget Your Supplements! Forgetting your supplements is a real danger. You don't want to start those cravings for nonfoods and junk foods again. And don't let nonfoods be your only choices. Here are some ideas for what you can eat in away-from-home situations.

On a Plane Ride. Take substantial snacks to substitute for whatever they serve on the plane that you won't want to eat. Drink lots of hot or cold water. Avoid the sodas, juices, and caffeinated drinks. Bring your own tea bags everywhere if you like hot drinks. *Note:* melatonin can really help with jet lag.

In a Convenience Store. Is there any food at a gas station or convenience store that you can eat? Yes. A package or two of pistachio nuts (which are not roasted in lots of rancid oil), a Balance Bar or a different 30-40-30 bar, a can of chili (always leave a can opener and plastic knives, forks, and spoons in your car), a pop-top can of tuna or chicken—anything but high-sugar or -starch foods, or junk fats, will see you through.

Hospital Food. Here is where a holistic doctor can be so helpful in backing you up to get the healthiest food possible. Hospitals are set up to deal with dairy and gluten allergies and diabetic diets. If you are planning a stay, call and speak to the dietitian and ask how you can get what you need. Ask your family members or your doctor to do it for you, if you are feeling too weakened to take on the job yourself. Your family can also help by bringing food in and making sure that you get whatever supplements you are allowed. (Hospital rules on this can vary a lot.)

If you haven't been able to stay on your Diet Cure while on your trip to see friends or family, on a vacation, or at the hospital, don't worry too much; you'll be home soon and right back to your eating and supplement plan.

WEEKS SEVEN THROUGH TWELVE

CUTTING BACK ON SUPPLEMENTATION

Reports should be getting solid. At some point you'll take off the training wheels and find you've been cured! Chapter seventeen advises you on gradually reducing your special supplements until you're just down to the basic supplements. Take your time. Everyone is different. Be sure to keep some of your old favorite supplements around, especially the amino acids and antistress supplements for hard times. If you get cravings after an illness, when you've been traveling, or during major stress, you may have become depleted and unbalanced again. But your supplements will shore you right back up. Review the amino acid chart on pages 122–123 if you've forgotten or want to be sure that you're taking the right doses, or to explore to see if there is a mood-lifting supplement that you need now that you did not need to take before. Regularly review the sections in chapters three and eleven on how to recognize and repair the damage to your adrenals caused by stress, because you never know when too much of it will hit you, or build up too high.

AFTER WEEK TWELVE

How will you be doing in a year or in five years? Six of the most impaired clients we ever had were interviewed nine months to three years after working with us for, at most, ten sessions. Three were anorexic, and three were overeaters or bulimics. Their nutritional counseling had been paid for through a scholarship arrangement with a county agency. The agency required the follow-up interviews as a way of determining if it should continue funding low-income county residents who wanted our clinic's help.

The interviews showed that all six had made major improvements early on in their work with us. Of the six, one anorexic had done poorly later. But all five of the others had not only sustained their original gains; they had gone on to make even more progress. The results of this small follow-up reflect the same success rate that I have found in every study that I have seen on nutritional therapy for addiction problems: approximately 80 percent. (You can read the details of our follow-up by turning to the Appendix.)

You can save yourself from a life of overeating, yo-yo dieting, moodiness, and ill health, and this book is a very good start. But we are learning more every day about new nutritional tools that will make your Diet Cure even better. For example, if mood swings and emotional overeating are big problems for you, you'll get lots more help in taking charge of your own mood chemistry (including those of you on antidepressants and medications) from my second book, *The Mood Cure*. Keep your eyes open. Read holistic health magazines. Keep taking good care of yourself, now that you know how, for good and all. I wish you the very best diet-cured life.

A Follow-up
of Six Recovery
Systems Clients

Six independently selected follow-up subjects were interviewed nine months to three years after their last session in Recovery Systems' outpatient eating-disorder treatment program. All subjects were severely disabled by anorexia, bulimia, and/or compulsive overeating when they were admitted. They received only nutritional counseling (including dietary supplements); most had already received extensive psychotherapy and twelve-step group support. Within two months, all subjects experienced dramatic initial improvement in mood, relief from obsessive eating, and weight normalization. At follow-up, five of the six had sustained or exceeded all the benefits they had received from the program.

The following section describes each client's symptoms as they appeared on admission, at discharge, and as they were reported in the follow-up interviews with psychotherapy graduate student and nutritionist Denise Heiden (now a doctor of Chinese medicine).

DANA S.

First visit: Dana was age 30, 5'7", and had been anorexic since age 15. Her weight fluctuated between 87 and 92 pounds. She had twice been hospitalized for treatment. She had had three years of psychotherapy.

Although she had graduated with honors from an Ivy League school, she was unable to work except as a babysitter. She ate nothing all day and drank milk and ate sweets at night. She was terribly anxious and depressed and was addicted to laxatives. She suffered constant negative obsessive thoughts about her body shape, weight, and about herself in general.

Dana started supplements on June 12.

By **June 18**, Dana was much more relaxed (which we attribute to GABA supplements) and less depressed (L-tyrosine supplements). She was able to eat two meals a day. B vitamins in nutritional yeast gave her energy. She drank this in water several times a day in the first few months. She had stopped using scales and was less obsessed with weight. She had gained three to four pounds (by our scale).

By **July 20**, she was eating three meals a day. Thyroid support (Gf Thyroid, by Systemic Formulas) helped increase her appetite.

July 30: Dana reported feeling "much clearer in the head." Her abdominal bloating was finally decreasing due to digestive enzymes and an herbal anti-parasite protocol to treat the parasites she had picked up in South America at the age of 15.

By **August 2, 1992,** Dana had gained ten pounds and her anxiety and depression were much reduced. Together with our medical consultant, we identified several major physical problems, including candidiasis, amebic cysts, and gluten intolerance, dating back to age 15, which had caused much of her digestive dysfunction and bizarre appetite.

August 13: Dana reported feeling "so much less insecure" and able to see things differently and more clearly.

August 17: Her bowels were now working better on their own (aided by aloe vera juice, magnesium, and flax oil).

By **August 30** she had gained five more pounds. Her parents said she looked good when she arrived back home to start teacher training (which she had been unable to do one month earlier). After that we had two final appointments.

Follow-up, three years later: Dana had no negative obsessions about her body, had maintained her weight gain, and was not depressed. She'd had no sugar binges and had learned to enjoy eating good food. She was working full-time, in graduate school completing an M.A., and living on her own, "None of which I could have done prior to Recovery Systems," she said. She had not been able to afford counseling, but had used Overeaters Anonymous successfully (another thing she previously had been unable to do).

ANDREA J.

First Visit: Andrea was 34. She had lived through a traumatic childhood. Her eating disorder began when she was 15 and using diet pills. Her food bingeing started at 16 and was out of control by 17. By age 24 she was using cocaine, sugar, and diet soda daily to control her appetite. This drug use continued until she entered a treatment program at St. Helena Hospital. Her compulsive eating and depression continued. By age 29 she had made two major suicide attempts.

When she came to us she had been in weekly therapy and Overeaters Anonymous for six years, yet her compulsive eating was so out of control that she was afraid she would die soon. After bingeing she frequently drove along the cliffs in West Marin trying to make herself drive off. An OA member brought her to us. She had been unable to work for some time and was living with friends. She could only afford the most minimal supplement program.

She stopped eating sweets, gluten-containing grains, and Nutra-Sweet in Week One. By the end of the week she had become binge-free and mostly craving-free on GTF chromium and L-glutamine three times a day.

By **July 30** she was depression-free and energetic on L-tyrosine three times a day. She had met with us five times initially, then five more times over the course of the next two years. She had no relapses.

March 25, the following year: Andrea reported, "I have never binged again, though I had struggled all my life with sugar bingeing. I went through an eating disorders treatment program and years of therapy and OA with no results. Now I am craving-free, depression-free, earning a living, present, and healthy."

Follow-up three years later: Andrea had maintained all of her improvements. She had been able to sustain a stable relationship and was going to college in addition to having developed her own successful business. She was still active in OA.

GREG E.

November: Greg, age 51, came to Recovery Systems with lifelong depression and an alcohol and drug addiction history starting at age 16. He had been in alcohol and drug recovery for ten of the prior twelve years after receiving intensive addiction treatment. But his depression and other compulsive behavior (food cravings, smoking, sexual obsessions) had continued. He was unable to concentrate or work and complained of a constant burning sensation across his temples, insomnia, and anxiety.

In the next twelve months, although he only came for two and a half of his six follow-up visits (four and a half visits total), his depression and anxiety were reduced dramatically. He cut his smoking from two and a half packs a day to half a pack per day, and he started school in a rehab program and loved it. His concentration improved and the burning sensation disappeared. Although he continued to have some food cravings, he was not overeating.

Follow-up, three years later: Greg was gainfully and happily employed for the first time in years. His depression had improved even further, as had his ability to concentrate. He was sleeping well and had little anxiety. He was not overeating. He continued to have mild sweet cravings. His sexual obsession continued (at that time, L-tryptophan and 5-HTP were not available, which we would use today to treat anyone with obsessive behavior).

CARLA V.

On admission: Carla came to Recovery Systems with lifelong depression, too despondent even to fill out our intake forms. Her mother had committed suicide, and alcoholism ran throughout her father's side of the family. She had been anorexic in the past and still ate very irregularly because eating made her so tired and she associated it with lifelong constipation. She was chronically fatigued and craved sugar constantly.

May 1, 1993: A month later she wrote about her progress to the funding agency, saying that her depression was gone and her energy much improved. She no longer needed naps and was alert until ten P.M. instead of being exhausted by six P.M.

May 12: Carla reported that she had stopped taking the nutritional supplements after two months. (We usually recommend taking them for three to six months.) Her energy had dropped after she stopped them, so we agreed that she would come back in to address low thyroid and other issues and get back on the supplements, but she did not return to do so.

Follow-up, two years later: Carla's depression had continued to improve, and her bowels had as well. She had no food cravings. But her energy had remained low. Stress and anxiety had become much worse, precipitating a nervous breakdown in 1995. She was undereating again in reaction to her stress and anxiety. She was finding psychotherapy helpful.

NATALIE G.

On admission: Natalie, age 25, was brought in by her mother because she had anorexia that had begun six months previously. She was low weight (thirteen-pound loss from a naturally slender frame), unkempt, weak, and very depressed. She was unable to leave the house. Her periods had stopped. She was obsessive, and her sleep was disturbed. Her mother and medical doctor were planning to hospitalize her if she did not respond to our program, because blood work showed alarming evidence of malnutrition.

For a few days she was too frightened to take the supplements, but on day six, April 10, she called to say she felt much better on them. Her mother confirmed that she was indeed eating again and feeling less depressed. Recovery Systems saw her three times. Grief counseling was recommended, but she refused.

Her last visit was **April 21, 1994,** although we continued to monitor her program through her mother by phone.

Follow-up, one year later: Natalie was free of the extreme depression. She had regained ten pounds, her energy was "excellent," her sleep was much better, she was worrying much less, she was able to go out, and she was using makeup and keeping clean again. She was menstruating regularly. She was eating regularly, and she had continued to explore nutritional supplements on her own very successfully. (Natalie's mother confirmed all of these sustained improvements.)

JANICE C.

On admission: Janice came to Recovery Systems at age 45. She had been obese since age 3. She had been addicted to alcohol and marijuana from adolescence until age 42, when she began using twelve-step programs successfully. She was the victim of violent and protracted childhood sexual abuse and had been working hard in therapy for several years to recover from it. She craved and overate sugar uncontrollably and was chronically exhausted. She became depressed and anxious, to the point of having panic attacks when she tried to go without sugar. She weighed more than three hundred pounds. (At age 16 she had weighed 380 pounds.) She was emotionally dissociated much of the time, a state that the bingeing promoted. She had irregular periods.

During her twelve-week program at Recovery Systems, Janice stopped craving and overeating foods, her period started again, and her energy and mood rose and stabilized. She was much less dissociated, which made her psychotherapy more effective. (She attributed this directly to her normalized eating.) She said that she was processing her traumatic past emotionally and moving on (her previous dissociation had made this level of psychotherapeutic work impossible). Her weight began to decrease, although she refused to weigh herself, and her clothes became loose and had to be replaced.

Follow-up, two years later: Janice had sustained all of these improvements! She had also continued to lose weight.

SUMMARY OF FOLLOW-UP

Of the six clients interviewed, all received dramatic benefit from the nutritional program within two months. At follow-up ten months to three years later, only one (Carla V.) had lost any benefits. Eighty-three percent had achieved and sustained a remarkable level of recovery.

ACKNOWLEDGMENTS

For someone like me, who is not as generous with praise as I should be, I am so happy to have this chance to express my gratitude and appreciation to Frances Lillian Ross, my mother, partner, and pal, whose brilliant sense of language made me love to speak and to write.

I am also most grateful to Helen Jones, courageous author and long-time friend, who believed in me when I needed it most; to Barbara Madore, whose early support made our clinic possible; to Dean and Liz Leith, kindred spirits whose generosity took us over the top; and to the valiant and beautiful Eileen Hinkson.

I am grateful to the following people for providing key steps in my understanding of eating disorders and nutritional therapy: Alex Schauss, Ph.D.; Lynn Elliott-Harding, R.N.; Joan Mathews Larson, Ph.D.; Krispin Sullivan, C.N.; William Timmons, N.D.; and Clara Felix.

To my agent, Faith Hamlin, who taught me how to propose a book, and to her associate Nancy Stender; to the winged feet of Nancy Peske, editor par excellence; to the exceptional vision of my editor at Viking, Janet Goldstein, and her colleagues Barbara Grossman and Susan Petersen Kennedy, who ordained the happy fate of this book, I give many thanks. To Stephen Morrison and Emily Murdock Baker at Penguin, many thanks for your help in monitoring the 2012 edition.

I was more than fortunate to have had around me colleagues, friends, and family who made it possible for me to finish the original text of this book despite the death of my mother. The contributions of my dear friend and colleague Genie Dreyfus on both the original and revised editions, which included daily support, computer research, and an intuitive ability to turn my illegible prose into computer clarity, are too numerous to catalogue. She and her brilliant husband, Jared, put together most of the wonderful information in chapters twenty and twenty-one (for both editions) from their own experience as master cooks (and master writers!). Another dear friend, Colleen Heater, did the great research on essential support for chapter twenty-one and held my hand throughout the writing of both editions. Timothy Kuss, Ph.D., my clinic's nutritional consultant since 1992, has been the mastermind behind many of our successful nutritional strategies. He compiled material for three of the book's most complex chapters. He is one of four superb clinicians who comprise the Board of Advisers for this book. I would like to thank the other three as well: Daniel Amen, M.D., with his extraordinary understanding of brain function; Kenneth Blum, Ph.D., my mentor in amino acid therapy; and Richard Shames, M.D., without whose care many of our clients would not have found their Diet Cures. And thanks to Sharna Rose, chef extraordinaire (and Genie Dreyfus, again!), who provided many scrumptious recipes out of their personal enthusiasm for *The Diet Cure*.

Because of the enormous clinical and administrative gifts of my colleagues, Recovery Systems has gone on without me, too often, these past months. Thanks to our spiritual and managerial leader, Patti Covell, and to our head nutritionist, Karla Maree, C.N., especially.

I also want to salute my two beloved brothers, Robert and Fred, their loving wives, Kay and Margo, and stalwart, darling Kass.

Final thanks go to my niece, Helen, and my nephew, Charley, whose piggy eraser and baseball games, respectively, kept me laughing during the 2011 revision process.

NOTES

Chapter 1. Depleted Brain Chemistry

1 Kenneth Blum, Ph.D., "Neuronutrition as an Adjunct to Addiction Therapy," *Nutrition Report* 7, no. 6 (1989).

2 Ryan S. King and Jill Pasquarella, *Drug Courts: A Review of the Evidence* (Washington, DC: The Sentencing Project, April 2009), p. 5.

3 Ernest L. Cowles, Ph.D., *Sacramento Probation Department, Adult Drug Court Program, 2006–2007 Executive Summary* (Sacramento, CA: Institute for Social Research, California State University, February 27, 2009); and Shannon M. Carey, Ph.D., and Mark Waller, *California Drug Courts: Costs and Benefits, Phase III: DC-CSET Statewide Launch, Superior Court of Sacramento County, Sacramento Drug Court Site-Specific Report* (Portland, OR: NPC Research, December 2008). Both available at http://www.carasac.org/DrugCourt Program.shtml.

4 Kenneth Blum, Ph.D., et al., "Clinical Evidence for the Effectiveness of Phencal in Maintaining Weight Loss in an Open-Label, Controlled, 2-year Study," *Current Therapeutic Research* 58, no. 10 (October 1997): 745–63.

5 Eric R. Braverman, M.D., et al., *The Healing Nutrients Within* (Laguna Beach, CA: Basic Health Publications, 2003), p. 240.

6 Henry David Abraham, M.D., and Anthony B. Joseph, N.D., "Bulimic Vomiting Alters Pain Tolerance and Mood," *International Journal of Psychiatry in Medicine* 16, no. 4 (1986–87): 311–6.

7 Walter H. Kaye, et al., "Serotonin Alterations in Anorexia and Bulimia Nervosa: New Insights from Imaging Studies," *Physiology and Behavior* 85, no. 1 (2005): 73–81; and Katharine A. Smith, M.A., MRCPsych, Christopher G. Fairburn, D.M., FRCPsych, and Philip J. Cowen, M.D., FRCPsych, "Symptomatic Relapse in Bulimia Nervosa Following Acute Tryptophan Depletion," *Archives of General Psychiatry* 56 (1999): 171–6.

8 Dean Wolfe Manders, Ph.D., "The FDA Ban of L-Tryptophan: Politics, Profits and Prozac," *Social Policy* 26, no. 2 (1995).

9 C. Cangiano, et al., "Effects of 5-Hydroxytryptophan on Eating Behavior and Adherence to Dietary Prescriptions in Obese Adult Subjects," *Advances in Experimental Medicine and Biology* 294 (1991): 591–3.

Chapter 2. Malnutrition Due to Low-Calorie Dieting

1 Cincinnati Grammar School Study Results, *Eating Disorders Review*, 1993.

2 Michael L. Dansinger, M.D., et al. "Comparison of the Atkins, Ornish, Weight Watchers, and Zone Diets for Weight Loss and Heart Disease Risk Reduction: A Randomized Trial," *JAMA* 293, no. 1 (January 5, 2005): 43–53.

3 National Institutes of Health Technology Assessment Conference Panel, "Methods of Voluntary Weight Loss and Control" (1992), Office of Medical Records, Bethesda, MD.

4 Traci Mann, et al., "Medicare's Search for Effective Obesity Treatments: Diets Are Not the Answer," *American Psychologist* 62, no. 3 (April 2007): 220–33.

5 David M. Garner and Susan C. Wooley, "Confronting the Failure of Behavioral and Dietary Treatments for Obesity," *Clinical Psychology Review* 11, no. 6 (1991): 729–80.

6 U.S. Department of Agriculture, U.S. Department of Health and Human Services, "Balancing Calories to Manage Weight," in *Dietary Guidelines for Americans 2010*, p. 8.

7 Dennis T. Villareal, M.D., et al., "Bone Mineral Density Response to Caloric Restriction–Induced Weight Loss or Exercise-Induced Weight Loss: A Randomized Controlled Trial," *Archives of Internal Medicine* 166, no. 22 (December 11–25, 2006): 2502–10.

8 Edward P. Weiss, et al., "Lower Extremity Muscle Size and Strength and Aerobic Capacity Decrease with Caloric Restriction but Not with Exercise-Induced Weight Loss," *Journal of Applied Physiology* 102, no. 2 (February 2007): 634–40.

9 Robert Garrison Jr., M.A., R.Ph., and Elizabeth Somer, M.A., R.D., *The Nutrition Desk Reference* (New Canaan, CT: Keats, 1995).

10 Mervat Nasser, *Culture and Weight Consciousness* (London: Routledge, 1997), p. 54.

11 K. S. Kendler, et al., "The Genetic Epidemiology of Bulimia Nervosa," *American Journal of Psychiatry* 148, no. 12 (1991): 1627–37.

12 L. K. George Hsu, *Eating Disorders* (New York: Guilford Press, 1990), p. 76.

13 Alexander Schauss, Ph.D., and Carolyn Costin, M.A., M.F.C.C., *Anorexia and Bulimia: A Nutritional Approach to the Deadly Eating Disorders* (New Canaan, CT: Keats, 1997).

14 A. Schauss and C. Costin, "Zinc as a Nutrient in the Treatment of Eating Disorders," *American Journal of Natural Medicine* 4, no. 10 (1997): 8–13.

15 Jane Wardle and Sally Beales, "Control and Loss of Control over Eating: An Experimental Investigation," *Journal of Abnormal Psychology* 97, no. 1 (February 1988): 35–40.

16 Robert Garrison Jr., M.A., R.Ph., and Elizabeth Somer, M.A., R.D., *The Nutrition Desk Reference* (New Canaan, CT: Keats, 1995), pp. 560 and 573.

17 Philip Gorwood, Amélie Kipman, and Christine Foulon, "The Human Genetics of Anorexia Nervosa," *European Journal of Pharmacology* 480, no. 1–3 (November 7, 2003): 163–70.

18 "Chemical Linked to Binge Eating," *New York Times*, May 28, 1993.

19 Katharine A. Smith, M.A., MRCPsych, Christopher G. Fairburn, D.M., FRCPsych, Philip J. Cowen, M.D., FRCPsych, "Symptomatic Relapse in Bulimia Nervosa Following Acute Tryptophan Depletion," *Archives of General Psychiatry* 56 (1999): 171–176.

20 Forest Tennant, M.D., Ph.D., *Carbohydrate Dependence: Is This Why I Can't Lose Weight?* (West Covina, CA: Veract Handbook Series, 1995).

21 Joseph Mercola, N.D. *Sweet Deception* (Nashville, TN: Nelson Books, 2006), p. 61.

22 Dennis W. Remington, M.D., and Barbara W. Higa, R.D., *The Bitter Truth About Artificial Sweetmers* (Provo, UT: Vitality House International, 1987), p. 29.

23 Joan E. Benson, Kathryn A. Engelbert-Fenton, and Patricia A. Eisenman, "Nutritional Aspects of Amenorrhea in the Female Athlete Triad," *International Journal of Sports Nutrition and Exercise Metabolism* 6, no. 2 (1996): 134–45.

Chapter 3. Unstable Blood Sugar

1 Joan Mathews Larson, Ph.D., with Keith W. Sehnert, M.D., *Seven Weeks to Sobriety: The Proven Program to Fight Alcoholism through Nutrition* (New York: Ballentine Books, 1997), p. 86; and Michael Murray, N.D., and Joseph Pizzorno, N.D., *Encyclopedia of Natural Medicine*, 2nd Edition (New York: Three Rivers Press, 1997), p. 549.

2 Thomas H. Maugh II and Patrick J. McDonnell, "Americanization a Health Risk, Study Says," *Los Angeles Times*, September 15, 1998, pp. A1 and A19. Study released September 7, 1998, by the National Research Council and the Institute of Medicine.

3 A. Janet Tomiyama, Ph.D., et al., "Low Calorie Dieting Increases Cortisol," *Psychosomatic Medicine* 72, no. 4 (April 16, 2010): 357–64.

4 Carey Goldberg, "The Simple Life Lures Refugees from Stress," *New York Times*, September 21, 1995, pp. B1 and B6.

5 Susan Mitchell, Ph.D., and Catherine Christie, *I'd Kill for a Cookie: A Simple Six-Week Plan to Conquer Stress Eating* (New York: Plume Books, 1998), p. 17.

6 Linda Rector Page, N.D., Ph.D., *Healthy Healing: A Guide to Self-Healing for Everyone*, 10th Edition (Del Rey Oaks, CA: Healthy Healing, 1997), p. 439.

Chapter 4. Unrecognized Low Thyroid Function

1 P. Chomard, et al., "Serum Concentrations of Total T_4, T_3, Reverse T_3 and Free T_4, T_3 in Moderately Obese Patients," *Human Nutrition, Clinical Nutrition* 39, no. 5 (September 1985): 371–8.

2 Stephen E. Langer, M.D., and James F. Scheer, *Solved: The Riddle of Illness* (New Canaan, CT: Keats, 1984), p. 156.

3 Susan Heavey, "FDA Panel Urges New Look at 'Silver' Teeth Fillings," *Reuters*,

December 15, 2010, http://www.reuters.com/article/2010/12/15/us-dental-mercury-idUSTRE6BE68Y20101215.

4   R. Maréchaud, "Low T₃ Syndrome," *La Revue du Praticien* 48, no. 18 (November 15, 1988): 2018–22.

5   A. P. Weetman, "Clinical Review: Fortnight review: Hypothyroidism: Screening and Subclinical Disease," *British Medical Journal* 314 (April 19, 1997): 1175.

6   Broda O. Barnes, M.D., "Basal Temperature versus Basal Metabolism," *JAMA* 119, no. 14 (1942): 1072–4.

7   Ronald A. Sacher and Richard A. McPherson, *Widmann's Clinical Interpretation of Laboratory Tests* (Salem, MA: F. A. Davis, 1991), p. 583.

8   Lewis E. Braverman, M.D., and Robert D. Utiger, M.D., editors, *Werner and Ingbar's The Thyroid: A Fundamental and Clinical Text*, 6th Edition (Philadelphia: J. B. Lippincott, 1991), p. 1331.

9   Steven E. Langer, M.D., *How to Win at Weight Loss* (Rochester, VT: Thorsons, 1987), p. 199.

Chapter 5. Food Addictions and Allergic Reactions

1   Christine Zioudrou, Richard A. Streaty, and Werner A. Klee, "Opioid Peptides Derived from Food Proteins: The Exorphins," *The Journal of Biological Chemistry* 254, no. 7 (April 10, 1979): 2446–9.

2   Kathleen DesMaisons, Ph.D., *Potatoes Not Prozac: Simple Solutions for Sugar Sensitivity* (New York: Simon & Schuster, 2008).

3   Zioudrou et al., "Opioid Peptides Derived from Food Proteins: The Exorphins."

4   A study published in the April 1996 issue of *Gastroenterology* found the prevalence in the United States of celiac disease is 1:250. This is similar to that reported from countries in Europe. Researchers concluded that CD is not rare in the United States and may be greatly underdiagnosed. See T. Not, et al., "Endomysium Antibodies in Blood Donors Predicts a High Prevalence of Celiac Disease in the USA," *Gastroenterology* 10, vol. 4 (April 1996): A1-1591.

5   Doris Rapp, M.D., *Is This Your Child?: Discovering and Treating Unrecognized Allergies in Children and Adults* (New York: William Morrow, 1992), p. 547.

6   National Institutes of Health National Digestive Diseases Information Clearinghouse.

7   Carl C. Pfeiffer, Ph.D., M.D., *Nutrition and Mental Illness: An Orthomolecular Approach to Balancing Body Chemistry* (Rochester, VT: Healing Arts Press, 1988).

8   Theron G. Randolph, M.D., and Ralph W. Moss, Ph.D., *An Alternative Approach to Allergies: The New Field of Clinical Ecology Unravels the Environmental Causes of Mental and Physical Ills* (New York: HarperPerennial, 1989).

Chapter 6. Hormonal Havoc

1 G. B. Phillips, M.D., "Relation Between Serum Sex Hormones and the Glucose-Insulin-Lipid Defect in Men with Obesity," *Metabolism: Clinical and Experimental* 42, no. 1 (January 1993): 116–20.

2 Michael T. Murray, N.D., *Premenstrual Syndrome: How You Can Benefit from Diet, Vitamins, Minerals, Herbs, Exercise, and Other Natural Methods* (Roseville, CA: Prima Lifestyles, 1997), p. 9.

3 Susan M. Love, M.D., with Karen Lindsey, *Dr. Susan Love's Hormone Book: Making Informed Choices About Menopause* (New York: Random House, 1997), p. 40.

4 Debra Waterhouse, M.P.H., R.D., *Outsmarting the Midlife Fat Cell: Winning Weight Control Strategies for Women Over 35 to Stay Fit Through Menopause* (New York: Hyperion, 1999), pp. 18–9.

5 Michael Murray, N.D., and Joseph Pizzorno, N.D., *Encyclopedia of Natural Medicine,* Revised 2nd Edition (New York: Three Rivers Press, 1997), pp. 744 and 910.

6 Elizabeth L. Vliet, M.D., *Screaming to Be Heard: Hormonal Connections Women Suspect and Doctors Still Ignore*, Revised Edition (Lanham, MD: M. Evans & Co., 2000), p. 88.

7 Ibid., 326.

8 Ibid., 84.

9 Ibid., 143.

10 Ibid., 181.

11 Ibid.

12 Jonathan V. Wright, M.D., and John Morgenthaler, *Natural Hormone Replacement for Women Over 45* (Petaluma, CA: Smart Publications, 1997), p. 56.

13 Love and Lindsey, *Dr. Susan Love's Hormone Book*, p. 123.

14 Kent Holtorf, M.D., "The Bioidentical Hormone Debate: Are Bioidentical Hormones (Estradiol, Estriol, and Progesterone) Safer or More Efficacious Than Commonly Used Synthetic Versions in Hormone Replacement Therapy?" *Postgraduate Medicine* 121, no. 1 (January 2009): 73–85.

Chapter 7. Yeast Overgrowth

1 Michael Murray, N.D., and Joseph Pizzorno, N.D., *Encyclopedia of Natural Medicine,* Revised 2nd Edition (New York: Three Rivers Press, 1997), p. 300.

2 Luc De Schepper, M.D., Ph.D., Lic.Ac., *Full of Life: How to Achieve and Maintain Peak Immunity: Combatting Chronic Fatigue and Other Immune-Suppressed Illnesses in the 90's* (Los Angeles: Tale Weaver Publishing, 1991), p. 81.

3 Elaine Gottschall, B.A., M.Sc., *Breaking the Vicious Cycle: Intestinal Health Through Diet* (Kirkton, Ontario: Kirkton Press, 1994), p. 10.

4 De Schepper, *Full of Life*, p. 72.

Chapter 8. Fatty Acid Deficiency

1 Artemis P. Simopoulos, M.D., and Jo Robinson, *The Omega Plan: The Medically Proven Diet That Restores Your Body's Essential Nutritional Balance* (New York: HarperCollins, 1997), p. 29.

2 P. Pietinen, "Fat Is Not the Enemy," The Diet Cure, http://www.dietcure.com /fat.html.

3 Dr. Mary Enig and Sally Fallon, *Eat Fat, Lose Fat: The Healthy Alternative to Trans Fats* (New York: Plume Books, 2006), pp. 60–3.

4 William S. Yancy Jr., M.D., et al., "A Low-Carbohydrate, Ketogenic Diet versus a Low-Fat Diet to Treat Obesity and Hyperlipidemia: A Randomized, Controlled Trial," *Annals of Internal Medicine* 140, no. 10 (May 18, 2004): 769–77.

5 Simopoulos and Robinson, *The Omega Plan*, pp. 79–80.

6 H. Okuyama, T. Kobayashi, and S. Watanabe, "Dietary Fatty Acids—the N-6/N-3 Balance and Chronic Elderly Diseases. Excess Linoleic Acid and Relative N-3 Deficiency Syndrome Seen in Japan," *Progress in Lipid Research* 35, no. 4 (December 1996): 409–57.

7 Charles Bates, Ph.D., *Essential Fatty Acids in Immunity and Mental Health* (Tacoma, WA: Life Sciences Press, 1987), p. 110.

8 Joan Mathews Larson, Ph.D., with Keith W. Sehnert, M.D., *Seven Weeks to Sobriety: The Proven Program to Fight Alcoholism Through Nutrition* (New York: Ballantine Books, 1997).

9 Timothy Kuss, Ph.D., *A Guidebook to Clinical Nutrition for the Health Professional: General Uses and Proven Applications of the Systemic Formulas* (Pleasant Hill, CA: Institute of Bioenergetic Research, 1992), p. 87.

Chapter 10. Nutritional Rehab for the Chronic Dieter

1 Glenn A. Gaesser, Ph.D., *Big Fat Lies: The Truth About Your Weight and Your Health* (Carlsbad, CA: Gürze Books, 2002).

2 *Consumer Reports*, June 1993, p. 350.

3 Thomas L. Halton, Sc.D., et al., "Low-Carbohydrate-Diet Score and the Risk of Coronary Heart Disease in Women," *The New England Journal of Medicine* 355 (2006): 1991–2002.

4 William S. Yancy Jr., M.D., et al., "A Randomized Trial of a Low-Carbohydrate Diet vs. Orlistat Plus a Low-Fat Diet for Weight Loss," *Archives of Internal Medicine* 170, no. 2 (January 25, 2010): 136–45.

5 Temple University Health Sciences Center, "Study of Obese Diabetics Explains Why Low-Carb Diets Produce Fast Results," *Science Daily*, March 26, 2005.

6 Christopher D. Gardner, Ph.D., et al., "Comparison of the Atkins, Zone, Ornish, and LEARN Diets for Change in Weight and Related Risk Factors Among Overweight Premenopausal Women: The A to Z Weight Loss Study—A Randomized Trial," *JAMA* 297, no. 9 (March 7, 2007): 969–77.

7   Magalie Lenoir, et al., "Intense Sweetness Surpasses Cocaine Reward." *PLoS One* 2, no. 8 (August 1, 2007): e698, http://www.plosone.org/article/info:doi/10.1371/journal.pone.0000698.

8   Nicole M. Avena, Pedro Rada, and Bartley G. Hoebel, "Evidence for Sugar Addiction: Behavioral and Neurochemical Effects of Intermittent, Excessive Sugar Intake," *Neuroscience and Biobehavioral Reviews* 32, no. 1 (2008): 20–39.

Chapter 11. Balancing Your Blood Sugar and Reviving Your Adrenals

1   R. A. Anderson, N. A. Bryden, and M. M. Polansky, "Dietary Chromium Intake. Freely Chosen Diets, Institutional Diet, and Individual Foods," *Biological Trace Element Research* 32 (January–March 1992): 117–21.

2   Robert C. Atkins, M.D., *Dr. Atkins' Vita-Nutrient Solution: Nature's Answer to Drugs* (New York: Simon & Schuster, 1998).

3   Michael T. Murray, N.D., *Diabetes and Hypoglycemia: Your Natural Guide to Healing with Diet, Vitamins, Minerals, Herbs, Exercise, and Other Natural Methods* (New York: Three Rivers Press, 1994).

4   Ibid., 97.

5   Artemis P. Simopoulos, M.D., and Jo Robinson, *The Omega Plan: The Medically Proven Diet That Restores Your Body's Essential Nutritional Balance* (New York: HarperCollins, 1998).

6   A. A. Papamandjaris, D. E. MacDougall, and P. J. Jones, "Medium Chain Fatty Acid Metabolism and Energy Expenditure: Obesity Treatment Implications," *Life Sciences* 62, no. 14 (1998): 1203–15.

7   William Timmons, N.D., *Practitioners' Manual* (San Diego: BioHealth Diagnostics, 1999), p. 48.

8   William McK. Jeffries, M.D., *Safe Uses of Cortisol* (Springfield, IL: Charles C. Thomas Publisher, 2004).

Chapter 12. Thyroid Solutions

1   Y. Ishizuki, et al., "The Effect on the Thyroid Gland of Soy Beans Administered Experimentally in Healthy Subjects," *Nihon Naibunpi Gakkai Zasshi* 67, no. 5 (May 20, 1991): 622–9.

Chapter 14. Hormone Help

1   Michael T. Murray, N.D. *Premenstrual Syndrome: How You Can Benefit from Diet, Vitamins, Minerals, Herbs, Exercise, and Other Natural Methods* (Roseville, CA: Prima Lifestyles, 1997).

2   J. Chen and J. Gao, "The Chinese Total Diet Study in 1990. Part II. Nutrients," *The Journal of AOAC International* 76, no. 6 (November–December 1993): 1206–13.

398 Notes

3 Michael Murray, N.D., and Joseph Pizzorno, N.D., *Encyclopedia of Natural Medicine,* Revised 2nd Edition (New York: Three Rivers Press, 1997).

4 T. Suzuki, H. Yoshida, and T. Ishizaki, "Epidemiology of Osteoporosis: Incidence, Prevalence, and Prognosis," *Nippon Rinsho* 56, no. 6 (June 1998): 1563–8.

5 R. Vettor, et al., "Gender Differences in Serum Leptin in Obese People: Relationships with Testosterone Body Fat Distribution and Insulin Sensitivity," *European Journal of Clinical Investigation* 27, no. 12 (December 1997): 1016–24.

6 Ching-Yi Hsieh, et al., "Estrogenic Effects of Genistein on the Growth of Estrogen Receptor–Positive Human Breast Cancer (MCF-7) Cells In Vitro and In Vivo," *Cancer Research* 58, no. 17 (September 1, 1998): 3833–8.

7 D. F. McMichael-Phillips, et al., "Effects of Soy-Protein Supplementation on Epithelial Proliferation in the Histologically Normal Human Breast," *The American Journal of Clinical Nutrition* 68, no. 6 (December 1998): 1431S–5S.

8 Alison M. Duncan, et al., "Soy Isoflavones Exert Modest Hormonal Effects in Premenopausal Women," *The Journal of Clinical Endocrinology and Metabolism* 84, no. 1 (January 1, 1999): 192–7.

9 Joan E. Benson, Kathryn A. Engelbert-Fenton, and Patricia A. Eisenman, "Nutritional Aspects of Amenorrhea in the Female Athlete Triad," *International Journal of Sports Nutrition and Exercise Metabolism* 6, no. 2 (1996): 134–45.

10 Robert Lustig, M.D., editor, *Obesity Before Birth: Maternal and Prenatal Influences on the Offspring* (New York: Springer, 2010), p. 377; and K. D. Setchell, et al., "Exposure of Infants to Phyto-Oestrogens from Soy-Based Infant Formula," *The Lancet* 350, no. 9070 (July 5, 1997): 23–7.

Chapter 15. Yeast Elimination

1 Timothy Kuss, Ph.D., *A Guidebook to Clinical Nutrition for the Health Professional* (Pleasant Hill, CA: Institute of Bioenergetic Research, 1992), p. 31.

Chapter 16. The Fatty Acid Fix

1 Timothy Kuss, Ph.D., *A Guidebook to Clinical Nutrition for the Health Professional* (Pleasant Hill, CA: Institute of Bioenergetic Research, 1992), p. 92.
2 Ibid.
3 Charles Bates, Ph.D., *Essential Fatty Acids in Immunity and Mental Health* (Tacoma, WA: Life Sciences Press, 1987), p. 69.

Chapter 17. Your Master Nutritional Supplement Plan

1 A. E. Czeizel, "Prevention of Congenital Abnormalities by Periconceptional Multivitamin Supplementation," *British Medical Journal* 306, no. 6893 (June 19, 1993): 1645–8.

2 Norra Macready, "Vitamins Associated with Lower Colon-Cancer Risk," *The Lancet* 350, no. 9089 (November 15, 1997): 1452.

3 Jason Lazarou, M.Sc., Bruce H. Pomeranz, M.D., Ph.D., and Paul N. Corey, Ph.D., "Incidence of Adverse Drug Reactions in Hospitalized Patients: A Meta-Analysis of Prospective Studies," *JAMA* 279, no. 15 (April 15, 1998): 1200–5.

4 Robert Garrison Jr., M.A., R.Ph., and Elizabeth Somer, M.A., R.D., *The Nutrition Desk Reference* (New Canaan, CT: Keats, 1995), pp. 597–8.

Chapter 18. Your Master Eating Plan—The Best Foods for Your Diet Cure

1 Yasumi Kimura, Ph.D., et al., "Meat, Fish and Fat Intake in Relation to Subsite-Specific Risk of Colorectal Cancer: The Fukuoka Colorectal Cancer Study," *Cancer Science* 98, no. 4 (April 2007): 590–7.

2 Renata Micha, R.D., Ph.D., Sarah K. Wallace, B.A., and Dariush Mozaffarian, M.D., Dr.P.H., "Red and Processed Meat Consumption and Risk of Incidence Coronary Heart Disease, Stroke, and Diabetes Mellitus: A Systematic Review and Meta-Analysis," *Circulation* 121, no. 21 (June 1, 2010): 2251–2.

3 Barbara V. Howard, Ph.D., et al., "Low-Fat Dietary Pattern and Risk of Cardiovascular Disease: The Women's Health Initiative Randomized Controlled Dietary Modification Trial," *JAMA* 295, no. 6 (2006): 655–66.

4 Artemis P. Simopoulos, "The Importance of the Ratio of Omega-6/Omega-3 Essential Fatty Acids," *Biomedicine & Pharmacotherapy* 56, no. 8 (October 2002): 365–79.

5 Patty W. Siri-Tarino, et al., "Saturated Fat, Carbohydrate, and Cardiovascular Disease," *The American Journal of Clinical Nutrition* 91, no. 3 (March 2010): 502–9.

6 Mark D. Wilson, Ruth D. Hays, and Stephen D. Clarke, "Inhibition of Liver Lipogenesis by Dietary Polyunsaturated Fat in Severely Diabetic Rats," *The Journal of Nutrition* 116, no. 8 (August 1986): 1511–8; and William S. Yancy, Marjorie Foy, Allison M. Chalecki, Mary C. Vernon, and Eric C. Westman, "A Low-Carbohydrate, Ketogenic Diet to Treat Type 2 Diabetes," *Nutrition & Metabolism* 2 (2005): 34.

7 U.S. Department of Agriculture, Economic Research Service, Food Availability (Per Capita) Data System, Added Food Fats and Oils 1909–1998.

8 R. B. Singh and M. A. Niaz, "Genetic Variation and Nutrition in Relation to Coronary Artery Disease," *The Journal of the Association of Physicians of India* 47, no. 12 (December 1999): 1185–90.

9 Brahma P. Sani, et al., "Interference of Retinoic Acid Binding to Its Binding Protein by Omega-6 Fatty Acids," *Biochemical and Biophysical Research Communications* 147, no. 1 (August 31, 1987): 25–30.

10 Gary Taubes, "Nutrition: The Soft Science of Dietary Fat," *Science* 291, no. 5513 (March 30, 2001): 2536–45; and Daniel McGee, et al., "The Relationship of Dietary Fat and Cholesterol to Mortality in 10 Years: The Honolulu Heart

Program," *International Journal of Epidemiology* 14, no. 1 (March 1985): 97–105; and S. M. Scanlon, D. C. Williams, and P. Schloss, "Membrane Cholesterol Modulates Serotonin Transporter Activity," *Biochemistry* 40, no. 35 (September 4, 2001): 10507–13.

11 Feng J. He, Ph.D., Caryl A. Nowson, Ph.D., Graham A. MacGregor, F.R.C.P., "Fruit and Vegetable Consumption and Stroke: Meta-Analysis of Cohort Studies," *The Lancet* 367, no. 9507 (January 28, 2006): 320–6.

12 Nicole M. Avena, Pedro Rada, and Bartley G. Hoebel, "Evidence for Sugar Addiction: Behavioral and Neurochemical Effects of Intermittent, Excessive Sugar Intake," *Neuroscience and Biobehavioral Reviews* 32, no. 1 (2008): 20–39; and Carlo Colantuoni, et al., "Evidence that Intermittent, Excessive Sugar Intake Causes Endogenous Opioid Dependence," *Obesity Research* 10 (2002): 478–88; and C. Erlanson-Albertsson, "Sugar Triggers Our Reward-System. Sweets Release Opiates Which Stimulates the Appetite for Sucrose—Insulin Can Depress It," *Läkartidningen* 102, no. 21 (May 23–29, 2005): 1620–2, 1625, and 1627; and A. B. Kampov-Polevoy, et al., "Sweet Preference Predicts Mood Altering Effect of and Impaired Control over Eating Sweet Foods," *Eating Behaviors* 7, no. 3 (August 2006): 181–7.

13 American Dietetic Association, "Inadequate Fruit and Vegetable Consumption Found Among U.S. Children," *ScienceDaily*, (March 2, 2009).

14 Elizabeth Somer, M.A., R.D., *The Essential Guide to Vitamins and Minerals* (New York: Collins Reference, 1995), p. 3.

15 Timothy Kuss, Ph.D., *A Guidebook to Clinical Nutrition for the Health Professional* (Pleasant Hill, CA: Institute of Bioenergetic Research, 1992), p. 78.

16 Brenda Biondo, "Is There Poison in Your Produce?" *USA Weekend*, August 15–17, 1997, p. 10.

17 Jane Higdon, Ph.D. "Soy Isoflavones," Oregon State University, Linus Pauling Institute Micronutrient Information Center, January 2006, updated by Victoria J. Drake, Ph.D, December 2009, http://lpi.oregonstate.edu/infocenter/phyto chemicals/soyiso.

18 Robert Lustig, M.D., editor, *Obesity Before Birth: Maternal and Prenatal Influences on the Offspring* (New York: Springer, 2010).

19 Samuel N. Nahashon and Agnes K. Kilonzo-Nthenge, "Advances in Soybean and Soybean By-Products in Monogastric Nutrition and Health," in *Soybean and Nutrition*, edited by Haney El-Shemy, (Rijeka, Croatia: InTech, 2011), p. 134.

Chapter 19. Shopping for Supplies for Your Master Plan and Planning Your Meals

1 "Interim Advisory on Alfalfa Sprouts," Food and Drug Administration Talk Paper, JN8-47, August 31, 1998.

Chapter 21: Essential Support

1 DiscoveryHealth.com, "Alternative Medicine Goes Mainstream," report on *JAMA* 1997 study, http://www.health.howstuffworks.com/wellness/natural-medicine/alternative/alternative-medicine-goes-mainstream.htm.
2 Ibid.

INDEX

in milk products, 78
and yeast overgrowth, 100–101, 102
Antibody tests
for food intolerance, 194
thyroid function test, 67, 68, 176
Antidepressants
amino acid substitutes. *See* L-tyrosine; Tryptophan
limitations of, 15
serotonin as, 8, 15
See also Selective serotonin reuptake inhibitors (SSRIs)
Antifungal regimen. *See* Yeast elimination
Anti-gliadin test, 194
Antimicrosomal test, 67
Antithyroglobulin test, 67
Anxiety
and adrenal exhaustion, 50–51, 165–166
amino acid therapy. *See* GABA (gamma-aminobutyric acid)
and hypoglycemia, 44
and low-calorie diet, 20
and menopause, 88
and thyroiditis, 69
Appetite loss
and adrenal exhaustion, 50
in eating disorders, causes of, 26–27, 35
restoring. *See* Zinc supplementation
Armour, 65, 183–184
Artichoke extract, 240
Artificial sweeteners
amino acid therapy for, 140–141
avoiding, yeast elimination, 228
health risks from, 39, 290
overeating caused by, 38–39
Asian food, foods to eat/avoid, 312–313
Aspartame, negative effects, 39
Atkins, Robert, Dr., 138–139, 247
Atkins Diet, 71, 72, 110, 272
pros/cons of, 139–140
Attention problems
ADHD, Feingold elimination diet, 78
See also Mental focus, loss of

Autoimmune disease
and low thyroid function, 58
and microwave cooking, 292
thyroiditis, 68–69
Avocados, 142, 160
dressing, recipe, 326, 330–331

Baby boomers, and dieting craze, 22–23, 29
Bariatric surgery, 137
Barley, intolerance to. *See* Gluten intolerance
Barnes, Broda, Dr., 65, 175, 187
Basal body temperature, thyroid function test, 65–66
Beans
benefits/types of, 281–282
cooking guidelines, 304
See also Legumes
Becker, Nathan, Dr., 185
Beriberi, 22
Bernstein, Richard K., Dr., 41, 143, 154, 160
Beverages
caffeinated, avoiding, 290–291
carbonated, avoiding, 285, 291
healthy types, 141, 163
minimum requirement/daily foods, 268
soft-drinks, avoiding, 283–284
water, 284–285
yeast elimination diet, 227, 230
Beyond Pritikin (Gittleman), 33, 113
Big Fat Lies (Gaesser), 28
Bile, and fat digestion, 114
BioHealth Laboratory, 362
Bioidentical hormones, 220–223
buying, sources for, 222–223
compounding, 220–222
hormone regimen in, 222
precautions about, 221
BioSET, 194
Biotin
blood sugar regulation, 156
yeast elimination, 232
Birth control pill
and hormone imbalance, 91
and yeast overgrowth, 101

Headaches
  and menopause, 88
  and sugar allergy, 78
Health Diagnostics and Research
      Institute, 131, 362
Health foods, sweeteners in, 42
Health food stores, 300
Health professionals, 356–361
  finding, resources for, 360–363
  ordering tests, 356
  types of, 357–359
Heart disease
  and low-fat diet, 33
  oils, types to avoid, 238–239
Hepatitis C, 234
Herbs
  menopausal symptoms, 213
  premenstrual syndrome (PMS), 212
  yeast elimination, 231–233
Herring, 237
High fructose corn syrup, health risks
      from, 29, 45–46, 283
Holistic medical doctors (M.D.), 357,
      360–361
Homeopathic remedies
  menopausal symptoms, 215
  thyroid recovery, 183
Homeopaths, 361
Hormonal events, and low thyroid
      function, 59–60, 65, 88, 90
Hormonal food craving, 207–210
  addictive foods related to, 207–208
  amino acid therapy, 208–209
  and estrogen/progesterone levels,
      85–86, 88
  food choices, 210
  vitamin/mineral supplements,
      209–210
Hormone imbalance, 83–96
  and adrenal exhaustion, 49, 93, 215
  causes of, 89–91
  determining, questionnaire section,
      xxx
  and eating disorders, 27, 144
  estrogen, signs of, 92
  and food cravings, 85, 88, 207–208
  and low thyroid function, 218
  and mood problems, 85–86
  premenstrual syndrome, 86, 89

pre perimenopause, 87–88
progesterone, signs of, 92
recovery from. See Hormone
      imbalance recovery
and soy products, 211–212
and stress, 215
testosterone (men), 84–85, 210
testosterone (women), 86, 93, 210
Hormone imbalance recovery, 207–223
  action steps, 223–224
  for endometriosis, 212
  high levels, reducing, 223
  for hormonal food cravings,
      207–210
  menopause approaches, 213–223
  for premenstrual syndrome (PMS),
      212
Hormone replacement therapy (HRT),
      94–96
  bioidentical hormones, 220–223
  health risks of, 94–96
  and low thyroid function, 62
Hormone testing, 216–219
  blood tests, 216–217
  hormones measured, 218
  importance of, 219
  results, actions to take, 222
  saliva testing, 217
Hospital food, 378–379
Hot flashes. See Menopause
      approaches
How to Win at Weight Loss (Langer),
      68–69
Hsu, L. K. George, Dr., 24
Hydrocarbons, and low thyroid
      function, 62
Hydrogenated vegetable oils, health
      risks of, 109, 238–239,
      277–278
Hydrolysates, 199
Hydrolyzed casein, for adrenal
      exhaustion, 168
Hydroxytryptophan (5-HTP). See
      5–HTP (hydroxytryptophan)
Hyperthyroidism, iodine therapy, 63
Hypoglycemia, 43–48
  and adrenal exhaustion, 48–53
  adrenals' reaction to, 43–44, 48
  carbohydrates/sugars addiction, 47

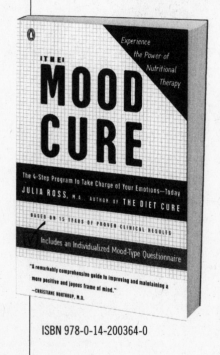